**MENSTRUAL PURITY**

_____

> Nostalgia Jewishness is a lullaby for old men gumming soaked white bread.
>
> J. GLADSTEIN, *modernist Yiddish poet*

**CONTRAVERSIONS**

**JEWS AND OTHER DIFFERENCES**

---

**DANIEL BOYARIN,**

**CHANA KRONFELD, AND**

**NAOMI SEIDMAN,** EDITORS

---

The task of "The Science of Judaism" is to give Judaism a decent burial.

MORITZ STEINSCHNEIDER,

*founder of nineteenth-century philological Jewish Studies*

# MENSTRUAL PURITY

## RABBINIC AND CHRISTIAN RECONSTRUCTIONS OF BIBLICAL GENDER

CHARLOTTE ELISHEVA FONROBERT

Stanford University Press • *Stanford, California*

Stanford University Press
Stanford, California
© 2000 by the Board of Trustees of the
Leland Stanford Junior University
Printed in the United States of America

Library of Congress Cataloging-in-Publication Data

Fonrobert, Charlotte Elisheva.
 Menstrual purity : Rabbinic and Christian reconstructions of Biblical gender / Charlotte Elisheva Fonrobert.
  p. cm. — (Contraversions—Jews and other differences)
 Includes bibliographical references (p.  ) and index.
 ISBN 0-8047-3725-8 (cloth : alk. paper) : ISBN 0-8047-4553-6 (pbk. alk. paper)
  1. Ritual purity—Judaism.  2. Menstruation.  3. Talmud, Niddah—Criticism, interpretation, etc.  I. Title.  II. Contraversions (Stanford, Calif.)
BM702.F66 2000
296.7'42—dc21                                                                    99-462388

♾ This book is printed on acid-free paper.

Original printing 2000
Last figure below indicates year of this printing:
09  08  07  06  05  04  03  02

Typeset by Keystone Typesetting, Inc. in Minion, with Copperplate display.

*This work is lovingly dedicated to my parents*
*Barbara and Wilfried Fonrobert*

## ACKNOWLEDGMENTS

IN THE PREPARATION OF this volume I have had the good fortune to benefit from the resources and faculty of the University of California at Berkeley, the Graduate Theological Union, and the University of Judaism. I owe a special debt of gratitude to Daniel Boyarin of the University of California at Berkeley. Dr. Boyarin has been a great teacher and colleague. His passion for scholarship and for intellectual integrity, as well as his philological and textual expertise, made this work possible.

I am also deeply grateful to Dr. Martin Jaffee who has carefully read the manuscript in its various metamorphoses. I benefited greatly from his comments during my year as a Hazel B. Cole Fellow at the University of Washington in Seattle. Both Dr. Boyarin and Dr. Jaffee have been extremely supportive of scholarship that asks questions about gender in rabbinic culture while at the same time requiring the indispensable textual and philological work that must form the basis for such a project.

Further, I owe a profound debt to the Lady Davis Fellowship, which enabled me to study in Jerusalem for a year, both at the Hebrew University and at the Hartman Institute. Of the people from whom I learned the most with respect to analyzing the dialectics of talmudic reasoning I would like to mention in particular Menachem Kahana and Yaakov Sussman at the Hebrew University, and Menachem Lorbeerbaum and Aaron Shemesh at the Hartman Institute. Without their teaching this work would have been impossible.

I would be remiss if I did not mention my teachers during my career as a graduate student, first and foremost David Biale and Clare Fischer, who provided invaluable emotional and intellectual support throughout my development as a scholar. I am also fortunate to have studied with the late Amos Funkenstein.

It was through numerous discussions with friends and colleagues that this work took its final shape. These friends are all pursuing their own intellectual and scholarly passions. I owe a great debt to my collegues Aryeh Cohen and Eliezer Slomovic, who provided me with invaluable insights with which to strengthen some of my analyses. Further, I would like to thank Sharon Koren, Jonathan Schorsch, Rochelle Tobias, Liz Shanks, Betty Brasky, Cornelius Schmaltz, M.D., and Ian Merles, all of whom are engaged in the process of learning. My students have made invaluable contributions to sharpening the arguments.

Finally, I would like to thank my editor Mary Severance, who astutely recognized the improvements the manuscript required, and Ann Klefstad, who copyedited it scrupulously. Louise Herndon did a superb job of proofreading the text, while Pamela Macfarland Holway saw it through to publication with humor and aplomb—and Victoria Scott's assistance.

This book is dedicated to my parents, who have had endless patience with my endeavors, which have led me into unexpected fields of research and to even less anticipated parts of the globe. They have had to endure the geographical distances between family members that are part of the academic world. It is my hope that this book will be a source of joy to them.

C.E.F.

**CONTENTS**

INTRODUCTION  *1*

**1** FRAMING NIDDAH  *15*

**2** THE WOMAN AS HOUSE: CONCEPTIONS OF WOMEN'S CORPOREALITY IN TALMUDIC LITERATURE  *40*

**3** READING RUPTURES IN THE MASSEKHET/FABRIC OF NIDDAH  *68*

**4** THE HERMENEUTICS OF COLORS AND STAINS: THE RABBINIC SCIENCE OF WOMEN'S BLOOD  *103*

**5** WOMEN'S MEDICINE IN RABBINIC LITERATURE: BETWEEN FEMALE AUTONOMY AND MALE CONTROL  *128*

**6** MENSTRUAL POLITICS IN EARLY CHRISTIAN LITERATURE  *160*

CONCLUSION  *211*

NOTES  *217*
BIBLIOGRAPHY  *301*
INDEX OF PRIMARY SOURCES  *319*
GENERAL INDEX  *323*

**MENSTRUAL PURITY**

# INTRODUCTION

> *What I want to say, Linda,*
> *is that there is nothing in your body that lies.*
> *All that is new is telling the truth. . . .*
> ANNE SEXTON, "Little Girl, My String Bean,
> My Lovely Woman"

> *One cannot relocate in any possible vantage*
> *point without being accountable for that*
> *movement. Vision is always a question of*
> *the power to see and perhaps of the violence*
> *implicit in our visualizing practices.*
> DONNA HARAWAY, *Simians, Cyborgs, and Women:*
> *The Reinvention of Nature*

THIS BOOK PRESENTS first a study of the classic rabbinic discourse on menstruation and of the range of meanings that talmudic literature accords to women's bodies in its discourse on Niddah, or the regulations appertaining to menstruation that are derived from biblical law. My study focuses on texts from the foundational period of rabbinic Judaism: those texts produced between the period from the redaction of the earliest rabbinic text, the Mishnah, to the end of the redaction of the Babylonian Talmud.[1]

The Babylonian Talmud, among its many volumes on a myriad topics, includes one fairly long volume or tractate—in Hebrew *massekhet*, or "fabric"[2]—on rules and laws pertaining to menstruation. To the modern Western mind, nurtured on centuries of a skeptical silencing of and distancing from thinking corporeality, particularly female corporeality, these texts craft a discourse that appears strange, obscure, graphic, or even bizarre. Like few other cultures, rabbinic Judaism in this tractate transforms blood and bodies into language, analyzes the nature of blood and pads, of births and abortions or miscarriages. One detects no sense of embarrassment, shame, or disgust in those pages of the Talmud, feelings familiar to those of us who have grown up in the cultural context of the West, which allows mostly only euphemistic, hidden references to bodies and their messiness. The texts in Tractate Niddah might just as well be about zoology, astronomy, physics, or mathematics, judging by their tone. We learn about the fine distinctions of colors of blood. We learn about a whole hermeneutics of bloodstains. We learn about complicated temporal calculations of menstrual cycles that could try anybody's patience. We learn about criteria for ritual purity and impurity as the rabbinic framework for thinking about menstruation. Inherited from biblical law, this aspect of the halakhic, or legal, discourse of menstruation had become a primarily theoretical issue after the destruction of the Temple in Jerusalem in 70 C.E., the reference point of the biblical notion of purity. Already at the time of the editing of the earliest of rabbinic texts, the Mishnah, this discussion was theoretical. And yet almost the entire rabbinic discourse on niddah, from the Mishnah on, is framed by and committed to just this aspect of the biblical discourse on menstruation.

**Overture on the Ethics of Reading Talmud**

Anyone who comes to read books or study texts does so within a specific, culturally determined psychological or emotional context, particularly in the case of religious or canonical texts that are claimed to be foundational by religious communities. Such texts are never just part of the distant past, long since gone. They continue to structure reality and to form ways to look at the world. Rabbinic literature is canonical in that it has been foundational to Jewish culture throughout its history since the destruction of Jerusalem. It makes claims on its students and constructs a voice of authority. These texts have a continuous life, down to the present, and are used and abused to justify structures of authority, as well as to critique such structures. Therefore, since readers of rabbinic texts tend to have an investment in the text of some kind or another, I want to reflect briefly on my desires in studying (and now teaching) rabbinic texts, and specifically those desires and perspectives that launched this particular project. I am hoping that such a reflection will provide a context for the following studies so that the reader may better understand why certain hermeneutic choices were made. Further, it is my belief that in the current polemical climate—both *within* the academy, where the politics of reading, writing, and representation are disputed, and *between* the academy and religious communities that have a stake in religious texts of whatever kind—only a precise articulation of one's own investments, as well as a self-critical reflection on the motivations behind them, will bridge differences and establish communities of readers and thinkers. There is, then, no neutral reading of rabbinic literature.[3] An objective reading is not possible, but a critical reading is possible.

My naive initial approach to those rabbinic discussions assembled in Tractate Niddah had been to find a tractate entirely devoted to menstruation as that aspect of a woman's life that I have lived with, at times angrily, at times gratefully. My primary desire was to enter into a world that was able to look at women's bodies *as women's bodies*, in their particular physiology and capabilities, and to find a world that inscribed women's bodies with cultural meanings that I could find meaningful; that is, a place different from the European culture that taught me to see the world in its often masculinist terms. At first glance, the rabbinic texts in Tractate Niddah held such a promise.

### Interlude on the Genesis of a Talmud Student

I encountered the Talmud first as the literary monument of the Jewish community, the community that the people among whom I grew up had attempted to erase from the face of this earth. The culture that claimed the Reformation, claimed the best of humanism, literature, and philosophy as its own, attempted to erase Jewish culture from the memory of humankind. Having been raised with the best of German literature as the horizon for the formation of my trust in the goodness and beauty of this world, I had to reconcile those fundamentals with the memory of two World Wars that this same culture unleashed in this century. One way to reconcile the impulse of creation and the impulse of destruction was to think that the former failed: Poetry and music had to fall and remain silent.[4]

However, a people does not own its literature. It does not even own its language, and that is the only reason why it is perhaps not possible to argue that the German language was buried in the concentration camps of Nazi Germany. The murderers spoke the language of Heinrich Heine, Franz Kafka, Walter Benjamin, Gertrud Kolmar, and Else Lasker-Schüler. To let the murderers speak the last word is to silence these voices—voices which have survived and are speaking today.

I studied my first page of *gemara* (talmudic discussion) at the same time that I encountered Walter Benjamin's work. It was Benjamin, then, who did not allow me to condemn the German language and its many voices and to rest comfortably with a judgment which would have allowed me to come to terms with the murderous past of the world in which I had grown up.

Therefore, the Talmud came to promise me something else: the understanding of what it was that those who spoke my language tried to murder. I hoped to unlock the secret of that otherness that seemed to have burned so brightly within a world of desired sameness, so that the people of sameness could not bear to see its light and obsessively set out to extinguish it. Within my sight, Jews—in the early eighties in Germany the word *Jude* was still inscribed with guilt and shame, with incomprehension, with insurmountable distance—came to embody what is now commonly called the "Other." The Talmud, to me then as now in many respects the greatest cultural, textual, and literary monument of Jewish culture, seemed to hide all the wisdom that would explain to me what had made *die Juden*—as bearers of Jewish culture—into the prime targets of the unleashed, murderous lust of those people who bore the culture that I was born into and inherited. If the Talmud was the founding literature of the Jewish community in exile, I expected it to explain to me this ultimate "otherness." The first time I saw a *daf gemara* (a leaf in the Talmud), I saw it as the surviving voice of those whose bodies had been burned to ashes and whose living communities had been erased from the maps of Europe. Violently disembodied words. Words printed on a page that could no longer be deciphered by those who had lived the words, but by me, who tried to cope with the unspeakable. Words that were not addressed to me, but to those who were gone forever. When I studied my first page of gemara at the age of nineteen at German institutions of higher education, I had never met a Jewish person. All the Jewish women, children, and men I had seen—in photographs in books and in museums—were dead. I wanted the gemara to become the redemptive voice for those who had been murdered.

Now, thirteen years of learning later, the gemara has become a fairly constant partner in dialogue for me. To study Jewish culture, specifically Talmud, in America and in Israel has given the voice of the gemara a very different sound. Within the context of American Jewish culture it has ceased to be the voice from the grave. I have had the opportunity to learn Talmud with people who live the words, whose life is circumscribed by *halakha*, and, over time I, too, have grown into such a life, having been absorbed by the text and the community. The voice of the dead has regained its body, in many different shapes and genders, in different communities of readers and students: the university, the synagogue, the Beit Midrash.[5] My love for the text is not just a love in the mind, but a love passionate with all the fluctuations, frustrations of distance, anger at rejection, and exaltation of intimacy that such love entails. The voices in the text are not merely voices from the past anymore, but also the voices of all those among whom I have studied and study the text. The printed text is not merely that which lies in front of me and waits for me to give it a contemporary voice by imposing my interpretation onto it. It is, rather, an open forum for dialogue and discussion which invites me, and every one of its students, to participate in it. The experience at the Beit Midrash has taught me the impossibility of the initial one-way street from me to the text. Rather, to learn gemara in the traditional *hevruta* style (with study partners) means to be drawn into and to reenact an ongoing conversation within the text that is not closed by virtue of being enclosed in a printed volume. In this way, I have changed seats, or rather, the seating arrangement has changed. Where the text ceases to be the fixed entity that I encounter from outside its fixation, there I am no longer sitting in the chair of her who came from beyond the boundaries of the *ethnos* which claims the Talmud as its cultural constitution. The Talmud has made me part of its world, of its own community, and seated me among those who participate in its heated debates.

### Interlude on the Genesis of a Woman Studying Talmud

That love for the Talmud came first. The ongoing reconstitution or redirection of myself in ethno-religious terms is a product of this love. However, with some delay, another starting point for a process of reconfiguring identities was conceived, creating with equal intensity difficult moments of alienation and moments of exaltation. This struggle is the struggle to become woman,[6] the struggle to fully come to life and language, the desire to reshape and remake the world in ways that will allow this to happen. This process was, of course, launched by the encounter with the literature of feminist criticism in its various forms and contexts, an uneasy encounter at first. That uneasiness derived from the fact that this literature asks its readers to position themselves, just like religious texts which demand that their readers position themselves with respect to their own authoritative claim. As such, the literature of feminist criticism asks for a commitment that can create, initially, a conflict of commitments. This conflict is particularly acute when one is trying to make one's home in a textual world such as the Talmud—which all of a sudden is reconfigured as a man's world, and one does not want to see it as such. Furthermore, uneasiness arises from the fact that entering the (European) university, studying, finding an intellectual home and staking out a territory in the intellectual world, all function for so many women, as for me, as an escape route from being "merely" a woman, in a sort of de Beauvoirian mode.[7] While being on the run, one does not like to be reminded of the impossibility of escape.

But feminist criticism, its various hermeneutic approaches, most fundamentally its hermeneutics of suspicion, and its fine-tuned methodologies of analyzing gender, turns into a powerful tool of both critical and constructive reading. As a tool to reconstitute meanings of texts, it creates possibilities of reshaping the world. The gift of feminist criticism, therefore, is a paradoxical one. On the one hand, it prohibits us from being easily at home in any given tradition or text, and keeps us from being blind to the refusal of such texts to allow women to be at home. It does not allow us to ignore dogmatic or rhetorical mechanisms of exclusions. Sometimes it will painfully prohibit us from finding ourselves as women even in the margins of such texts. At the same time, it allows us to remake our home in different, more meaningful and life-sustaining terms. The ongoing challenge, however, is to find a critical balance between commitments, between the commitment to texts that one loves with all their faults, which have sustained and continue to sustain identities of communities and individuals, my own no less, and the commitment to making this world a better world, for men and women alike.

## Return to the Overture

The following chapters attempt to find such a critical balance. On the one hand, rabbinic texts present a multiplicity of voices, construct a textuality of collectivity, craft webs or fabrics (*massekhtot*) of discourse that continue to be woven, texts that remain alive. On the other hand, the feminist literature of the last thirty years teaches us to see the limitation of that collectivity and its multiplicity of voices. The textual collectivity is composed of male voices, the product of either structures of discipleship between master and students or of the Beit Midrash[8] as the central institutions of rabbinic learning and discussion during the talmudic period. Both institutions were famously exclusive of women.[9]

My initial desire had been to look for the woman in the texts on niddah. With one hundred and forty-three pages of talmudic discussion on the language of women's bodies and on the attempt to articulate this language, it seems justifiable to expect to find a woman's voice.[10] However, this tractate is no different from others in that the hermeneutic and analytic voices in these pages are primarily the voices of men. We do find a series of narratives about women presenting evidence of their blood to rabbinic experts for evaluation, a practice still common today, which will require a closer examination in the talmudic context. But first, even these narratives are not necessarily about "real" women and their practice. Second, they present women as functioning within a cultural system that the rabbinic texts are only beginning to institute, hence already as only on the receiving end of rabbinic discourse, rather than as participants in creating the discourse. Women, therefore, appear in Tractate Niddah only as reflected in the discussions of men or as speaking in stories told by men.

But as feminist literary criticism teaches, the question is more complex than the gender of the speakers or authors of the discourse.[11] We must turn our analysis on the structures of authority engendering rabbinic discussions and engendered by rabbinic texts. Who does systematically have the authority to speak about women's bodies? Is there a uniformly gendered perspective constructed in the multivocal discussions? What sort of thinking do the texts want to engender in order to institute or maintain certain authority structures? What possibilities of thinking are excluded from the texts? What do the texts allow the reader to see and how? What do they keep from sight? What are the mechanisms that stabilize exclusions? If we ask questions such as these the actual gender identity of individual speakers ultimately turns into a subsidiary question. For example, in Chapter 2 I will focus on the metaphorical construction of women's bodies in Tractate Niddah in terms of architectural or domestic structures as the dominant linguistic feature of women's corporeality in rabbinic texts. The questions I want to pursue here are what cultural function or discursive effect such a construction has, and how we read the rabbinic thinking of gender.[12] Similarly, in part of Chapter 3 I will analyze what kind of halakhic or legal analogies for women's bodies the rabbis allow into the discussion. The metaphorical construction and such analogical links, supporting and illuminating each other, are two sides of the same coin.

This coin is what I will call the dominant androcentric perspective of talmudic discussions. In the case of rabbinic literature, I understand and use the term *androcentrism* as an analytically descriptive term. On a most basic level, an androcentric perspective on the world and human culture is one in which the literary subject as the projecting center of perceiving is gendered male, explicitly or not. In other words, we are not merely dealing with a textual culture that creates explicit hierarchies, but one that imagines a certain directionality of perceiving. The male subject may be qualified in multiple ways, but in an androcentric body of literature the imagining, perceiving, speaking, and knowing subject is predominantly marked as male. Often, this marking is hidden or only implied, which may make it much more powerful and convincing.[13] But directions of perception may be reconstructed, particularly in texts that deal with gender or sexual difference, even where the gender marking of the perceiving subject of the text remains hidden. To stay with the examples cited above: if women's bodies are metaphorically represented in terms of architectural, domestic structures, they are turned into mere functions, instrumentalized by the (male) perceiving subject projected in the texts, especially when such a metaphorical construction is only performed on women's bodies. Women are imagined as dwellings of their husbands, but not vice versa. Thus one major task of our readings of texts in Tractate Niddah is to find textual and discursive mechanisms that enable the construction of such a perspective, and enable the reader of such texts to remain ignorant of the gender marking of projected perspectives.

Finally, literary feminist criticism has developed and taught methods of "reading against the grain" of the gender ideologies of texts. Depending on the nature of the texts to be analyzed, "reading against the grain" can take various forms, just as its goals can be variously formulated. One may, for example, search for lapses in ideological coherence of a text or a set of texts, or one may interrogate texts with respect to traces of possible choices not made. One can locate what appears to be the "repressed" of a text; one can emphasize what the text hides, embedded in overt rhetorical structures; or one can highlight what are only moments of disturbance in the overall dominant ideology of the text.[14] What characterizes most of such readings is the highlighting of the cultural, textual, or rhetorical constructedness of gender.[15] The assumption is that once the constructedness of sexual difference in a text is revealed, alternative readings and alternative cultural choices may open up. Such methods are highly self-conscious or self-critical; they focus on the process of "reading" as an act of re-inscribing the text, re-appropriating or even re-writing it.[16] Adapting some of these strategies, I will focus in chapters 3 through 5 on some of the moments of disturbance in the various genres of the talmudic discussions of menstruation.[17] These moments of rupture in the androcentric fabric allow me to read a counter-discourse in those discussions.[18]

This politicized aspect of feminist literary criticism is perhaps its most contested one. It is caught between accusations of polemic and apologetic politics, both within the institutional confines of the academy as to the politics of reading, and between academic scholars and religious communities with respect to undermining dogmatic positions and structures of authority. Often in such acrimonious debates, especially with respect to rabbinic texts, the texts are represented as victims of readers and their mis- or forced readings. A reader of rabbinic texts is accused of polemical misrepresentations of the texts when she is pointing out a gender bias in the sources. Or readers may be represented as (involuntary) victims of the texts and their inherent authority structures. In accusations of apologetics a reader of rabbinic texts may be said to not take women's desires for autonomy seriously.

A critical balance in this climate can only be the product of respect for what can be learned from both sides. Ultimately, readings that enrich the meanings of rabbinic texts also enrich our own understanding of ourselves.

**A Short Note on Reading Tractate Niddah Historically**

The following chapters will not primarily read rabbinic texts as historical texts[19] but will study their discourse on menstruation, the construction of women's bodies as objects of talmudic discussion, and the lasting discursive effects of these discussions on thinking gender. I do not intend, however, to read them out of historical context. The talmudic discussions, as foundational texts for the rabbinic version of Jewish culture, do have a historical context in the cultural world of late antiquity. As is well known, it is extremely difficult to make an argument for a specific historical context for any of the individual text-units, due to the long history of each of the larger collections of rabbinic texts.

For the purposes of this book, I am defining the parameters of the historical and cultural context for the rabbinic discussions on menstruation in the widest possible terms. One such context that offers itself is the tradition of Greco-Roman gynecological literature, beginning with the pre-Aristotelian Hippocratic texts of the late fifth and early fourth century B.C.E. Aristotelian texts, and specifically gynecological texts by authors such as Soranus and Galen in the second century C.E. are also potential contexts. The former body of texts were composed centuries before the earliest rabbinic text was redacted into a collected whole. They turned into classical textbooks of medical literature with a diachronic tenacity even up until the second century C.E. I do not believe that we will be able to prove that the rabbis of the Mishnah or Talmud knew any specific texts from this body of literature or whether they knew of its existence at all. Nonetheless, I will show that two kinds of correlation can be drawn. On the one hand, the Mishnah tries to conceptualize a discourse of women's bodies in its Tractate Niddah at roughly the same time that Soranus and Galen attempted to develop a more focused gynecological vocabulary. We can look at both bodies of texts as products of a cultural impulse to make women's bodies accessible to language, to epistemology and the inquiring male mind.

On reading and comparing some of the arguments in the Greco-Roman gynecological literature and in the talmudic discussions, one cannot help noticing some convergences and parallels. For example, Chapter 3 describes how a talmudic dialectical discussion of the Mishnah resembles a debate between Hippocratic and Aristotelian notions of the physiology of menstruation. How is such a parallel to be understood? Did the rabbis know these theories? Is this a chance parallel, considering that there are not that many ways to interpret the physiology of menstruation? Again, I do not think that these questions can be resolved with certainty. But I will suggest the possibility of a rabbinic engagement of such debates in their cultural environment, by means of which they absorbed notions circulating in late antique culture. Taking such a possibility into account adds to our understanding as to how the rabbis located themselves in relationship to the larger cultural context of late antiquity.

Further, still defining the historical cultural context of the rabbinic texts by the widest possible parameters, I will also draw into the discussion texts that have traditionally been in the domain of scholars of early Christianity. Some of the early Christian texts intersect with rabbinic texts in their claim for biblical heritage—that is, in their hermeneutic link with the same textual fundament as rabbinic literature, the Bible. That hermeneutic link can obviously look very different from the rabbinic one, but it is exactly through this link that we can relate some of the early Christian texts that deal with menstruation, biblical notions of menstrual impurity, and interpretations of these notions, to the rabbinic discourse. Moreover, and more importantly, we will see that sometimes texts are too easily classified as unambiguously Christian texts. As to the discussions on menstruation, menstrual impurity, and rituals around this discourse we are extremely fortunate to have one important text, the *Didascalia Apostolorum*. A third century Syriac text, it polemicizes against a group of Jewish women who converted to Christianity but insisted on a Christianized observance of rituals concerning menstrual impurity. The author of this text engages in a prolonged debate with these women in ways that allow us to retrieve the arguments that the women brought forward in defense of their practice.[20] This text is important in various ways: first, it is one of the few texts, if not the only one, in late antique post-biblical cultures in which women themselves produce reasons for why they wish to observe a form of menstrual withdrawal.[21] Second, we can read this text in the margins of rabbinic culture, since the women clearly come from a Jewish context of halakhic interpretations of biblical tradition.

But they appear to come from a halakhic context that is not familiar to us from rabbinic literature. Hence, this text broadens the Jewish hermeneutic choices that existed in the cultural context of the rabbis. And finally, the women in the *Didascalia* allow us to think about how ethnic religious identities were constituted when women are at the center of the debate. Commonly, discussions of late antique religio-ethnic identities focus on ethnic markers such as circumcision, which reinforce constructions of male identities as the center of conflicts over the constitution of ethnic or religious identities in the culture of late antiquity. In contrast, the women in the *Didascalia* can help us to refocus this discussion so that gender is made to figure into it as a major factor.

These are the two major discourses in the cultural world of late antiquity which intersect with rabbinic culture. They will help us to illuminate some of the hermeneutic choices in the rabbinic texts. This latter historical contextualization can also be defined in terms relevant to this introduction on the ethics of reading Talmud. Since the Christian texts on menstrual impurity intersect with the rabbinic discussions by virtue of their hermeneutic link to biblical sources, scholars of early Christianity have sometimes commented on the rabbinic texts in various forms of anti-Jewish rhetorics, which will be discussed in more detail in the last chapter of this book. A more sophisticated juxtaposition of rabbinic and Christian texts on menstruation will allow us to challenge those models of reading Christian literature which reconstruct the emergence of Christianity as a liberation of Jewish women from the bonds imposed on them by the patriarchal rules and regulations of their "native" culture.[22]

## Coda to the Overture

I want to conclude the overture to the book with a few notes on writing about rabbinic texts, especially talmudic texts. To the person who is not initiated into the labyrinths of talmudic argumentation, most of its discourse may seem extremely obscure and hard to comprehend. The dense design of talmudic textuality is partially intended by the rabbis and anonymous editors who designed these labyrinths. A famous midrash relates the following reflection on the "readership" of rabbinic texts. God rejects Moses' request to receive the Mishnah, the first rabbinic document of what the rabbis call oral Torah, in writing. The reason is that

> since the Holy One, Blessed Be He foresaw that the Gentiles would translate the [written] Torah and read it in Greek [the Septuagint] and thereupon they would declare "We are Israel" . . . , the Holy One, Blessed Be He said to the nations: "You aver that you are my children? I cannot tell! Only they who possess my *arcana* [מסטורין] are my children." Which are these? The Mishnah. (Tanhuma, Ki' Tissa', par. 34)[23]

This text, most likely a product of polemics against the Pauline Christian interpretation of the (written) Torah and its subsequent claim of representing biblical Israel, marks rabbinic interpretations of the written Torah as belonging to "Israel" alone. The midrash indicates that certain forms of textuality are at the intersection of hermeneutic arguments and are overdetermined by identity politics. The post-talmudic period of Jewish culture down to the present age indicates how effective the crafting of rabbinic textuality as arcana was in terms of supporting a strong identity as a minority culture.

The difficulty of making talmudic discussions accessible to the noninitiate is corroborated by the fact that the terms of textual analysis, produced in centuries of yeshiva learning, and adapted in modernity by academic scholars of talmudic texts, are highly specialized.

However, since I intend here to make some of the rabbinic discussions accessible to students and scholars of feminist criticism, and to students of the complex interaction between cultural groups in late antiquity as well as scholars of rabbinic text, I want to provide a few notes on some of the terms recurring in these pages.

The earliest collection of rabbinic legal traditions, edited into a continous whole at the end of the second century or the beginning of the third century C.E., is the Mishnah. Other than being subdivided into individual massekhtot (by and large thematic tractates), the smallest textual unit of the Mishnah is an individual mishnah.[24] An individual mishnah often addresses a single issue or a rabbi's opinion on a given subject. An individual mishnah can list more than one opinion, carefully structuring these opinions as actual disagreements. The number of opinions may range from one to four.

A companion document to the Mishnah is the Tosefta (or "Supplement"), redacted a few decades later than the Mishnah. The Tosefta is largely parallel to the Mishnah. It comments upon the Mishnah, expands it, abbreviates it, or provides additional information.[25] The smallest text-units in the Tosefta I will refer to as *baraita*.[26] These texts, along with the early collections of midrashim,[27] or rabbinic exegetical works, are mostly of Palestinian origin. Later rabbinic traditions, beginning with the Talmud, endow these texts with the highest degree of authority, as they were the product of the earlier generations of rabbis, designated the *tannaim* in talmudic scholarship.

Both the Mishnah and the Tosefta are by and large elliptical texts.[28] They primarily present the opinion of individual rabbis on a given subject, but they hardly ever explain why such opinions are held. The discourses are structured as disagreements on issues, with one to (rarely) four differing opinions. Hence these texts, though carefully arranged, are basically a collection of statements rather than argumentations.

The Talmuds (*Talmudim*), both the Palestinian and the Babylonian Talmud, the latter of which is much more central to this book, have their origin in the elliptical nature of those earlier texts. The Talmudim, known also as the gemara to the Mishnah,[29] follow the basic structure of the Mishnah and present a discussion of it, attempting to analyze the reasons for opinions stated in the Mishnah. The rabbis who are presented as discussing the Mishnah in the gemara are called the *amoraim*. It is the gemara that presents itself as argumentation (of the Mishnah) and creates the dialectical structure that the Talmud is famous for.[30] The basic unit of the gemara is the *sugyah*, often translated as pericope, which is a self-contained unit of talmudic argumentation on an individual mishnah. The sugyah is a multilayered text that may cite any genre from biblical verse, mishnah, baraita, midrash, or individual statements of post-mishnaic rabbis, and sometimes also extended narrative, known as *aggadot*. Sugyot, which can have various lengths and complexities of argumentation, have been constructed and edited anonymously. Unfortunately, we do not know anything with certainty about either the editors or the process of editing. But it is the sugyot that present the idiosyncratic genius of the Babylonian Talmud in particular. They are characteristic of what is known as talmudic literature. Sugyot are mostly self-referential in terms of rabbinic literature and cross-referential in terms of other sugyot.

# 1 FRAMING NIDDAH

PERHAPS MORE THAN other aspects of rabbinic literature, the laws concerning menstruation have been caught in the current battle of polemics and apologetics on gender relations in Jewish culture. Rabbinic texts on the impurity of menstruation are inscribed with halakhic readings of the centuries following the Talmud. The social and religious institutions they engender, such as the *miqveh*, are an essential if often contested part of Jewish culture today. Debates on the role of women in Jewish cultures of the past and of the present often focus on the issue of menstrual impurity and the significance of the ritualization of menstruation for women.

The contemporary debates produce by and large two extreme positions. Sometimes the ritualization of menstruation and its designation as menstrual impurity with the concurrent requirement of purification are evaluated as an index of the sexism of traditional Jewish culture.[1] This polemical position depicts the psychological consequences of this ritualization as ranging from absolutely crippling to somewhat damaging. A more apologetic position emphasizes the positive aspect of the ritualization of women's bodies and its affirmation of women's physiology. This position classically focuses on the psychological health inherent to the ritualization of menstruation.[2] By requiring a married couple to abstain from marital intimacy for a certain amount of time, the sexual life of a couple is affirmed and regulated. The periods of withdrawal that are created teach a couple to fall in love with each other regularly.

Simultaneously, the apologetic position has adapted to the force of feminist criticism and its challenge to write and create a Jewish culture that does justice to women's desire for spiritual and religious fulfillment. The flourishing literature by orthodox women and for orthodox women on Jewish womanhood and its emphasis on the meaningfulness of rituals such as menstrual separation attests to this. Often, the argument is made that the observance of menstrual rituals, especially the immersion in the miqveh at the end of the period of menstruation, connects women with previous generations of Jewish women. Thus the observance of menstrual rituals can be represented as a form of Jewish women's heroism.[3]

The debate that focuses on the practice of menstrual rituals may not be productive, since it produces two juxtaposed positions: criticism of the practice or defense of it. I want to focus in this book on the discourse on menstruation, rather than on the practice of it. Focusing on the discourse concerning menstruation allows us to read the practice in the larger context of culture. It allows us to refine our understanding of the function of gender in Jewish culture and to reflect on such questions as: Who is speaking for whom? Who is allowed to speak? Who is producing meanings? What are the effects of creating certain meanings for gender relations?

In the next few chapters I will present studies of the foundational literature on niddah—that is, the rabbinic texts of late antiquity. These texts of the past can only be read through layers and layers of historical and cultural readings that have accumulated around them. In the current chapter, therefore, I want to collect a few archaeological fragments of these layers that inevitably inflect our readings of the rabbinic texts.

### Niddah: The Politics of Etymology

The fundamental problem begins with language, and with the ways menstruation is conceptualized in the language of the rabbis. Some feminist studies begin with a reflection on etymology of the term *niddah* itself, and what the etymology signifies concerning the cultural inscription of menstruation.[4] However, as Moshe Greenberg has pointed out most recently in his review of etymological suggestions: "Recent studies of the etymology of נידה '(menstrual) impurity' are inconclusive" ("Etymology," 69).[5]

There are two choices as to the verbal root of the word and two choices as to the referent of the action described by the verb. Concerning the root, the first option is *n-d-d*, "to depart, flee, wander." The second option is *n-d-h*, "to chase away, put aside," a cognate from the Akkadian *nadu*, "to throw, cast down."[6] Barukh Levine suggests that the Akkadian cognate "to cast, hurl, throw" offers an additional connection: "It represents a variation of *n-z-h*, 'to spatter,' . . . a connection suggested by Rashi in his comment to Numbers 19:9 [and the ashes of the heifer shall be kept outside the camp in a clean place, and it shall be kept for the congregation of the children of Israel for the *water of sprinkling*: it is a purification offering]."[7] Furthermore, Milgrom defines the biblical term *niddah* as expulsion or elimination.[8]

With respect to the second set of options, the choices between referents of the action described in the verbal root, we enter a more contentious area. According to Levine, "it does not connote impurity in and of itself but, rather, describes the physiological process of the flow of blood" (*Leviticus*, 97). Similarly, Jacob Milgrom regards the physiological process of discharging menstrual blood as the referent of *niddah* as expulsion. But he continues: "*niddah* came to refer not just to the menstrual discharge but to the menstruant herself, for she too was 'discharged' and 'excluded' from her society by being banished to and quarantined in separate quarters" (*Leviticus 1–16*, 745).[9] Levine, however, maintains that when the term is applied to the menstruating woman herself, rather than to menstruation itself, it means "one who is spilling blood."[10]

Clearly there is a significant difference between these two explanations, with different implications for our perception of the menstruous woman in biblical culture and subsequently in rabbinic literature. Basically, the practice of banning a menstruating woman, except to exclude her from the Temple precinct, is not warranted by our textual sources,[11] and even Jacob Milgrom has to resort to the practice of menstrual exclusion in other cultures to provide evidence for his statement. The term נדה cannot be proven to have its roots in the sociocultural practice of banning or ostracizing women. Such a practice was not implemented by the priestly sources in the biblical texts, nor is it referred to in the rabbinic texts. The term *niddah* does not have an inherent meaning, in and by itself, of "the ostracized woman" or "abhorrence and repulsion," nor can we reconstruct its original meaning. Rather, it acquires different meanings and connotations in different contexts. Greenberg points out that in the priestly stratum of the biblical texts, including the chapter on the impurity of genital discharges (Lev. 15), the term *niddah* bears the specific sense of menstrual impurity, whereas in post-biblical usage, specifically in "*Mishnaic* Hebrew the concrete sense 'menstruant' prevails" ("Etymology," 76).[12] Meaning depends on context.

In the context of rabbinic texts, the meaning of the term *niddah* is primarily "a woman who menstruates." We do not find any texts or statements that indicate any valuation of the term, or that use the concept of *niddah* in any moralizing context,[13] such as Ezra[14] or the prophet Ezekiel[15] might have suggested to the rabbis. We can also observe that rabbinic literature does not anywhere indicate or allude to a practice of women's public segregation.[16] The literature maintains almost uniformly a careful distinction between a practice of ostracizing women or banishing them from the life of the community, and the practice of separating husband and wife in terms of intimacy within the household. The former would put the menstruant into an adverse relationship to the community as a whole, and the act of separating her from the community would consequently isolate her socially as a menstruant woman,[17] which is not indicated in any way in rabbinic texts. The latter, however, sets only husband and wife sexually apart, without necessarily even banning the wife from the normal life of the household as a whole. Again, there is no indication of such a practice, either in legal discussions or in narrative texts.[18] The separation that rabbinic literature delineates is exclusively that between husband and wife, the married couple itself, and not between the menstruous woman and the community or the household. This is expressed clearly in the following passage in the Babylonian Talmud:

אמר ר' עקיבא כשהלכתי לגליא היו קורין לנדה גלמודה מאי גלמודה גמולה דא מבעלה

Rabbi Akiva said: When I went to Gallia they used to call a niddah *galmudah*.
What is a *galmudah*? She who is weaned from (*gemulah da*) her husband. (bRosh Hashana 26a)

This little account is part of a *baraita*, an earlier authoritative tannaitic source in which Rabbi Aqiva is represented as introducing an unknown term for the menstruous woman. Those in the Talmud who transmit this textual source are not sure what the term *galmudah* means. It is an extremely rare term in talmudic literature. The question the Talmud asks—What is a *galmudah*?—is answered with a pseudo-etymological wordplay by rearrangement of letters, a classic midrashic technique and quite common in rabbinic literature: "She is weaned (*gemulah da*) from her husband!"[19] As Rashi, the canonical commentator on the Talmud, explains, she is separated (מובדלת) from her husband, but not from society. This point is also emphasized by Yedidyah Dinari, who argues that "it has to be assumed that the whole explanation of 'what is *galmudah*?' is introduced only to emphasize that she is only weaned from her husband, but not from anybody else" ("Customs Relating to the Impurity of the Menstruant," 313).[20]

Rabbinic literature addresses a situation after the destruction of the Temple, the reference point of holiness of the biblical discourse of purity and impurity. The biblical text establishes explicitly, "Thus shall you separate the children of Israel from their impurity, so that they will not die in their impurity *when defiling my tabernacle* that is in your midst" (Lev. 15:31). People had to be in a status of purity if they wanted to approach the Temple in Jerusalem or if they handled food or items that were dedicated to the Temple. Shaye Cohen points out that the synagogue does not replace the Temple in this respect since "in the Mishnah and the Talmudim the synagogue has no inherent sanctity; sacred rituals are performed there, but the building has no sanctity at all. It is certainly not a temple; even a leper is permitted to enter" ("Menstruants and the Sacred," 285). Further, there is no evidence that women should be kept separate from "holy books" because of a potential supposed danger of transferring their menstrual impurity to them.[21] On the contrary, there is at least one tannaitic source that—almost in passing—explicitly allows the menstruous woman to read Torah: "Men and women with irregular genital emissions, menstruants, and parturients are permitted to read the Torah, and to study Mishnah, Midrash, laws and homilies"(tBer 2:12).[22]

In sum, the context of rabbinic literature as the primary semantic field of the term *niddah* does not support the meaning of ostracism and banning. The literature does not reflect or even allude to a practice of excluding menstruating women from social life. On the contrary, some of the texts indicate or even emphasize that menstruating women are not to be excluded from social life. In rabbinic literature, therefore, the primary range of meaning of the term *niddah* seems to be simply "the woman who is menstruating."

### The Conceptual Frame: Sexual Taboo Versus Ritual Impurity

Obviously, the rabbinic discussions of menstruation are built on biblical law, not merely biblical language. As self-evident as this point is, it needs to be reiterated as part of constructing the frame for the following readings. The rabbis do not merely institute a legal discourse, they also choose to inherit one. Thus, when we read gender in rabbinic culture, one of the aspects to be considered is the intersection between rabbinic literature and biblical texts. Rabbinic gendering is framed by its hermeneutic of biblical texts. This is particularly the case with niddah.

The two *conceptual* contexts for biblical menstruation are, on the one hand, the priestly system of purity and impurity and, on the other, the lists of prohibited sexual relationships. Both contexts are conceptually independent from each other. Lev. 15, the biblical chapter on the impurity of genital discharges, discusses the transference of a status of impurity from one person to another through sexual intercourse or touch, either from male to female or from female to male. A person with a certain kind of genital discharge could transfer a status of impurity to a thing or to any other person, not just to his or her spouse. The consequence of contracting a status of impurity is the requirement of certain rituals of purification, including a bird offering to be brought to the Temple. Lev. 18 and 20, on the other hand, provide lists of sexual relationships prohibited by punishment of *karet*, extirpation, which the rabbis read as death at the hand of God in the form of premature death.[23] Included in these lists is the prohibition of sexual relations during a wife's menstrual period (Lev. 18:19 and 20:18).

These two contexts are conceptually independent from each other in that Lev. 15 is contingent on a specific social-institutional structure, the existence of the central Sanctuary, whereas Lev. 18 and 20, the lists of sexual taboos, are not. As already mentioned, at the time of the redaction of the Mishnah, that is, at the end of the second century C.E. and the beginning of the third, this question has clearly no practical, halakhic relevance. With the destruction of the Temple in Jerusalem by the Romans in 70 C.E. the *axis mundi* and point of reference for the practice of a large number of the purity and impurity regulations had vanished, since it had been the Temple that served as the space of holiness to be separated from impurity.[24] However, menstruation as included in the list of sexual taboos structures the relationship primarily between husband and wife, but not between the husband or wife and other people. This conceptual context continues to be practically relevant today, since it is not contingent on the existence of the Temple. In post-Temple times, most of the halakhic regulations and observances still practiced today concern the prevention of sexual relations between husband and wife during the wife's menstrual period. For example, the prohibition on a man touching his wife is not based on the fear of her menstrual impurity, but on the notion that touching her will lead to sexual relations at a time when they are biblically prohibited to each other. Similarly, a man may not touch any woman other than his wife, again not because of her potential impurity, but because of rabbinic concepts of touch and the loss of male sexual self-control. This distinction is important for gauging the nature of menstrual laws in Jewish practice. These contemporary halakhic precautions of not touching are meant to prevent husband and wife from accidentally becoming too intimate. They are not fully spelled out in rabbinic texts. Obviously, this practice can be regarded as quite problematic as to rabbinic concepts of touch and male sexuality. However, what is important here is that this practice has nothing to do with the woman's supposed impurity. Rather, it is based on a definition and circumscription of the erotic during a period when sexual relations are prohibited.[25]

Conceptual clarity is important, since in the polemical or apologetic discussions about menstrual regulations in rabbinic discourse this issue is often raised. Sometimes the argument is made that the entire practice of niddah rests purely on the notion of women's impurity, and therefore is denigrating to women but not men, and thus it is an inherently sexist practice.[26] It needs to be clarified that just as a man with an ir/regular discharge is no longer a source of impurity in post-Temple times, neither are women who have their menstrual periods. Or, at the very least, the biblical definition of such a man or woman as a source of impurity has become irrelevant in post-Temple times. Menstruous women do not transfer a status of impurity to anybody else through touch, not even to their husbands. However, even though a reading of the observance of niddah as rooted in a perception of women as inherently impure is not entirely correct, to argue the opposite would be no more correct. The opposite reading would be to focus merely on the conceptual, biblical-halakhic framework and to argue that the practice of niddah in post-Temple times only has to do with the prohibition of sexual relations between husband and wife during the wife's menstrual period, and has nothing to do with women's impurity. As we shall see, neither of these positions is entirely correct, nor are they entirely wrong.

### Discursive Framing in Rabbinic Literature

Rachel Biale has suggested that, "beginning with the talmudic material and continuing through the medieval period, we see the transfer of the focus of the laws of *niddah* from the realm of ritual impurity to the sphere of marital and sexual relations . . . we observe a gradual fundamental transformation in the laws of *niddah*; the meaning and focus of these laws shifts from the fear and control of impurity to the regimentation of sexual relations" (*Women and Jewish Law*, 158). It is not quite clear how Biale envisions the shift or the "transfer of focus." For what she does not reflect upon is the fact that the rabbinic discourse of menstrual *impurity* versus the "regimentation of sexual relations" does not simply vanish, in spite of its halakhic-practical irrelevance. With respect to other purity and impurity regulations one might argue that they eventually do vanish, since of all the mishnaic tractates in the order of "Purities" we have a talmudic discussion only for the tractate on the regulation of menstruation. As far as Tractate Niddah is concerned, the Babylonian Talmud provides a gemara for the whole tractate, whereas the Palestinian Talmud provides a gemara for the first three chapters of the mishnah only.[27]

There has been considerable, albeit inconclusive, speculation on the reason for the absence of a talmudic discussion for the rest of the mishnaic order of "Purities." The traditional argument, that these other tractates remained without a gemara because they had lost relevance for the praxis, is not necessarily compelling, since the Babylonian Talmud, for example, provides a gemara for those tractates that deal with sacrifices in the Temple. Even Tractate Niddah does not have practical relevance in most of its details.[28] They continue to inquire under what circumstances a woman in her menstruation transfers the status of impurity to objects and other persons. Thus, though we might think of a "transformation" (Biale, *Women and Jewish Law*, 158) in terms of the practical applicability of the discussions, there is not therefore a "transfer of focus" from one to the other, at least not in terms of continuing production of halakhic literature and discourse on the aspect of impurity of menstruation. Here parts of the textual constellations in the Mishnah as well as of the discussions in the gemaras could ultimately be studied as if the Temple had not been destroyed, because the texts do not make the destruction an issue. Ultimately, Biale's historical reasoning fails to account for the discursive energies behind the continuing discussions of the status of impurity of the menstruous woman.

Thus rabbinic literature does not neatly fit this conceptual framework of the biblical texts. We are faced with the counterintuitive phenomenon that the majority of the mishnaic and talmudic Tractate of Niddah deals with questions of menstrual impurity. As also noted by Judith Hauptman, the mishnaic Tractate Niddah "shows very little interest in the home life of the couple when she is a niddah" (*Rereading the Rabbis*, 160). It focuses on just that conceptual context from biblical law that has lost its historical reference point. Of course, according to the logics of talmudic literature, beginning with the Mishnah, this is not necessarily a counterintuitive phenomenon, since much of the Mishnah deals with laws related to the Temple cult.[29] However, Mishnah Tractate Niddah focuses exclusively on one of the two conceptual framings from the biblical text. Tractate Niddah is part of the Order of Tohorot, or Order of Purities. The thirteen tractates of this order deal with all kinds of aspects of ritual impurity, beginning with the classification of what kinds of vessels can contract ritual impurity, including tractates on regulations pertaining to the miqveh and the impurity of men with irregular genital emissions, and ending with a short tractate on the transmission of impurity to the fruit from stalks, peels, or kernels. By focusing exclusively on the conceptual framework of impurity, most of the Mishnah Tractate Niddah seems to be a theoretical, halakhic text which discusses Jewish law as an abstract construct.

As an example, we need only consider the opening chapter of this tractate. It is concerned with the discussion of the possible retroactivity of menstrual impurity. Such a discussion has relevance only for how the woman's potential status of im/purity would affect objects that must be handled in a status of purity, that is, objects related to the Temple, such as the heave-offering to be given to the priests. If a woman has handled such objects close to the onset of her menstruation she might have been in a status of impurity earlier than she thought. Clearly, this discussion is applicable only with the existence of the Temple and its cultic implements, a condition that no longer applies at the time of the redaction of the Mishnah.

In the mishnaic text, therefore, the other conceptual framework of the Bible seems to have atrophied. Allusions are hidden in other contexts, almost buried in lists: Sexual relations with a woman who is niddah are listed among the 36 transgressions punishable by premature death, if done deliberately (mKer 1:1, bKer 2a). A famous mishnah in Tractate Shabbat mentions that "for three transgressions women die in childbirth—if they are not punctilious with respect to niddah, to hallah (the offering of dough to be separated from bread), or to the lighting of lamps [on the eve of Shabbat]" (mShab 2:6, bShab 31b). Here it is left open what exactly the observance of niddah entails, but presumably the allusion is to the prohibition of sexual relations. Further, it appears in a list of those behaviors and transgressions committed by a wife that would provide the grounds for a divorce, which also included sexual relations with her husband while being niddah (mKet 7:6).[30] Finally, a mishnah in mShev 2:4 discusses how a man should behave if his wife starts to menstruate at the moment of intercourse.

### The Anecdotal Evidence of the Sexual Taboo in Talmudic Literature

The Talmud provides only scanty, anecdotal references to the prohibition of sexual relations during the wife's menstrual period, again primarily outside of Tractate Niddah. Again, the references seem to be buried in other contexts. Thus, in the context of dealing with marital behavior the Babylonian Talmud includes a brief remark attributed to a rabbi of the end of the third century:

> Rabbi Yitzhaq said in the name of Rav Huna: "All those labors which a woman performs on behalf of her husband, a *niddah* performs for her husband, except for the mixing of the cup [of wine],[31] the making of the bed, and the washing of his face, hands and feet." (bKet 61a, bKet 4b)[32]

As all the talmudic commentators point out, "all these are matters of contact and affection and, therefore, lead to transgression" of the biblical prohibition of sexual relations.[33] The issue of this rabbinic ruling is the definition of what constitutes erotic stimulation, obviously within a relationship in which the wife is subservient. Such erotic stimulations are to be avoided during the period in which the couple is prohibited from having sexual relations.

The other two anecdotes will begin to hint at what we can read as a discursive obfuscation in rabbinic discussions of menstruation. This obfuscation is the result of intertwining the two conceptually different contexts. Both anecdotes are revealing.

A brief but famous reference in Tractate Niddah of the Babylonian Talmud, found in the midst of moralizing explanations of biblical rules, attributes to Rabbi Meir, a rabbi of the second century, the question of why the Torah prohibits a menstruous wife to her husband. The answer is that "the Torah said that she will be in the status of impurity for seven days, so that she will be beloved to her husband as in the hour of her entering the Huppah [the wedding canopy]" (bNid 31b). This passage has gained particular fame in the contemporary polemic and apologetic literature. Polemics against the ritual of niddah typically use it to point out that the whole practice is geared toward the desire of the husband. Apologetic literature, on the other hand, typically uses this passage to point out how good, and psychologically wise, the practice of periodic sexual abstinence is for a marriage to preserve mutual erotic desire. My primary interest here is not to judge between the two positions as to their accuracy. Rather, what we will note immediately here is the linguistic framing of the sexual prohibition. According to the text,

אמרה תורה תהא טמאה שבעה ימים כדי חביבה על בעלה כשעת כניסתה לחופה—

"the Torah said that she will be *in the status of impurity* for seven days so that she will be beloved to her husband. . . ." Here the language of "impurity" is not used to indicate a concrete ritual status, but more loosely as an expression for the wife's sexual inaccessibility. "She is in the status of impurity" means only "the husband will not be able to have sexual relations with her," since she is menstruating. This is a merging of two different halakhic concepts.

This is repeated in the other anecdotal reference, which can be found in parallel versions in both the Palestinian and the Babylonian Talmuds, this time concerning the wife of Shmu'el, a famous rabbi of the first generation of talmudic teachers at the beginning of the third century.[34] The version of the Palestinian Talmud presents a a conversation between Shmu'el and his wife. By contrast, the Babylonian Talmud has a much briefer version that eliminates the wife's direct speech and merely reports an inquiry of Shmu'el submitted to his colleague about a woman's potential claim. The Palestinian version is as follows:

> Shmu'el wanted to sleep with his wife.
> She said to him: I am *in the status of impurity* [טמאה אני].
> But the next day she said: I am *in the status of purity*. [אני טהורה]
> He said to her: Yesterday you were *in the status of impurity*, today you are *in the status of purity*!?
> She said to him: Yesterday I did not have the same strength as today.
> He went to ask Rav, who said to him: If she gave you a plausible reason to her words [and she did], she can be believed. (pKet 2:5, 26c; also quoted in Tosafot, bKet 22b, ד"ה ואפילו)[35]

This story is quite revealing as to the anxiety that occurs when women take halakhah into their own hands, and what this implies for the relationship between men and women, between rabbis and women, and between husbands and wives. I agree with Hauptman that it is important to acknowledge that "the purity rules, which some say treat women like objects, in this case give a wife a measure of control over the couple's sex life" (*Rereading the Rabbis*, 248). However, rather than postulating that "the deliberate, even savvy inclusion of anecdotes like these shows that the Talmudic rabbis do not take themselves too seriously," (249)[36] I would suggest reading a narrative like this symptomatically, as a symptom of the rabbis' or the redactors' anxiety about women making legitimate *halakhic* arguments to their own advantage. In such instances, women's discourse is curtailed by repeatedly framing it as an issue of their believability, even in a case such as this where a rabbi rules in favor of the woman. This framing will be discussed in greater detail in Chapter 4, in a close reading of another such story in which a woman is represented as taking the halakha into her own hands, also a narrative dealing with niddah. The two narratives are linked exactly by the framing of women's halakhic discourse as an issue of believability.

As to my current argument, however, we can again make the observation that in this narrative the woman is represented as employing the language of im/purity to indicate that she is sexually unavailable to her husband. When Shmu'el's wife says טמאה אני/טהורה אני—"I am in the status of im/purity"—

what she really is saying is "I am menstruating and, therefore, am sexually prohibited to you."³⁷ This text merges the two conceptual frames of forbidden sexual relations and impurity, and deploys the language of purity more loosely as an equivalent expression of sexual inaccessibility.

## The Linguistic Obfuscation of Niddah in Rabbinic Literature

Having discussed the scant anecdotal evidence in the talmudic texts, we can now advance a larger claim. The anecdotal evidence provides the few references in talmudic texts in which menstruation is discussed with respect to the sexual prohibition inherited from biblical law. From the point of view of practice or observance, it is exactly this issue that remains applicable for the rabbis. At the same time, Tractate Niddah, both the Mishnah and the discussions in the gemara, focus primarily on the issue of ritual im/purity, which in post-Temple times no longer has practical relevance. Finally, we have begun to observe that the anecdotal evidence in the two Talmuds in some sense merges the two conceptual frameworks. Whereas they are really "about" menstruation as sexual prohibition, the two anecdotes employ the language of im/purity as an index of the sexual inaccessibility of the woman, solely with that meaning in mind. אני טמאה comes to mean "I have my menstrual period (and therefore cannot have sexual relations with you, my husband)."

Based on these observations, I want to suggest how the conceptual framework of menstruation, inherited from biblical law, can be put together with our observations about the discursive framework of menstruation in rabbinic literature, and its contextualization in the mishnaic Order of Purities. In rabbinic literature, we can observe a sliding of the two conceptual frameworks into each other, primarily on a linguistic level. On the one hand, the rabbinic texts continue to distinguish *halakhically conceptually* between the two. That is, the system of impurity follows certain rules of the production and transference of a status of impurity. In and by themselves, these are completely independent from the issue of the sexual prohibition. On the other hand, the rabbis employ the language of impurity as *an expression* describing the woman's condition in which she is prohibited from having sexual relations.

This happens within the mishnaic (and subsequently talmudic) tractate on niddah as well. Certain parts of the tractate, such as the first chapter mentioned above, quite clearly deal with questions about impurity as if the Temple still existed, hence as a theoretical concept. However, in the later chapters the mishnaic tractate turns to issues that we will discuss in more detail in the following chapters of this book. Therefore, I want to introduce an exemplary issue at this point, with respect to the *language* that the Mishnah (and subsequently the Talmud) employs. In its later chapters the mishnaic tractate discusses the difference between colors of blood. It also introduces the question of bloodstains, and gives criteria for how to read bloodstains depending on their size, shape, or location. Thus, "five colors of blood are *impure* [טמאים] in a woman" (mNid 2:5), or "a woman who sees a bloodstain on her flesh close to her genitalia is *impure* [טמאה], but if it is not in the vicinity of her genitalia, she is pure [טהורה]" (mNid 8:1). The primary meaning of such texts is that such colors, or such stains, indicate that the blood is most likely uterine or menstrual. They, consequently, indicate that the woman is in a status of impurity. Hence, (theoretically) precautions would have to be taken with respect to Temple-related foods and tools or vessels.

But these texts also have a secondary meaning that allows them to slip into contemporary handbooks on Jewish law of menstruation.[38] Their secondary meaning is that certain colors of blood or certain stains indicate that the blood is most likely uterine or menstrual and therefore prohibits the woman having sexual relations with her husband. In other words, the above-mentioned phrase—"five colors of blood are impure in a woman"—comes to also mean—"five colors of [genital] blood indicate that she has her menstruation, and therefore cannot engage in sexual relations with her husband."

What this means is that, after all, Mishnah Tractate Niddah is not merely about ritual purity and impurity with respect to the Temple and the items related to it. That would have made the entire tractate irrelevant for later halakhic discussions. Rather, the tractate also develops indexes as to how menstruation as such can be recognized and thus rule out sexual relations with the husband. It is this merging of two conceptual frameworks into each other, the linguistic obfuscation, which makes Tractate Niddah one of the most difficult tractates in the Talmud.

To sum up, the linguistic slippage introduced by the rabbis obscures what biblically and halakhically are two different conceptual frameworks for discussing menstruation. Rabbinic texts employ the phrase אני טמאה to say "I am menstruating." The expression gets separated from its technical meaning of requiring meticulousness about Temple items, and comes to mean "I am not available sexually to my husband." Technically, a menstruating woman is not a source of impurity to other people in post-Temple halakha, no more and no less than a man with a genital emissions. Like him, she does not transfer a status of impurity to other people. Linguistically, however, she is called "impure."

This obfuscation allows for the coining of the phrase *taharat ha-mishpaha*, or "family purity," in popular literature on Jewish law, as an umbrella term for the laws regulating sexual relations between husband and wife during her menstrual period. In spite of its widespread use in current linguistic habits,[39] this phrase is never used in talmudic literature. The concept of "family purity" has been rightly criticized for instrumentalizing women's menstrual cycles as a function of family and making women's bodies alone responsible for the potential impurity not only of women themselves, but of the entire family. Beyond that, the term actually is a halakhic and conceptual misnomer, since the relevant laws of niddah do not concern ritual purity or impurity. Hence, this term is inapplicable for reading rabbinic discussions of menstruation. Reading against the grain of convention entails pushing aside layers of assumptions that keep us from understanding the texts of the past.

**The Midrashic Reason for the Commandment of Menstrual Separation**

Our readings of the rabbinic discussions of menstruation need to be framed by another conceptual context of reading. As is common in biblical law, the laws concerning menstrual impurity do not provide any etiological reason other than the need for the ritual purity of the central sanctuary. Neither does the list of prohibited relationships provide any reason why certain relationships are prohibited. Rabbinic texts, on the other hand, do reflect on the divine reason for establishing the *mitzvat niddah*, the commandment of sexual abstinence during menstruation. They construct a mythological *ai-*

*tion* to account for the fact that the Bible proscribes certain relations. A construction of such reasons betrays something about the general perception of menstruation and women's bodies in rabbinic texts.

There are only a few such passages in rabbinic texts. They appear mostly in midrashic literature, but not within the framework of the mishnaic and talmudic Tractate Niddah. Thus, in a midrash ascribed to Rabbi Yehoshua, a Palestinian rabbi from the beginning of the second century, the "commandment of niddah" is interpreted as a divine punishment for the first woman's act of disobedience, since by her disobedience she became complicit in the death of the first man:

ומפני מה ניתן לה מצוות נדה על ידי ששפכה דמו שלאדם הראשון לפיכך ניתן לה מצוות נידה

[the students asked him:] and why was she [the generic woman] given the "commandment of niddah"? [Rabbi Yehoshua answered] because she spilled the blood of the first *adam*, therefore she was given the "commandment of niddah." (*Midrash Bereshit Rabba*, Albeck and Theodor, 160)

The midrash reasons by analogy. The first woman committed a transgression by disobeying the creator, the consequence of which was the expulsion of the first man and woman from the Garden. This expulsion brought about the introduction of death ("spilling of blood") into human life. Therefore, God punished her with a commandment having to do with blood. Similarly, Rabbi Yehoshua interprets the other commandments incumbent especially upon women, that is, the commandment of separating the first portion of dough (*mitzvat challah*) and the commandment of lighting the sabbath lamp (*mitzvat ner shel-shabbath*), as divine punishments for the first woman's disobedience, again by analogical reasoning:

מפני מה ניתן לה מצוות חלה אמר להן מפני שקילקלה את אדם הראשון שהיה חלתו שלעולם לפיכך ניתן לה מצוות חלה ומפני מה ניתן לה מצוות נר שלשבת אמר להן על ידי שכיבת נשמתו שלאדם הראשון לפיכך ניתן לה מצוות נר שבת

Why was she [the generic woman] given the "commandment of challah"? [Rabbi Yehoshua answered] because she spoiled the *first adam* who was the "challah" of the world [at creation]. Therefore she was given the "commandment of challah." And why was she given the "commandment of lighting the sabbath lamp"? [Rabbi Yehoshua] answered: on account of the extinction of the soul of *the first adam*, therefore she was given the "commandment of lighting the sabbath lamp." (ibid.)

The midrashic motif of blaming the first woman for the first man's death reappears in various rabbinic texts. The Palestinian Talmud offers the midrash, possibly citing from our midrash (Boyarin, *Carnal Israel*, 91 n.24), without, however, attributing it to Rabbi Yehoshua. Here the formulation is more explicit, in that the text adds the emphasis that וגרמה לו חוה מיתה לפיכך מסרו מצות נדה לאשה—"Eve caused his [the *first adam*'s] death, therefore he [God] gave the 'commandment of niddah' to the woman" (pShab 2:6, 5b). An even more extreme version of the midrashic interpretation as punishment[40] reads the mitzvat niddah as the woman's expiation for Eve's act of murder:

ולמה נצטוו הנשים על המצות הללו אלא אמרו חכמינו שאדם היה תחלת ברייתו של עולם ובא חוה ושפכה דמו . . . ואמר הקב"ה תנתן לה מצות דם הנדה שיתכפר לה על אותו הדם ששפכה

And why are women given these commandments (the triad of *niddah*, *challah* and lighting the shabbat light)? Since our sages said that *'adam* was the beginning of the creation of the world and [then] Eve came and spilled his blood . . . and the Holy One Blessed Be He said: She shall be given the commandment of the blood of *niddah* so that it can serve as her expiation for the same blood which she spilled. [Tanh. Buber, *Noah*, 1:14b; cp. ibid. *Metzora*, 17:27a and AdRN B 9, 13a][41]

From the traditional, historical perspective this latter version of the motif is most likely a more recent one. The date of the redaction of the Tanhuma as well as of Avot di-Rabbi Nathan is in dispute among scholars, but the consensus seems to be that they are post-talmudic, though both contain earlier traditions.[42] However, the Palestinian Talmud cites the midrashic motif in connection with the mishnah mentioned above, which states somewhat matter-of-factly that "for three transgressions women die at the time of childbirth: if they are not careful in the observance of niddah, of challah, and of the lighting of the [shabbat] light" (mShab 2:6).

Feminist scholars have mostly interpreted this mishnah as a threat to women (Baskin, "Separation of Women," 7–8; Wegner, *Chattel or Person?*, 155; R. Kraemer, *Her Share of the Blessing*, 100). However, this mishnah can be seen in the context of the rabbinic concept of divine punishment as "measure against measure." This is meted out against men and women alike (see Urbach, *The Sages*, 436–44). The discussion of this mishnah in the Babylonian Talmud (bShab 32a–34a) reflects on situations in which any person's transgressions might lead to an "analogous" punishment, such as for instance the transgression of either parent that could explain the death of children (see Boyarin, *Carnal Israel*, 92–93). Hence the midrashic trope of measure for measure has to be read on the background of certain questions: What could possibly explain the death of women in childbirth? the death of children? This logic cannot be reversed, such that if women transgress they will necessarily die, or that if men neglect the study of Torah their children will die. This is further corroborated by the statement that the possibility of death as a retribution for heedlessness in the practice of the commandments incumbent upon a woman is not arbitrary, but is active only at the time of childbirth. So many women died in childbirth that this raised the ultimately inexplicable question of theodicy: "Why?" Hence it is in particularly dangerous moments that humans can be divinely tested as to their transgressions. Such moments, which also apply to men, are the crossing of a bridge, or the crossing of a river on a ferryboat, for instance (bShab 32a). At the same time, the rabbis are theologically careful to allow for the cause-and-effect relationship to not be inevitable: ואלו הן פרקליטין של אדם תשובה ומעשים טובים ואפילו תשע מאות ותשעים ותשעה מלמדים עליו חובה ואחד מלמד עליו זכית—"Repentance and good deeds can serve as advocates for a person at the time of divine testing, even if the relationship is one [good deed] to nine hundred and ninety-nine [bad deeds]" (bShab 32a).

The other Palestinian appearances of our motif seem to presuppose this connection, since they all cite the mishnah before offering the explanation for why the woman was given these commandments. Hence, the midrashic trope of punishment by analogy: the woman's expiation for Eve's misdeed is emphasized. If she practices the commandment carefully, she achieves expiation. If, however, she is not heedful in the commandment having to do with blood she may die in childbirth, just as her foremother has caused the death of the first man, and thus in some sense spilled his blood. Obviously, these preceding versions are highly problematic not only as to their view of women's mythological role in the origin of human civilization, but also as to their punitive framing of the rabbinic ritualization of menstruation.

On the other hand, the Babylonian Talmud offers a more positive assessment of the divine intent behind the commandment, here attributed to a nameless person:

כדדרש ההוא גלילאה עליה דרב חסדא אמר הקדוש ברוך הוא רביעית דם נתתי בכם על עסקי דם הזהרתי אתכם ראשית קראתי אתכם על עסקי ראשית הזהרתי אתכם נשמה שנתתי בכם קרויה נר על עסקי נר הזהרתי אתכם

As a certain Galilean expounded in front of Rav Hisda:[43] The Holy One Blessed Be He said: I have put into you [plural] a quarter of a *log* of blood.[44] [By analogy] I have cautioned[45] you [plural] in matters having to do with blood. I have called you "firstling." [By analogy] I have cautioned you [plural] in matters having to do with the first [portion of the dough]. The soul which I have given you is called lamp. [By analogy] I have cautioned you [plural] in matters having to do with a lamp. (bShab 31b/32a)

Here the three women's commandments are interpreted as human obligations in response to God's gift of life. These commandments, which interestingly the Babylonian Talmud understands—at least conceptually—as incumbent upon the community as a whole and not just upon the woman or women,[46] are interpreted as reminders that life is God-given. Therefore, the Galilean constructs them as an expression of the positively defined relationship between the divine as creator and the human as the created, embodied being.

Both these midrashic interpretations, punitive and positive, aim at probing the divine intent behind the biblical commandment. The former is based on a clearly sexist reading, which marginalizes the mitzvat niddah along with the other two commandments as not only merely women's commandments, but also as an explicit divine punishment. The latter interpretation, on the other hand, binds the commandment into the collectivity of the community as a whole, thereby turning it into one of the corporeal practices of the community in its relationship to the divine.

Daniel Boyarin discusses these two midrashic interpretations in his analysis of the various late antique readings of the garden story with respect to their implications for the portrayal of women's origin and role. He argues that Rabbi Yehoshua's midrash and its variation in the Palestinian Talmud are exceptional in rabbinic literature. At least, according to Boyarin, this midrash has to be contextualized with other midrashic interpretations of the garden story, in which the first woman is not interpreted to be the source of all evil.[47] Thus he claims that "open misogyny like that of Rabbi Yehoshua is rare indeed in the rabbinic corpus, certainly by comparison with Philo, on the one hand, or Patristic culture on the other" (*Carnal Israel*, 90). He emphasizes in a footnote that "to the best of my knowledge, the two texts cited here from a single place in *Genesis Rabba* are the only examples of such misogynistic diatribe in all of the classical rabbinic literature" (*Carnal Israel*, 90 fn.23).[48] To Boyarin, these texts are "exceptions to the cultural pattern" (89) of rabbinic androcentrism versus Greco-Roman misogynism. With this claim he endeavors to contextualize the force of Rabbi Yehoshua's midrash over and against those polemical analyses that have extracted a text like this from the multiplicity of midrashic interpretations and then written off the whole of rabbinic discourse as systematically and endemically misogynist.[49]

Whereas the latter is clearly a distortion because of its selective reading, Boyarin's assessment here is not without its own difficulties, since he attempts to marginalize the misogynist text within rabbinic literature. But how are we to extrapolate from the texts to a "cultural pattern"? Does the quantitative rarity of a trope, in our case the interpretation of the commandment of niddah as punishment for the first woman's murder of the first man, in the literary corpus mean that it lies outside the "cultural pattern"? Can we judge, based on the criteria of textual quantity, what is endemic to the discourse or even to the "culture," extrapolated from the text, and what is not?

I would like, therefore, to take a slightly different approach. These two midrashic interpretations, the Palestinian and the Babylonian, represent the only attempts in talmudic literature to probe the divine intent behind the mitzvat niddah. Indeed, the phrase *mitzvat niddah*, referring to the prohibition of sexual intercourse during a woman's menstrual period, appears only in these two contexts, never in the mishnaic or Palestinian and Babylonian talmudic Tractate Niddah or elsewhere in classical rabbinic literature. As a stenographic formulation it pertains only to one aspect of the regulations concerning menstruation, that is, the prohibition of sexual intercourse, and has a function only in the context of the discussion of the triad of women's commandments and their reasons. The halakhic discussion of menstruation, however, is not dependent on either of these midrashic interpretations, nor are they its necessary framework. In this respect, both Rabbi Yehoshua's interpretation and that of the unnamed Galilean are mere theological *opinions*, of which hypothetically many more could have been produced. But Rabbi Yehoshua's midrash does not, therefore, transform the halakhic discourse on menstruation into an ideological misogyny. This is all the more true for rabbinic literature as a whole, as Boyarin argues in his chapter.

Nonetheless, I want to resist the relativization of the misogynist elements as necessarily external to the "pattern" of rabbinic culture. As a culture, it harbors these elements, just like any other culture in late antiquity. Here we may recall the famous passage from Pliny's second-century *Natural History*, which indicates the cultural choices in the rabbis' environment at a time when the mishnaic tractate on niddah was in the process of being redacted. Pliny writes:

> Nothing could easily be found that is more remarkable [*magis monstrificum*] than the monthly flux of women. Contact with it turns new wine sour, crops touched by it become barren, grafts die, seeds in gardens are dried up, the fruit of trees falls off, the bright surface of mirrors in which it is merely reflected is dimmed, the edge of steel and the gleam of ivory are dulled, hives of bees die, even bronze and iron are at once seized by rust, and a horrible smell fills the air; to taste it drives dogs mad and infects their bites with an incurable poison. (Pliny, *Natural History*, vol. 7, 15: 64)

Pliny continues with a few more such "remarkable" facts. Pliny's documentation is repeated in various texts in the Roman world.[50] Lest we think that the Babylonian Talmud was entirely immune to such folklore, we find the following passage:

> Our sages taught [in an anonymous *baraita*]:
> Three things should not pass [between two men] nor should [two men] pass between [two of] these. These are: a dog, a palm-tree and a woman. And there are those who say, also a pig. And there are those who say, also a snake.

This citation can be found in a long list of twosomes considered to be dangerous, which as twosomes will activate the realm of demons and spirits. These demonic fantasies are characteristic of the Babylonian Talmud. After providing a brief remedy for passing between these twosomes, the gemara continues to add anonymously to the citation in Aramaic:

> [Concerning] two men between whom a woman in her menstrual period passed [אשה נדה]—if it was the beginning of her niddah, she kills one of them, if it was the end of her niddah, she causes a rift between them.(bPes 111a)

This text falls into the category of folk literary genre.[51] But it is part and parcel of the Babylonian Talmud's polyphonic text, which, as Galit Hasan-Rokem states, carries "many diverse, even conflicting, messages synchronically" ("Narratives in Dialogue," 110). Thus the Babylonian Talmud does attempt to develop a halakhic discourse of menstruation that sets up the biblical prohibition of menstrual sex as one of the cornerstones of marital life. At the same time, it integrates in different contexts fragments such as the above. In its Plinian overtones such a view would undermine the very endeavor of discussing menstruation as a "respectable" halakhic discourse.

However, part of the talmudic polyphony is also the midrash of the unnamed Galilean, which actively contests elements that marginalize the ritualization in the rabbis' larger theological understanding of Torah as a gift. In fact, it is possible to read the midrash of the unnamed Galilean in the Babylonian Talmud, the later text, not only as undermining the infamous mishnah to which it is attached (Boyarin, *Carnal Israel*, 91), but also as rewriting the Palestinian tradition attributed to Rabbi Yehoshua. Here, the Babylonian Talmud does not necessarily profess concern for women, but is concerned that to designate one set of biblical commandments as divine punishment does not cohere with the general theology of Torah.

In either case, the halakhic discourse on the implications of the biblical mitzvat niddah is not dependent on the midrashic opinion of either Rabbi Yehoshua or of the unnamed Galilean. Neither one serves as a prologue for the tractate that actually deals with the menstrual regulations. What we can say at most is that a Rabbi Yehoshua would study the tractate in a quite different light than the unnamed Galilean in Rav Hisda's *Beit ha-Midrash*. Both would frame the talmudic discourse on menstruation very differently.

∽

I have attempted to trace in this chapter the particular "face" that the rabbis give to their discussions of menstruation. The difficult tension in talmudic literature that I have tried to unravel is the tension between linguistic conventions and the halakhic or practical reality behind such linguistic conventions. There is an obfuscation that springs from the slippage from the language of impurity into the conceptual framework of the prohibited sexual relations. An understanding of this tension is crucial, not just generically for the reading of rabbinic texts on menstruation, but crucial also for clarifying the use of the language of (ritual) impurity in the context of menstruation. It is this language that has been caught most between polemics and apologetics with respect to the rabbinic discussions. The language of impurity with respect to the menstruating woman undergoes a change in that it is employed more loosely than in the biblical priestly context. In some of the rabbinic narratives women are represented as indicating their sexual inaccessibility by saying: "I am impure." The rabbis did not create a language particular to sexual inaccessibility. Rather, they continued the biblical language and readapted it. On this basis we can read many of the following texts as discussions on the beginnings or ends of menstrual periods, or on the distinction between menstrual and other kinds of blood.

As a concluding moment, I want to revisit the connection between biblical law and the rabbinic discussion. The rabbis did not simply inherit biblical law. They chose to inherit it in a particular way. If we read rabbinic texts for their constructions of women's bodies and of gender, we cannot merely read them synchronically, such as in their contexts in late antiquity. Particularly with regard to niddah, we need to take the diachronic perspective into consideration.

Here I want to take Boyarin's suggestion into consideration: to read hellenistic Jewish, Paulinic, and rabbinic claims of inheriting biblical law as contesting hermeneutics.[52] Boyarin suggests, in *Carnal Israel*, reading the rabbis' hermeneutics of biblical texts as a hermeneutics of resistance against the parallel claim of early Christians and the larger discourse of dualism of body and spirit. The rabbis resisted Paul's decorporealized understanding of the biblical Israelite community and the bodily rites biblically prescribed for it, or at least contested Paul's vision of a disembodied Judaism (232). According to Boyarin the rabbinic resistance against the disembodiment of biblical Israel, ethnically defined, is exemplified dramatically in the interpretation of the rite of circumcision: "In one stroke, by interpreting circumcision as referring to a spiritual and not corporeal reality, Paul made it possible for Judaism to become a world religion" (233). Boyarin claims that "for *the Jews* of late antiquity . . . the rite of circumcision became the most contested site of this contention, precisely because of the way that it concentrates in one moment representations of the significance of sexuality, genealogy, and ethnic-specificity in bodily practice" (emphasis added, 7). This statement may be true for *male* Jews of late antiquity. But is it true for women? Or could it have been true for women, since we have no historical evidence for how Jewish women thought about this cultural conflict?[53] In other words, what happens when the female body is the center of the debate? How do women's bodies figure into this debate? If we agree that the rite of circumcision lies at the center of the contestation of Jewish ethnicity, what could this definition of ethnicity do for Jewish women?

I am not contesting the centrality of the debate on circumcision in the literary sources that have been preserved, since that is reflected in the texts and cannot be contested.[54] Rather, my agenda is to retrieve the female body as a potential site of resistance to the prevailing androcentrism of rabbinic gender politics. This presents an effort to engage in what Ilana Pardes calls a "reversal of canonical hierarchies" (*Countertraditions*, 13). That is to say, we don't need to accept the concern about circumcision and its inherent assumption of the male body as the representative Jewish body as the center around which the understanding of Jewish culture evolves in late antiquity, *even though* Greco-Roman male intellectuals such as Tacitus defined the *difference* of Jewish culture through its inscription on male bodies, and *even though* Jewish male intellectuals debated the significance of circumcision for their understanding of Jewish culture. In spite of and against the textual evidence we have to at least try to conceive of how Jewish women might have argued about their "Jewishness" as an ethnic identity, and how Greco-Roman intellectual women would have perceived the difference of Jewish culture in a debate with or against their female Jewish colleagues. Such debates may never have taken place. We do have, however, some scant evidence about a reading of niddah as constituting women's Jewish identity. The Babylonian Talmud mentions:

> One [unspecified] time the [Roman] government decreed that they [the Jews] should not observe the Shabbat, and that they should not circumcise their sons, and that they should have intercourse with *niddot* [their wives during their menstrual periods]. (bMeilah 17a)

Leaving the problematic question of the historicity of this text aside for a minute, this text provides the rare mention of women in a list of items that the Talmud understands to be the essentials of Jewish culture. Further, the Talmud envisions the Romans as equally understanding these to be the essentials of Jewish culture. Based on such an understanding, the Romans would outlaw such practices in order to annihilate Jewish culture. At the margins of the interethnic debate on Jewish identity women come into view, if only doubly reflected through male identity politics. But Jewish women's identity is considered to be constituted through the punctilious observance of menstrual abstinence from sexual intercourse.

What do we gain from this? Does it mean that Jewish women in late antiquity constructed their Jewish identity primarily through the observance of niddah? Does that mean that we can reconstruct such women's perspectives? None of these questions can be answered with any certainty. What we can do, however, is to take a heuristic step in the enterprise of decentering the androcentrism of our sources and of our own understanding of the emergence of rabbinic Judaism. This may be possible, if we interrogate closely the discussions of women's bodies and women's blood in rabbinic texts.

# 2 THE WOMAN AS HOUSE

## CONCEPTIONS OF WOMEN'S CORPOREALITY IN TALMUDIC LITERATURE

THE PREVIOUS CHAPTER lays out the rabbis' desire to preserve and enact the biblical community of Israel as an ethnically distinct, embodied community distinguished by corporeal practices as the grounds for understanding the rabbinic discourse on menstruation. Any understanding of how gender ideologies function in rabbinic texts and factor into the production of the talmudic discussions needs to be grounded in such an understanding. The rabbinic understanding of corporeal practices and the body's role in the constitution of the Jewish community are products of the rabbis' biblical hermeneutics as much as the other way around, as will be shown in the following pages. The purpose of this chapter is to discuss through close readings of talmudic texts the ways in which the rabbis turn women's bodies into objects of rabbinic discourse. I want to focus our attention on the rhetorics of the talmudic literature, on the metaphors it employs to make the female body readable and speakable. The question I ask is what kind of implications a particular choice of metaphors carries along with it. How does rabbinic culture conceptualize gender? How we situate women in the larger network of rabbinic culture depends in part on how we read and understand the discourse of the female body, particularly in Tractate Niddah. As we will see in this chapter, the dominant group of metaphors are spatial metaphors, metaphors related to the house. First, the obvious needs to be emphasized. Rabbinic discourse objectifies women's bodies and by extension women themselves. In reflecting on the function of the metaphorization of the female body in the larger context of rabbinic culture we can draw on Page duBois's work on Greek literature. In her analysis of metaphors of women's bodies—such as field, furrow, stone, oven, and tablet—in classic Greek literature, duBois writes:

> Aristotle makes clear the motive of domination implicit in the Greeks' penchant for metaphorizing, for analogizing, the woman's body. To compare a human body to an inanimate thing might be seen as a practice of abuse, unless the status of such a thing—the field of the fathers, for example—might not in some way have higher social status than a human being.... To use these metaphors in this way, as the Greeks do, is eventually to instrumentalize the female, to reduce her to the status of a thing, an object to be manipulated, to be filled up, broken into, erased. (*Sowing the Body*, 34)

In the following pages we will see that like the Greeks, the rabbis also metaphorize the woman's body and compare it to an inanimate thing, the house. We should keep in mind that Greek and rabbinic literature are not driven by the same logic of sexual difference. What we need to trace is whether "the desire, expressed by metaphor, to control, name, and produce the female by analogy" (duBois, *Sowing the Body*, 34) produces the same mechanics of domination as the Greek literature analyzed by duBois. For this task it is crucial to consider the larger context of the metaphorization. We need to question whether the metaphorization forms the basis of a stable androcentric perspective. Are the metaphors the predominant categories of representation of the female body? Or is this form of representation challenged by other counter-hegemonic perspectives?

Thus the development of the metaphorization of the female body from biblical to talmudic literature will concern us here. In the next chapter, however, I will try to show that, interestingly, the commodification of women's bodies, predominant certainly in the Mishnah as well as in the talmudic discussions based on the Mishnah, is at war with itself in the discussions in the Babylonian Talmud. The texts betray a self-consciousness about their own androcentric, exclusionary nature. This internal self-criticism needs to be traced very carefully in the texts before we can evaluate it.

Let me begin with a few general observations to frame the textual analyses. First of all, during approximately the same period of the cultural history of late antiquity in which rabbinic literature develops its own language of the body, and the female body in particular, the Greco-Roman medical literature of Rufus, Soranus, and Galen makes a massive effort to develop a uniform map of the medicalized body and a uniform anatomical terminology (Lloyd, *Science, Folklore, and Ideology*, 158). The contemporaneity of the flourishing Greco-Roman gynecological literature with the burgeoning discourse on women's bodies in rabbinic culture needs to be taken into consideration as a possible cultural context for the rabbis to develop their own medical language.[1]

Second, though it was absent almost entirely from the biblical scene, the nature and mysteries of the female body in its corporeal specificity occupy a large part of the rabbinic discussions on menstruation. Already the *tannaim* (the rabbis of the mishnaic period), and certainly the *amoraim* (the rabbis in the gemaras), use the biblical purity and impurity regulations to think women's bodies in their corporeal specificity and to turn women's bodies into discourse. This may not have been the intent of the rabbis. My argument is about the *effect* of the discussions. Here the rabbinic hermeneutic desire is no longer directed toward the biblical text but toward the female body. From the rabbis' hermeneutic desire for the biblical text then emerges a hermeneutics of gender which is characteristically rabbinic and rooted in the cultural world of the rabbis.

Finally, on the level of discursive effect rather than authorial intent, the texts can be positioned in constellation with current theoretical debates on gender, especially if we turn the focus of our attention to the aspect of the talmudic discussions that is concerned with the creation of a female halakhic body, quite distinct from the male halakhic body. The framework of the regulations of menstruation turns into an occasion for the rabbis to think about gender difference as based in bodies and to reflect on how gender differentiation is produced by corporeal differences and their signification. It is on this level that feminist critical theory is most fruitfully engaged with rabbinic texts. What I am thinking through in this chapter is how current feminist thinking about the body and its role in the production of gender difference can contribute to our reading of the rabbinic configuration of the female body and its role in the production of gender difference in rabbinic culture.

One cautionary remark has to be made: feminist theory, ever since Simone de Beauvoir's magisterial *Second Sex*, has a specific location in Western discursive practices, as a critique of Western metaphysics. Therefore, it cannot simply be *applied to* the reading of gender difference in talmudic literature. Rather than thinking a unilateral relationship of feminist theory with rabbinic literature as its object, I wish to consider the rabbinic literary construction of female corporeality as a contribution not only to our study of gender in history, but also to our feminist thinking about the body. This is what I would call de-objectifying the text. The text does not simply make meaning by itself. We make it mean. This is not to say that the talmudic discussions present us with a proto-feminist theory of women's corporeality. My interest is not to judge rabbinic literature as producing either a misogynist or a proto-feminist discourse, as if it simply *is* one or the other, rather than *being read* by us as such. Rather, I want to use rabbinic literature for thinking through issues vital to feminist critical theory of difference/s today, just as my reading of rabbinic literature will be informed by feminist hermeneutics. Currently one of the most crucial issues in feminist critical theory is our thinking about sexual difference in positive or constructive terms without falling into the trap of essentializing female bodies, female embodiedness, and women. Furthermore, the question is how to think about female embodiment and how to conceptualize knowledge as effects of specific bodies, against the effacement of the female body in Western intellectual tradition.[2] In collaboration with such an effort it might be worthwhile to consider how talmudic discourse—as a discourse that does not cultivate the metaphysics of the universal mind equated with the male, from which the body, equated with the female, is structurally excluded[3]—conceptualizes female corporeality in distinction from male corporeality. Since rabbinic anthropology considers the material reality of the body as primary, and not secondary to the spiritual reality of the mind or the soul,[4] it is based on the very notion of embodied sexual differentiation. A differentiation, I hasten to add, which is not simply a mimetic reproduction of presumably "real" sexed bodies, but which the texts creatively produce.

Prepared by these preliminary reflections, we may now turn to the textual emergence of the female body in talmudic literature.

### "In Her Body": The Biblical Gender Constellation

The following observation is the foundation of my analysis of rabbinic thinking and discourse on women's bodies in the context of the impurity/purity system: the rabbinic conceptualization of female bodies as different from male bodies is not rooted in the perception of the male body as normative—ontologically or biologically—and female bodies as substandard to the male body, as Aristotle would claim.⁵ Rather, as we will see, the rabbinic conceptualization of the difference between male and female bodies quite literally hinges on a single letter in the biblical text, or, one could say, on the difference between two letters in the text. Lev. 15, the foundational document on the impurity of bodily discharges, decrees that a man is in the status of impurity when he has a discharge "*from* his body" (מבשרו, Lev. 15:2), whereas the woman is in the status of impurity when she has a discharge "*in* her body" (בבשרה, Lev. 15:19). It is the difference between these two letters, or prepositions in the English translation, which to the rabbinic sages establishes the male body in terms of surface, as exteriority, and the female body in terms of space, as interiority.⁶

The following two verses establish the impurity of genital discharges in the priestly code:

איש איש כי יהיה זב מבשרו זובו טמא הוא

> When any man has a discharge, his discharge [being] *from* his body, he is in the status of impurity. (Lev. 15:2)⁷

ואשה כי תהיה זבה דם יהיה זובה בבשרה שבעת ימים תהיה בנדתה

> When a woman has a discharge, her discharge [being] blood *in* her body, she shall remain in her status of separation for seven days. (Lev. 15:19)

These two verses establish a basic symmetry between man and woman with respect to their discharges. Both verses begin with the general introduction of the case of a man or woman who has a genital discharge. In both cases, the paragraph introduced by these verses proceeds to make a distinction between common and uncommon discharges.⁸ The chapter is structured chiastically.⁹ It discusses first the impurity caused by an uncommon discharge of the man (Lev. 15:2–15), then proceeds to the impurity caused by a *common* seminal discharge (Lev. 15:16–18), stays with the common discharge when it begins to discuss the woman (Lev. 15:19–24), that is, menstrual bleeding, and reverts to the uncommon discharge in her case (Lev. 15:25–30). In the case of the uncommon discharge both count seven clean days after their discharge ceases (Lev. 15:13.28), both are to take two turtledoves or two pigeons to the priest, and in both cases "the priest shall offer them, the one as a sin offering, and the other as a burnt offering. Thus the priest shall make expiation on his/her behalf, for his/her discharge, before God" (Lev. 15:15.30).[10]

In the case of common discharges, the symmetry seems to break down, since the woman is in a status of impurity for seven days, whereas the man with a seminal discharge is in the status of impurity only until the evening (Lev. 15:17). This could perhaps be explained by the different nature of the discharges and would not essentially disturb the symmetry, since menstrual bleeding can last for several days, versus a seminal discharge, which is a one-time, momentary event.[11] But furthermore, in the case of menstrual bleeding the woman's status of impurity shares some of the more severe consequences of an uncommon discharge, which the seminal discharge in the man does not.[12]

Nonetheless, the categorical distinction is upheld between the uncommon discharge, as more severe with respect to the status of impurity it causes, and the common discharges, for both the man and the woman.[13] Thus the passage on the status of impurity caused by genital discharges establishes a symmetry of gender, though not equity, based on the physiological differences between man and woman. This would seem to present an almost direct contradiction of what Elizabeth Grosz has presented as a Western modeling of gender difference based on corporeality:

> Those regulating and contextualizing the body and its pleasures have thus far in our cultural history established models which do not regard the polluting contamination of sexual bodies as a two-way process, in which each affects or infiltrates the other. Such a model involves a dual sexual symmetry that is missing in patriarchal structures. It is not the case that men's bodily fluids are regarded as polluting and contaminating for women in the same way or to the same extent as women's are for men. It is women and what men consider to be their inherent capacity for contagion, their draining, demanding bodily processes that have figured so strongly in cultural representations, and that have emerged so clearly as a problem for social control. (Grosz, *Volatile Bodies*, 197)

The priestly text of Lev. 15 seems to suggest itself as a case of a dual sexual symmetry, in spite of its location in a patriarchal culture: men's bodily fluids transfer a status of impurity to anyone, including the woman who has sexual relations with him (Lev. 15:7), just as women's bodily fluids transfer a status of impurity to anyone, including the man who has sexual relations with her. A man's seminal discharge during intercourse transfers his status of impurity to the woman (Lev. 15:18), just as women's bodily fluids during intercourse transfer her status of impurity to him (Lev. 15:24).

The point is not that to claim the priestly writers had some concept of gender equity in mind when they structured the regulations of the impurity of genital discharge. Nonetheless, it is important to acknowledge this symmetry, where corporeality and its inscription are the basis for impurity regulations at the originating moment of niddah in Jewish culture.

### The Prohibition of Sexual Relations

This symmetry is subsequently thrown out of balance with the prohibition of sexual intercourse with a menstruous woman in Lev. 18:19—"Do not come near a woman during her period of impurity to uncover her nakedness"—and 20:18—"If a man lies with a woman in her infirmity and uncovers her nakedness, he has laid bare her source and she has exposed the source of her blood; both of them shall be cut off from among their people." As a collection of laws dealing with the subject of incest and other forbidden sexual unions, Leviticus 18 and 20 do not prohibit sexual relations with a man who has an uncommon discharge.[14] The list in Lev. 18 bespeaks the androcentric perspective of the priestly writer, in that it is rhetorically addressed directly and exclusively to an imaginary male audience. The prohibited relationships listed are those prohibited to a man. The chapter lists all those female relatives "he" may not have sexual relations with, and adds other sexual relations, such as with a menstrous woman, with another man, or with animals. Since the imaginary audience of the text is male, and sexual intercourse with any man is prohibited to a man, it never occurred to the editor of the list to specify the prohibition of sexual relations with a man who has an uncommon discharge, since the imaginary subject of such a prohibition would have been a woman.

Nonetheless, the text does not entirely objectify the woman with regard to the prohibition of sexual intercourse during her menstrual period. Namely, the restatement of the prohibited sexual relationships in Leviticus 20 is not directly addressed to the imaginary male audience, since it is formulated in the third person, while also adding the divine retribution for the transgression of the prohibition. In spite of the overall androcentric perspective also of this chapter, the reformulation of the prohibition of sexual intercourse during a woman's menstrual period reintroduces a dual perspective, in which both the man and the woman, in the case of a transgression of the prohibition, are active participants in the sexual act and are punished accordingly: "he laid bare her source and she exposed the source of her blood. Thus both of them shall be cut off from among their people" (20:18). Hence, the prohibition is incumbent upon both of them.[15] However, what we do not find here is the woman incurring guilt for sleeping with a man who is in the status of impurity, and in this the text remains committed to its primary androcentrism.

## Inside and/or Outside

The rabbinic approach to the biblical text latches on to a surface feature which is not its most prominent aspect, and which is, indeed, almost hidden in the textual crevices. Thus the basic gender symmetry of the impurity of bodily discharges is fundamentally disturbed, in fact unhinged, by the rabbinic ingenuity of midrashic reading.

As we have seen, in the two verses Lev. 15:2 and Lev. 15:19, which are intended to be introductory formulas to the sections that deal respectively with the male and the female discharges, the formulation in the case of the man is מבשרו—"from his body," whereas in the case of the woman it is בבשרה—"in her body." This difference is often glossed over by contemporary biblical commentators, beginning with the translations. More often than not, translations do not account for the difference of preposition. Whereas the Septuagint translates the pronouns fastidiously [ἐκ τοῦ σώματος αυτου and ἐν τῷ σώματι αὐτῆς], modern translations often ignore the difference between the prepositions or the linguistic parallelism as to the origin of the discharge: "When any man has a discharge, his discharge being *from his member*, he is impure" and "When a woman has a discharge, her discharge being blood *from her body*, she remains in her menstrual impurity seven days" (Milgrom, *Leviticus 1–16*, 902–3; cf. Levine, *Leviticus*, 93–97).[16]

Whereas both Milgrom and Levine agree that the reference to the man's body (Lev. 15:2) is traditionally read euphemistically as penis,[17] only Milgrom suggests that the term בבשרה might therefore equally be read as a euphemism for the woman's genitals,[18] as in the case of the man, which nonetheless would not account for the difference of preposition.[19] There is no compelling reason to read just one element of the linguistic parallelism euphemistically, and not the other. Furthermore, there is no compelling reason to disregard the difference of prepositions.[20] It is this difference of preposition that allows for the emergence of a complex architecture of the woman's body in the rabbinic discussions.

### The Rabbinic Female Body as Architecture of the Interior

Sifra, one of the oldest halakhic Midrashim, which has variously been regarded as a commentary on or criticism of the Mishnah and was edited close to it in the second half of the third century (Stemberger, *Einleitung*, 257), explains these two verses in the following manner:

מבשרו—עד שתצא טומאתו חוץ לבשרו

"From his body"—[he is in the status of impurity only] when his impurity appears outside his body. (Sifra, 1, מצורע פ׳ זבים פרק 75a)

בבשרה—מלמד שהיא מטמאה בפנים כבחוץ

"In her body"—[this formulation] teaches that she is in the status of impurity [or: renders somebody or something else impure][21] [when the blood is still] inside just as [when it appears] outside. (Sifra, 4, מצורע, פ׳ זבים פרשה 78a)

Why does the midrashic commentary make this fundamental distinction, one that engenders far-reaching consequences in rabbinic halakhic discussions? For if we hold that the woman enters a status of impurity when the blood is still inside her body, it will be difficult to determine the chronological beginning of her status of impurity. When the blood exits from her body, it has already been inside her body. How long? Where? How far back in time from the point that the blood appears "outside her body" has she been in the status of impurity? These are questions that account for one of the most complicated discussions in talmudic literature, in the opening sugyah of Tractate Niddah in the Babylonian Talmud, which I will discuss later.

We have observed that the midrashic commentary Sifra can make its case linguistically, based on the difference of prepositions. Sifra underlines the deliberateness of the biblical writer employing this linguistic feature by making the following argument: since hypothetically it might have been possible to think in terms of a symmetry between the woman and the man, and since, therefore, it might have been possible to hold that either the man is in the status of impurity already when his discharge is still inside—like in the case of the woman, or that the woman is only in the status of impurity when her discharge of blood appears outside—like in the case of the man, the scriptural text deliberately made an explicit distinction by crafting its formulations with the different prepositions. According to Sifra, the biblical text prohibits making such a hypothetical argument from gender analogy, even though it considers the possibility. As an element of its logic, however, it dismisses this possibility. One can only fantasize what would have happened had Lev. 15:19 read מבשרה or had Lev. 15:2 read בבשרו. In the former case much of the talmudic discussions in Tractate Niddah would have been impossible.

But the biblical text says what it says. Whether one holds that the rhetorical difference is only an arbitrary one, as some biblical commentators would have us believe, or whether one holds that the biblical text's formulation was quite deliberately crafted, Sifra presents us with a reading which is a possible reading, albeit not the only possible reading. It underscores what could be called the rabbinic architecture of the woman's body. With such an exegetical notion as their basis, the rabbis, in various contexts, proceed to construct the interior of the woman's body, while not admitting the possibility of thinking the interior of the male body.

Thus we learn in the Mishnah:

משל משלו חכמים החדר והפרוזדור והעליה דם החדר טמא נמצא בפרוזדור
ספקו טמא לפי שחזקתו מן המקור

The sages crafted a metaphor concerning the woman: [there is in her] a chamber,²² a vestibule²³ and an upper chamber. Blood from the chamber is in the status of impurity. If it is located in the vestibule, it is in the status of impurity if there is a doubt, since the assumption is that it derives from the source. (mNid 2:5)

The concern of this mishnah is to determine the status of her bleeding in relation to these locations in the female house. Menstrual blood is biblically defined as deriving "from the source" (Lev. 20:18). Our mishnah, however, considers the possibility that a woman's genital bleeding may not always derive "from the source" and may, therefore, not always be menstrual bleeding. This is the presumption for the metaphoric architecture. The rabbis speculate on various sources for bleeding in the various rooms in the woman's body. The blood from the chamber is in the status of impurity,²⁴ whereas the status of blood located in the vestibule²⁵ carries a halakhic status of doubtful impurity, rather than being considered as nonmenstrual blood, "because the assumption is that it derives from the source" (mNid 2:5). The Tosefta elaborates on this mishnah and clarifies what the practical consequences of a halakhic status of "doubtful impurity" would be. Employing the same metaphors as the Mishnah, it comments that "on account of the blood which is located in the vestibule they burn the *terumah*²⁶ and they declare in its case a liability with respect to the purity of the Temple and things related to the Temple" (tNid 3:9). Here the Tosefta makes explicit the practical consequences of the status of doubtful impurity which the bleeding brings about, as relevant to Temple practices only and not to the question of intimate relations with the husband, a point that corroborates what I have discussed above.

Neither the Mishnah nor the Tosefta discuss the case where blood derives from the "upper chamber," but the assumption is that it is in the status of purity, as the Palestinian Talmud makes explicit in its interpretation: "This is [what] the Mishnah [implies]: The blood of the chamber is in the status of impurity, but the blood of the upper chamber is in the status of purity" (pNid 2:4, 50a).²⁷

Both the Babylonian and the Palestinian Talmud in their exegetical comments on this mishnah attempt to locate the rooms in terms of their relative interiority or exteriority:

רמי בר שמואל ורב יצחק בריה דרב יהודה תנו בי רב נדה בי רב הונא אשכחינהו רבה בר רב הונא דיתבי וקאמרי החדר מבפנים והפרוזדור מבחוץ ועלייה בנוייה על שתיהן ולול פתוח בין עלייה לפרוזדור

Rami bar Shmuel and Rav Yitzhaq the son of Rav Yehudah studied [the tractate of] Niddah at Rav Huna's school.[28] Rabbah the son of Rav Huna found them sitting and saying: the chamber is within, the vestibule is without and the upper chamber is built above them, and a pathway[29] connects the upper chamber and the vestibule. [bNid 17b]

רב יהודה בשם שמואל החדר לפני' מן הפרוזדור העלייה נתונ' על גבי החדר עד חצי פרוזדור ופתיח' של עלייה פתוח לפרוזדור

Rav Yehudah [said] in the name of Shmu'el: The chamber lies more inside than the vestibule. The upper chamber is located on top of the chamber [reaching] towards half of the vestibule, and an opening of the upper chamber opens into the vestibule. [pNid 2:4, 50a]

Both interpretations largely agree on the relative location of the internal chambers, with the one exception that the Palestinian Talmud specifies the location of the upper chamber with respect to the vestibule differently. The remainder of the short exegetical sugyah in the Palestinian Talmud is concerned with the last part of the mishnah, according to which the blood located in the vestibule (פרוזדור) is doubtful as to its origins, and hence doubtful as to its status of impurity. Its exegetical argument is concerned with the question whether the mishnah then would think of the blood in the vestibule from the opening to the upper chamber on inwards, or from there on outwards.

רב נחמן בר רב יצחק שאל לרב חונה מתני' בשנמצ' מפתח עליה ולפנים א"ל אם בשנמצא מפתח עליה ולפנים בודאי היא אלא כן אנן קיימין בשנמצא מפתח עליה ולחוץ

Rav Nachman the son of Rav Yitzhaq asks Rav Huna:[30] Does the mishnah [on the blood in the vestibule] refer [to the blood] which is located [in the vestibule] from the opening to the upper chamber on inwards? Rav Huna answered: If it is located from the opening to the upper chamber on inwards, it is in a status of certainty [i.e., it certainly derives from the source and is therefore impure]. Rather, we interpret [the mishnah] this way: [the mishnah refers to the situation] when the blood is located [in the vestibule] from the opening to the upper chamber on outwards. (pNid 2:4, 50a)

Here the Palestinian Talmud further subdivides the vestibule into its internal and external half, divided at the mark of the opening of the upper chamber into the *prozdor* or vestibule. It suggests that blood in the former is certainly derived from the (inner) chamber and therefore menstrual blood, whereas the latter remains in question. As can easily be seen, neither the Babylonian nor the Palestinian interpretations are entirely unambiguous, since the point of reference of their respective relative location remains unclear. Thus, ever since, commentators have attempted to define the referents of the metaphors, that is, to determine which room stands for which reproductive organ. Maimonides and the Meiri, two medieval scholars with some knowledge of their era's medical science, consider as referents the uterus for the chamber, the vagina for the vestibule, and the cavity that contains the ovaries and the fallopian tubes for the upper chamber, while the pathway would refer to the fallopian tubes themselves.[31] Among modern commentators, Albeck (*Shishah Sidrei Mishnah 1–6*, 383)[32] suggests that the chamber is the uterus, the vestibule the vulva, and the upper chamber possibly the vagina. Finally Meacham, who discusses the various possibilities for referents extensively ("Mishnah Tractate Niddah," 224–31), adds the bladder as a possible referent for the upper chamber.[33] The only agreement between all these commentators is that the chamber refers to the womb or the uterus.

The search for the referents of the metaphors, however, produces a major hermeneutic impasse. Basically, the choice of referents is culled from the sphere of the various medical or scientific-anatomic knowledges of the commentators, none of which are either accurate or objectively mimetic themselves.[34] The attempt to ascribe accuracy, defined in such terms, to the late antique rabbis has to remain fruitless by definition, even if we assume that they had relatively advanced medical knowledge.[35] For all that one is able to conclude in the end is that the rabbis did perhaps not exactly know what they were talking about, because we cannot identify the rabbinic metaphors in terms of our current scientific-medical knowledge. The attempt to identify the anatomical referents, then, has reached an impasse.

Let us take a different approach. We will focus on the rhetorical choice of metaphors, that is, the choice of architectural metaphors, or more generally spatial metaphors, for the interior of the woman's body. What do these rhetorical choices imply for the construction of gender in rabbinic culture and what purposes do they serve? Do these metaphors function to enhance the construction of gender differences as radical difference? If this is the case, can we draw conclusions not only about linguistic and semantic structures, but also about the embeddedness of these in the larger cultural and social context?[36]

Of the metaphors for the interior of women's bodies we find more. The most prominent architectural metaphor in Mishnah Niddah besides the one discussed so far is the following:

כל הנשים מטמאות בבית החיצון שנאמר דם יהיה זובה בבשרה אבל הזב ובעל קרי אינן מטמאין עד שתצא טומאתן לחוץ

> All women are in the status of impurity [when blood is][37] in the outer room, since it is said "her discharge being blood in her body" [Lev. 15:19], whereas the man with an uncommon discharge and the one with a seminal emission are in the status of impurity only when their impurity [appears] outside [their body]. (mNid 5:1)

As does the halakhic midrash in Sifra, the Mishnah notes the rhetorical distinction in Leviticus between "in her body" (Lev. 15:19) and "from his body" (Lev. 15:2), without, however, adducing the biblical proof-text in the case of the man. As we have previously seen, the halakhic midrash in Sifra derives from the biblical verse a fairly simple distinction between external and internal, between inside the body in the case of the woman and outside the body in the case of the man. The Mishnah, on the other hand, in its own midrash on the same verse, again develops the interior of the woman's body into an architectural trope. Here, the Mishnah remains consistent with its own linguistic construction of the female body in terms of architectural metaphors. Again, the question remains, in relation to what is the "outer room" exterior? Or how, if at all, is this part of the woman-house related to the previous metaphors? Is it an additional part of the building described previously, or is it a term that comprises parts of those other parts of the building? In the commentary literature only the Meiri suggests an explicit correlation between the two metaphors—that is, that the בית החיצון is, in fact, the פרוזדור or vestibule (*Beit ha-Bechirah*, 145).³⁸ If it is a more general term, the "outer room" is perhaps considered exterior with reference to the בית הרחם, the "house of the womb."³⁹

Rhetorically, this metaphor strikingly represents a space that is an interface,⁴⁰ simultaneously internal and external. The strict distinction between exterior and interior collapses in this metaphor. Even though the Mishnah projects a stable juxtaposition between exterior (in the male case) and interior (in the female case), the Babylonian Talmud recognizes the ambiguity suggested by the choice of metaphor and highlights it. Again in an exegetical sugyah, it first adduces a disagreement between two *amoraim* who are famous partners in debate in the Talmud:

הי ניהו בית החיצון
אמר ריש לקיש כל שתינוקת יושבת ונראת
א״ל רבי יוחנן אותו מקום גלוי הוא אצל שרץ
אלא אמר רבי יוחנן עד בין השינים
איבעיא להו בין השינים כלפנים או כלחוץ
ת״ש דתני רבי זכאי עד בין השיבים בין השינים עצמן כלפנים

[The anonymous editorial voice asks:]
Which is the "outer house" [of which the Mishnah talks]?
Resh Laqish said: everything which appears [or can be seen] when a little girl sits.⁴¹
Rabbi Yohanan responded: That place is [that much] exposed [even] with regards to a *sheretz*!⁴²
[Instead] Rabbi Yohanan interpreted: as far as [the space] between the 'teeth.'⁴³ (bNid 41b)

According to Resh Laqish the "outer house" is completely exterior, as that which is exposed and can be seen. Resh Laqish's illustration raises some important points that underline the dominant androcentric perspective of the talmudic texts on women's bodies. His introduction of vision as a means of definition is meant to stabilize the ambiguity of the metaphor. What duBois demonstrates for classical Greek literature applies in our case also: "It is always men (except for Sappho) who see women and define them in metaphor and 'theory'" (*Sowing the Body*, 64). The imagined spectator in

Resh Laqish's case is, in spite of the passive formulation—"everything which appears"—the man. It is a little girl whom Resh Laqish imagines squatting because a child is nominally not an object of sexual fantasy and can be seen, even with her genitalia exposed. Resh Laqish's statement itself works as an interface: he simultaneously guards the laws of modesty by choosing an asexual object of his gaze, and circumvents them by looking where men are not supposed to look.

Rabbi Yohanan's seemingly bizarre objection is that Resh Laqish's definition does not adequately fit the biblical expression "*in* her body," adduced explicitly by the mishnah as *terminus interpretivum* of "outer house." Rabbi Yohanan's rhetorical question alludes to the complex of rabbinic laws of impurity according to which the touch of a sheretz conveys a status of impurity only to external organs, but not internal ones. He argues essentially that Resh Laqish resolves the ambiguity of the metaphor while focusing too much on only one of its elements, the חיצון of בית החיצון.[44] Instead, Rabbi Yohanan seems to intend an interpretation that locates the "outer house" more internally: it extends inwards toward the space between the "teeth" שיניים.[45]

The metaphor of the teeth raises another important set of questions: Do the rabbis equate the vagina with the mouth, as the Hippocratics already do? And if so, do they develop the notion of the parallel between the lower and the upper mouth? Ann Hanson has analyzed the rhetorics of the Greek gynecological writings, especially their deployment of metaphors for women's sexual organs. Among other sets of metaphors she points out that "the gynecology of the [Hippocratic, Ch.F.] *Corpus* contains a number of passages in which the two *stomata*, upper and lower mouths, show similar or parallel responses" ("Medical Writers' Women," 328).[46] The Babylonian Talmud does, in a different context in Tractate Niddah, employ the term פה or "mouth" for the woman's vagina, when it discusses a scenario where הרוק בתוך הפה—"the spittle is still in the mouth" (bNid 16b)—that is, the blood is still inside the vagina.[47] However, it appears to me that in talmudic texts both "mouth" and "teeth" are less specific and more randomly deployed metaphors than in the Hippocratic texts, whereas the architectural metaphors are much more omnipresent and present a much more elaborate system. In the rabbinic case, פה or mouth acquires the general meaning of "opening," and appears in phrases such as פי הארץ "the opening of the earth" and פי הבאר, "the opening of the well." Similarly, the metaphor of "teeth" is used in other phrases for protrusions of any kind.[48] The rabbis do not develop this set of metaphors as fully as they do architectural metaphors. In Tractate Niddah, each of them appears only once and both times more or less in passing.[49]

To Rabbi Yohanan's and Resh Laqish's disagreement the Talmud adds the following brief afterthought:

> The question was raised: Is [the space] between the 'teeth' [itself] considered to be interior or exterior?
> Come and hear as Rabbi Zakhai taught: [Rabbi Yochanan said] "as far as [the space] between the 'teeth,'" [implying that] the space between the "teeth" [itself] is considered to be interior. (bNid 41b)

The second part of this discussion, a talmudic supercommentary on the disagreement between Rabbi Yohanan and Resh Laqish, asks even further, whether that space between the teeth, which served as Rabbi Yohanan's *terminus ad quem*, is itself to be considered as exterior or interior. This confirms that the "outer house" would then be imagined as some sort of interface between the interior and the exterior of the woman-house.

By now what in Lev. 15 could have been read as a symmetrical relationship between male and female bodies, the physiology of male and female discharges, and the impurity ascribed to them, has vanished into the spaces of the woman who is the house. The woman's body has been rendered as diametrically opposed to the male body, as the embodiment of interiority versus the male embodiment of exteriority.

### Architectural Metaphors in Rabbinic Literature in General

The architectural metaphors of the interior are not restricted to Mishnah Niddah and its discussion in the Talmud. They are distributed throughout all of rabbinic literature and thus seem to be firmly inscribed in the rabbis' linguistic and cultural imagination. A famous metaphor can be found in midrashic literature that employs it in connection with pregnancy. The midrashic commentary on the story of creation records Rabbi Chisda's midrash, according to which God "constructed within her [the woman] more storage rooms than in the man, wide below and narrow on top so that she would be receiving embryos" (BerR 18:3; Albeck and Theodor, *Midrash Bereshit Rabba*, 163).⁵⁰

Here, another text enhances this discussion significantly. In the context of a discussion on the number of parts in the human body, traditionally 248,⁵¹ the Talmud attributes to the *amora* Shmu'el the bizarre story of an experiment conducted by Rabbi Yishma'el's students who boiled a prostitute:

> A story about the students of Rabbi Yishma'el who boiled a prostitute who had been condemned to burning by the king [i.e., the Roman government]. They examined and found in her 252 [parts].⁵² He said to them: Perhaps you examined a woman, because Scripture adds two hinges and two doors in her case [הוסיף לה הכתוב שני צירים ושני דלתות]. (bBekh 45a)

This story already troubled Julius Preuss in 1911, not so much because of its aspect of violence, but because this is the only report in all of rabbinic literature of such experimentation. Reading the story as a historical report, he assumes that the students are boiling a corpse (*Biblical and Talmudic Medicine*, 46). In terms of the midrashic logic of the narrative, this is possible, since execution by burning in halakhic theory is not by burning at the stake, but by pouring molten lead into the mouth of the condemned.⁵³ In other words, a corpse would be left after execution for the students to experiment with.⁵⁴ It needs to be noted, however, that the story allows for the possibility that the students acted as executioners on behalf of the Roman government. The story is most likely not a historical report, but is spun out of the *baraita* which the Talmud proceeds to cite as a proof-text for Rabbi Yishma'el's statement at the end. But whether one reads the story as a historical report, as Preuss does, or as a rabbinic midrash on the following midrash, in the end does not really make any difference with respect to its violence. In spite of its midrashic element, this is a climactic representation of that aspect of talmudic discourse which instrumentalizes women's bodies. It is ultimately this instrumentalization that enables that which women are excluded from, the study of Torah:⁵⁵ the prostitute's corpse is boiled in order to prove the fundamental tannaitic tenet of the 248 body parts. It is then perhaps not accidental that the story employs a prostitute for the experiment, the most instrumentalized of women.

The baraita on which this story is a midrash provides the proof-texts for Rabbi Yishma'el's explanation that Scripture adds two doors and two hinges to women:

> It is taught:
>
> Rabbi Ele'azar says: just as there are hinges [צירים]⁵⁶ for a house, so are there hinges for a woman, as it is said: "and she [Eli's daughter-in-law] bent down and gave birth, since her labor pains [ציריה] came upon her" (1 Sam. 4:19).
>
> Rabbi Yehoshu'a says: just as there are doors (דלתות) to a house, so there are doors to a woman,⁵⁷ since it is said: "[Cursed be the day on which I was born] since it did not shut up the doors [דלתי בטני] of my mother's womb" (Job 3:10).
>
> Rabbi Aqiva says: just as there is a key [מפתח] to a house, so there is to a woman, since it is said "and he [God] [יפתח] opened her [Rachel's] womb" (Gen. 30:22). (bBekh 45a)⁵⁸

Each of the body parts particular to women are derived midrashically through wordplay from biblical verses related to birthing. The referents for the individual metaphors are again ambiguous and difficult to identify. What is striking, however, is the insistence on comparison between the woman and the house: just as a house, so the woman. The association of house and the pregnant woman, the birthing woman, connects these midrashic readings with the preceding metaphor of the woman as (grain-)storage bin.

For the gender politics of this text we should draw on an intertext that is in the background of the framing discussion of the sugyah. The Mishnah in a different context states as a rule that מאתים וארבעים ושמונה אברים באדם, "there are 248 body parts in a person ['adam]" (mOhal 1:8), and then it proceeds to list them. To these body parts certain rules of impurity apply. What the Mishnah, however, implies is that the "normative" human being possesses this fixed number of limbs. In light of our baraita this mishnaic normative human being is clearly gendered and is male. The baraita, again, highlights the androcentric perspective of the Mishnah. The Talmud introduces, defines, and concretizes female difference around the birthing motif, interestingly as surplus, in direct opposition to the Aristotelian model of sexual difference, which defines the female as lacking.⁵⁹ However, this leads to no advantage concerning the representation of women in the cultural language of the rabbis, since the female body as surplus serves in the story to underline the equivalence between woman and house. Thus, whereas Aristotle and his successors may speak the language of women's exclusion from the equation human = male, the rabbis speak the metaphorical language of women's confinement to the house.

## The Opened Door

A metaphor that complements that of the house is the פתח פתוח, the "open door" that the Babylonian Talmud employs to refer to a suspected loss of virginity. The "open door" is used exclusively in the context of the woman's sexuality. In a discussion of marital laws the Babylonian Talmud (bKet 10a–b) introduces a list of five cases⁶⁰ in which a bridegroom brings his claim of his bride's nonvirginity before a rabbi. In all of these cases the rabbinic authority rules against the husband's claim.⁶¹ Within this list of cases the most common claim of the husband is that he did not find blood. However, in two cases the bridegroom's claim is formulated as finding a פתח פתוח—an "open door." In the first case the rabbi's answer is: אסבוהו כופרי מברכתא חביטא ליה—"strike him with spiked palm-switches, [for] is Mavrakhta prostrated before him!?" (bKet 10a). Rashi explains this obscure exclamation as a metonymy: "The prostitutes of this city whose name is Mavrakhta⁶² lie prostrate before him frequently to be unchaste, since he seems to be an expert in the matter of an opened door."⁶³ That is, since the bridegroom is promiscuous enough to recognize the difference between sexual intercourse with a virgin and a woman with sexual experience, he is the one who ought to be punished. Hence, the claim of the "opened door" backfires on the groom who raises it. In and of itself, the metaphor of the "opened door" corroborates the exclusivity of a husband's claim on his wife's reproductive capacity, which is representative of a unilateral relationship. The husband has exclusive rights to his "house," to his wife's reproductive capacity, but not vice versa. Even though this story seems to hold the husband accountable as well, it does not undermine this fundamental relationship. It ultimately only punishes his excess.

The second case, which also aims at disparaging the husband's claim of prior "inhabitance" of his bride, illustrates even more explicitly the relationship between the man and his wife as one who enters his house. Rabban Gamliel answers the groom who brought this claim before him:

שמא הטיתה אמשול לך משל למה הדבר דומה לאדם שהיה מהלך באישון
לילה ואפילה היתה מצאו פתוח לא היתה מצאו נעול
איכא דאמרי הכי אמר ליה
שמא במזיד הטיתה ועקרת לדשא ועברא אמשול לך משל למה הדבר דומה
לאדם שהוא מהלך באישון הלילה ואפילה היתה במזיד מצאו פתוח לא היתה
במזיד מצאו נעול

Perhaps you moved it aside! I will tell you a parable: To what can this matter be compared? To a man who walks in the deepest darkness of the night.[64] If he moves aside he finds it opened, if he does not move aside he finds it closed.[65]

There are those who say that this is how [Rabban Gamliel] answered him:

Perhaps you intentionally[66] moved it aside and thus tore away the door and the bolt. I will tell you a parable: To what can this matter be compared? To a man who walks in the deepest darkness of the night, and if he moves aside intentionally he finds it opened, if he does not move aside intentionally he finds it closed. (bKet 10a)

The point that both versions of this story make is that the man did not "find" the door opened, but that most likely he himself opened it, without being aware of it according to the first version of the story, or by being too forceful according to the second version. Again, the validity of such a claim is undermined because of mistaken sensation on behalf of the bridegroom. At the same time, his exclusive right of habitation is not questioned. Rather, it is reinscribed. In the second version of the story Rabban Gamliel's parable adds the metaphor of the door bolt, whose referent clearly is the concept of the hymen. In both cases, the *mashal* or illustrating parable functions as a metaphor, since it is an illustration of the metaphor of the bridegroom's claim, that is, the (opened) door. The woman is once again the house, closed as a virgin, to be opened by her groom for his exclusive habitation.

## The Metaphoric Body in Greco-Roman Medical Literature

In order to sharpen our understanding of the cultural implications of the rabbinic metaphoric process it might be helpful to briefly reflect on the way Greco-Roman medical literature metaphorizes the female body to construct the difference of male and female corporeality. Though it would be difficult if not impossible to determine direct influences on rabbinic literature, Greco-Roman gynecology is its cultural matrix. The rabbinic construction of the female body takes place at about the same time as the flourishing of Greco-Roman gynecological literature.[67] The divergences and convergences between the two textual traditions will help us to understand how rabbinic culture produced notions of sexual difference.

The Hippocratics laid the foundation for Greco-Roman gynecological literature during the last decades of the fifth and the first decades of the fourth century B.C.E. and remained popular, to become one of the major sources for the gynecological literature of the second century C.E.. They liken the woman's body to a ploughed and seeded field and the uterus to an upside-down jug (Hanson, "The Medical Writers' Women," 317).[68] Froma Zeitlin writes with respect to the metaphor of the jug:

> Throughout the Hippocratic corpus and the works of the later, more sophisticated anatomists, the woman's uterus is likened to an upside-down jar, furnished with two ears or handles. The *stathmos* or *puthmen* (Latin *fundus*) is the base or bottom of the jar, located now on top; the *stoma* (Latin *os*), or mouth, lies at the bottom; and the neck (the *auchen*, *trachelos*, or Latin *cervix*) opens in a downward direction. It too has a mouth and neck. This nomenclature is also pertinent to the widespread idea of a correlation between woman's sexual and oral appetites.... Popular and medical notions insist on a symmetry between a woman's two orifices, the mouth and the belly, reflected in prescriptions for gynecological therapy. ("The Case of Hesiod's Pandora," 65)

In her analysis of the construction of the female body in the Hippocratic writings, Ann Hanson points out that "the major concern [of this metaphor] is the management of liquids—irrigation, retention, and release at the proper time.... a man's body has few drainage problems, because his flesh is hard, dense, and nonabsorbent, like thickly woven cloth, while a woman's body is like the fleece used in agricultural hydroscopy to discover moisture hidden beneath the earth's surface" ("Medical Writers' Women," 317). She emphasizes the potency of the image of the upside-down jug, "as the verb μίγνυμαι, a verb for the mixing of liquids within a container and a verb for intercourse implies" (325). Ann Carson agrees with Hanson on the analysis of the Hippocratic preoccupation with woman's wetness and fluidity, that the woman's wetness established the structural difference from the male body. This has to be read in the context of both Platonic and Aristotelian philosophical anthropology. In both Platonic and Aristotelian philosophy the notion of woman's wetness is closely bound up with the notion of her formlessness, that is, her inability to be contained, and, therefore, her inability to be "someone."[69] Where the Hippocratic writers are concerned with the leakage of woman, with her wetness as opposed to the dryness of man, her interior is likened to a reservoir, to an upside-down jug, and menstruation is one of the means to unscrew the bottle and release excess fluids. The metaphor aids the construction of sexual difference, which in Aristotelian philosophy construes the woman as lesser than the male.

A few centuries later, during the time of the *tannaim*, the gynecologist Soranus in Rome reflects on the nature of the metaphoric process:

> The uterus (μήτρα) is also termed *hystera* and *delphys*. It is termed *metra*, because it is the mother of all the embryos borne of it or because it makes mothers of those who possess it; or, according to some people, because it possesses a metre of time regarding menstruation and childbirth. And it is termed *hystera* because afterwards[70] it yields up its products, or because it lies after all the entrails, if not precisely, at least broadly speaking. And it is termed *delphys* because it is able to procreate brothers and sisters.[71] (Temkin, trans., *Soranus' Gynecology*, 8)

Thus Soranus shows beautifully—via almost midrashic etymology—the metaphoric constructedness of the woman's anatomy. The names he chooses for the uterus are purely functional terms. Their matrix is the woman's repoductive capacity. This choice of metaphors corroborates Rousselle's argument that Greco-Roman gynecological literature could be read as a succession of "fertility manuals" concerned with the guaranteeing optimum reproduction (Rousselle, *Porneia*, 74).

Overall, the Greco-Roman texts mobilize *webs* of metaphors different from those found in rabbinic literature. That does not mean that we cannot find metaphoric crossovers. The rabbis, as we have seen above, can sometimes employ the metaphor of mouth for the vaginal orifice. Greek literature can also make use of metaphors that construct the association of women with the household.[72] However, we can observe the difference in emphasis, particularly in the gynecological contexts.

∽

Talmudic literature on menstrual impurity does not configure sexual difference in Hippocratic terms, since according to its biblical-textual foundation both man and woman "leak." But in its metaphoric configuration of the woman's body in architectural terms it creates a Hippocratic effect. That is, the rabbinic configuration of the female body corresponds more to the Hippocratic model than the Aristotelian. Since the Hippocratic writers thought of the woman as a completely different creature and not simply a substandard man, her "otherness allowed her body to be defined more by its own parameters" (Dean-Jones, *Women's Bodies*, 85–86). The biblical legislative discourse on the impurity of genital discharges engenders bodies in rabbinic literature which are wholly different from each other. Indeed, not only does the woman have a metaphoric relationship with the interior, she *is* the interior. The woman herself has become "house," linguistically attested as early as in mishnaic Hebrew. According to mYoma 1:1 the high priest before the Yom Kippur services at the Temple is to be separated from his "house(hold)." The Mishnah itself then offers a midrashic exegesis in the name of Rabbi Yehuda, according to which the biblical term has to be read specifically " 'his house' [Lev. 16:6]—that is, his wife."

In Babylonian Aramaic the designation of the wife of some rabbis as "his house" appears frequently.[73] The statement ascribed to Rabbi Yossi, presumably a second-generation Palestinian *amora*, is especially interesting:

אמר רבי יוסי מימי לא קריתי לאשתי אשתי ולשורי שורי אלא לאשתי ביתי ולשורי שדי —"Rabbi Yossi said: During [all] my days I have never called my wife 'my wife' and my ox 'my ox.' Rather, [I have called] my wife 'my house' and my ox 'my field.'" (bShab 118b, also cited in bGit 52a)

Rashi comments on why Rabbi Yossi names his wife "my house": שכל צרכי הבית על ידה נעשים והיא עיקר הבית וכן שור עיקרו של שדה—"Because all the needs of the house are done by her hands and she is the essence of the house. Similarly, the ox is the essence of the field" (ad bGit 52a).[74]

However, we also have to consider two mishnaic expressions that seem to employ the metaphor of house for the husband. One is the euphemism for marital intercourse: לשמש את ביתה—to serve her house (e.g. mNid 2:7, mMikv 8:4). The other is related: מותרת/אסורה לביתה—she is allowed or forbidden to her house (in certain circumstances). The latter is usually translated with "to her husband," to the effect that marital intercourse is prohibited. However, I remain unconvinced. mMikv 8:4 reads: "The woman who 'serviced her house'—ששמשה ביתה—and went down and immersed, but did not 'clean her house'—כבדה את ביתה—is as though she did not immerse." All the rabbinic commentators understand the referent of the second part clearly to be her genitalia. Hai Gaon reads: כבדה את הבית את אותו מקום = כלומר שלא קינחה—"'but did not clean her house' = that is to say, she did not wipe that certain place [her genitalia]."[75] Thus the parallelism in this particular mishnah leads me to believe that in both cases the Mishnah understands the referent of the "house" to be her genitalia, rather than in the first case her husband and only in the second part her genitalia. Rashi's comment on mNid 2:7 might suggest that he understands the referent of "her house" to be the husband, since he translates לשמש את ביתה [she is about to 'serve her house'] = עם בעלה "with her husband" (bNid 11a). However, we can also read his comment to supplement the mishnaic phrase: [she is about to serve her house] " . . . with her husband." Thus, the husband is not "her house." Rather, we might understand the metaphor to express that she employs or "services" and "prepares" her body and especially her sexual organs for the purpose of marital intercourse.

Having seen the pervasiveness of the designation of the wife as "house," I want to conclude this chapter by summoning into the conversation one recent reader of this aspect of the rabbinic discourse, and in particular the latter equation. In his essay "Judaism and the Feminine," the French Jewish philosopher and ethicist Emmanuel Levinas comments on this equation: "The house is woman, the Talmud tells us. Beyond the psychological and sociological obviousness of such an affirmation, the rabbinic tradition experiences this affirmation as a primordial truth" ("Judaism and the Feminine," 31–32). Thus "woman" is the space that "man" inhabits. Levinas most explicitly does not read the talmudic construct as just that, as a historically conditioned cultural construct. What Levinas means by "psychological and sociological obviousness" is expressed more clearly in his comment on the role of women in the biblical world, in which he draws this correlation between women and interiority as an essential, if not ontological one: "But the world in which these [biblical] events unfolded would not have been structured as it was—and as it still is and *always will be*—without the secret presence, on the edge of invisibility, of these mothers, wives and daughters; without their silent footsteps in the depths and opacity of reality, drawing the very dimensions of *interiority* and making the world precisely habitable" ("Judaism and the Feminine," 31; emphasis added).[76] He moves outside of the text and declares its fundamentally androcentric perspective to be an eternal and metahistorical truth. Levinas does not merely repeat the androcentric confining moment of the talmudic discourse, but intensifies it. Thereby, he assigns the task of making this world habitable to "these women" in a structure that not only was in the biblical past but "always will be," apparently his sense of "primordial truth," simultaneously relieving men from the responsibility of making the world habitable and structurally excluding women from the exterior. This entails Levinas's inability to conceive of "these" (biblical) women as other than by their relationship to the men in their lives, as other than "mothers, wives and daughters."

The metaphorization of the interior of the female body in talmudic literature would seem to corroborate Levinas's reading, since it configures the female body as the space the man enters and where he dwells. As we have seen in this chapter, women are represented as house, in the context of the discourse of anatomy, around associations of pregnancy/birth and sexual relations between husband and wife. In this respect, talmudic discourse (and all the more so Levinas's, as its reader) shares in what has marked much of the Western philosophical discourse.

The latter has undergone critiques from various perspectives of feminist theory in recent years. Many aspects of those critiques apply to the metaphorical domestication of the female in talmudic literature as well. Thus, Alice Jardine notes that "all of the words used to designate this space (now unbound)—nature, Other, matter, unconscious, hyle, force—have throughout the tenure of Western philosophy carried feminine connotations (whatever their grammatical gender)" (*Gynesis*, 88). The French feminist philosopher/psychoanalyst Luce Irigaray is much more forceful in her critique. In her essay on "Love of the Other" in *An Ethics of Sexual Difference* Irigaray claims that this relationship to women is not only a feature of androcentric culture, that is, a historical characteristic of an explicitly androcentric perspective, but is the essential property of a male relating to the world: "*To inhabit* is the fundamental trait of a man's being. Even if this trait remains unconscious, unfulfilled, especially in its ethical dimension, man is forever searching for, building, creating homes for himself everywhere: caves, huts, women, cities, language, concepts, theory, and so on" (141; her emphasis). Her use of "man (l'homme)" is, of course, deliberate. Hence, by his continuous effort of surrounding "himself with envelopes, containers, 'houses'" (142), his relationship with the world is a proprietary one. Besides Irigaray, other French feminists have targeted the signification of space as feminine or, vice versa, femininity as space, prominently Hélène Cixous and Julia Kristeva. Cixous writes in the essay in which she develops the notion of *écriture féminine* that because woman "has been made to see (= not-see) woman on the basis of what man wants to see of her . . . she has not been able to live in her 'own' house, her very body" (*The Newly Born Woman*, 68).

It should be noted here also that both Cixous and Irigaray move beyond the strategy of critique to a constructive mode. This latter mode might prove to be critical for rereading of rabbinic texts. For example, Verena A. Conley, one of the interpreters of Cixous's work, has described Cixous's strategy in terms that are fitting in the context of this chapter: "Cixous displaces the old phallocentric architectural metaphor of woman-as-house. She suggests the proximity of the mother-as-house but without doors, with open arches overlooking the sea" (*Hélène Cixous*, 36). Similarly, Irigaray contrasts the (male) mode of inhabiting with that of perception: "To perceive—is this the usual dimension of the feminine? Of women, who, it seems, remain within perception without need of name or concept. *Without closure*. To remain within perception means *staying out in the open*, always attuned to the outside, to the world. Senses alert" (*An Ethics of Sexual Difference*, 141; emphasis added). The question mark and the cautious "it seems" are perhaps engendered by the fact that women's relating to the world has never been thought, which is, of course, Irigaray's project. Whereas the former, male mode has been the characteristic mode of most of cultural history, dominated by patriarchal economies, the latter, female mode has to be carved out from within the former mode.[77]

To conclude, and to lead us into the next chapter, we need to underline one erroneous aspect of Levinas's reading of talmudic literature. Both Levinas and Morna Joy, in her reading of him, essentialize the "*Jewish* concept" of the feminine. Levinas engenders his equation of women and interiority from what "*the* Talmud" tells us, melding the heterogeneity of talmudic literature into the one single authorial voice. Joy, on the other hand, claims that "Levinas remains true to Jewish heritage. For, though in Judaism 'the feminine figures among the categories of Being,' a woman exists only in relation to a man. Her manifest destiny is to tend the hearth, to secure the amenities of life, to provide the ineluctable support that makes men's deeds possible" ("Levinas: Alterity, the Feminine, and Women," 20; emphasis added). For Joy it is "Judaism," extrapolated from any historical, social reality of the past, which confines women to the interior, though the referent of Judaism is far from obvious: does she mean biblical or rabbinic Judaism, medieval halakhic or mystical Judaism, modern orthodox, conservative, liberal, reform, or reconstructionist Judaism?

Against such essentializing extrapolation, however, which silences those differences from within talmudic literature and within "Judaism," I want to focus on one such moment of difference, which disturbs the talmudic metaphoric imagination of the woman's body even within talmudic literature, so much so that it resurfaces repeatedly in the Babylonian Talmud's discussions of menstrual impurity. It is our task as readers of talmudic literature not to succumb to constructing uniformity where there is doubt, contradiction, ambiguity, and difference. That which has proven to be a fairly omnipresent perspective of talmudic literature finds a counterdiscourse.

## 3 READING RUPTURES IN THE MASSEKHET/FABRIC OF NIDDAH

IN THE PREVIOUS CHAPTER I have shown that we can identify the treatment of women's bodies as architectural constructs as the dominant discourse of rabbinic culture. As the earliest text, the Mishnah introduces the more elaborate and detailed architectural terminology in its tractate on laws concerning menstruation. Both the Palestinian and Babylonian Talmud continue this discourse, and in their discussions of the specific mishnayot continue to build the "female" house. The Babylonian Talmud elsewhere cites tannaitic texts that employ similar linguistic constructions, and in the language specific to it—Babylonian Aramaic—deploys the designation of wife as house. The metaphoric construction may have its roots in the Mishnah, but it is subsequently shared by all the major texts, since both the Babylonian and the Palestinian gemaras adopt the metaphor into their own cultural vocabularies. From the Mishnah on we cannot really discern either chronological (tannaitic versus amoraic) or geographic (Babylonian versus Palestinian) differences with respect to this linguistic convention. The dominant metaphoric construction of women's bodies and physiology is one more aspect of a cultural perception that is frequently summarized with the citation of this famous biblical verse: כל כבודה בת מלך פנימה—"Every honorable king's daughter is within" (Ps. 45:14, according to the Hebrew text). The king's daughter—the Jewish woman—belongs inside the home.[1]

At the same time, the Babylonian Talmud in its discussion of menstruation and its physiology introduces a consideration that undermines this dominant discourse of androcentrism. This consideration is the conceptualization of the female body as a sentient being, as already "inhabited" by the feeling subject. This chapter will be built on a discursive analysis of a crucial sugyah that introduces this conceptualization and then develops strategies to contain its potential force, strategies of taming. To remind the reader, *sugyah* designates a self-contained basic unit of talmudic discussion and is developed and shaped especially in the Babylonian Talmud.² An analysis of talmudic constructions of gender that takes this unique textuality seriously needs to move beyond citing individual opinions of rabbis or even individual textual units, such as a mishnah or a baraita, as evidence of talmudic gender ideologies. Such units cited in a sugyah are always discussed from various angles, dissected and reassembled, recontextualized by juxtaposing them with yet other such textual units and tested for contradictions and agreements. In the framework of a talmudic sugyah, where such individual textual units serve as building blocks of an often unresolved argument,³ they can turn into oscillating, multileveled, and slippery units of meaning. An analysis of talmudic gender politics has to embrace the entire structure of an argument, that is, the sugyah. These remarks by way of introduction to this chapter are important, since I will read one argument introduced into such an argumentation as a rupture in the talmudic discourse on niddah *as a whole*. However, if multivocality and disagreements (מחלוקות) or negotiations of such disagreements (שקלא וטריא) are the very essence of talmudic literature, we have to be extremely cautious in making distinctions between overt or culturally endorsed differences of opinion and those suggestions that may have an effect on talmudic discourse as a whole.⁴

What I want to explore in the following pages is whether and how we can read a counterdiscourse in Tractate Niddah of the Babylonian Talmud. By counterdiscourse, in this context, I mean a discourse within the framework of the larger, dominant one which *conceptually* contradicts it.⁵

The first question is how to identify a counterdiscourse that would transcend the dialectics of the typical talmudic argumentation. In the specific context of Tractate Niddah we can use gender as a *hermeneutic* category to distinguish between types of discourses. Types of discourses on gender can be distinguished in part by asking questions such as these: Is sexual difference, the difference between male and female, constructed hierarchically? Is the notion of sexual difference as such rendered mute by either an objectification or instrumentalization of women or women's bodies? Is sexual difference perhaps even erased altogether through constructions of femininity in masculine terms? Or is sexual difference discussed in terms that allow for different, complementary subject positions to emerge? Taking these questions into account, the argument in this chapter is that we can, indeed, identify a counterdiscourse. If the dominant discourse identified in the previous chapter falls in the category of the objectification or instrumentalization of women as dwellings of their husbands, in this chapter I analyze a discussion in Tractate Niddah which allows for thinking about women as (different) subjects of the discourse.

We have to be even more careful with our evaluation of such a counterdiscourse, once identified, however, especially as to its relationship to the dominant discourse. Does it merely supplement the dominant discourse and remain an integral part of it? Or does it undermine or even critique the dominant discourse and thus limit its power to define reality? Do we attribute even intentional (self-)critique of the dominant discourse? Whether we end up doing anything on the scale from bad apologetics to injustice to the text depends on how we answer these questions. A helpful model is Mieke Bal's concept of *symptom* as *involuntary signs* (*Lethal Love*, 82). If the dominant discourse of niddah displaces women, the conceptualization of women's bodies as sentient, however briefly considered, "reinstates the repressed side of the text" (Bal, *Lethal Love*, 72). Keeping this in mind, I want to analyze the texts to demonstrate the possibility of identifying a counterdiscourse, while answering the second set of questions along with the textual analysis.

### The Rupture in the Fabric/Massekhet of Niddah

אמר שמואל בדקה בקרקע עולם וישבה עליה
ומצאה דם עליה טהורה שנאמר בבשרה עד
שתרגיש בבשרה

> Shmu'el ruled: If a woman examined the ground and after sitting on it, found on it some blood, she remains in the status of purity [contra the evidence], for it is said [in the biblical verse Lev. 15:19] "in her body," [meaning, she is not in the status of impurity] unless she *feels* "in her body." (bNid57a, beginning of the sugyah; emphasis added)

The Babylonian Talmud begins the sugyah with quite a different reading of the term "in her body" in our verse in Lev. 15:19, the material from which it fashions female corporeality. It is attributed to the name of Shmu'el,[6] one of the great authorities of the first generation of Babylonian amoraim. This little case, simple as it seems at first sight, is rather complex. First of all, Shmu'el seems to discuss only one specific case: the woman sits on the ground, rather than anywhere else. The context in which this case is raised is a mishnah that discusses a woman's status of im/purity when a blood spot is found on her body or on her garments. According to this mishnah the answer to the question of whether a woman is considered to be menstruating depends on where on her body the blood is found, that is, whether we can reconstruct the most likely source of the blood.[7] When the sugyah begins with the above text, Shmu'el seems to add only one more case scenario in addition to the considerable number of comparable ones mentioned in the Mishnah. Thus the implication seems to be that in this case, and in this case specifically, when the woman sits on the ground, she remains in the status of purity, even though the evidence would seem to indicate differently.

However, the halakhic midrash that Shmu'el attaches to the case to explain his reasoning introduces the general principle of the woman's sensation (הרגשה) as the determining factor of her status, which does not fit the particularity of his case scenario. That is, if in this case she remains in the status of purity because she did not have a sensation that would indicate menstruation, this could apply to the case in the mishnah to which the sugyah is attached, the case in which blood is found on a woman's body or clothing. However, this mishnah has just declared the location of the spot to be the determining criterion by which to derive the woman's status.

Attached to the particular circumstances of his own case scenario, Shmu'el's midrash takes an interesting and counterintuitive twist. Given the fact that he uses a midrashic reading of Lev. 15:19, we would have expected Shmu'el to employ the verse differently to strengthen his ruling. It might have seemed more logical for him to argue that since the biblical phrase states explicitly "in her body," a woman is in the status of impurity only if the blood is "in her body," but not when it is "on the ground." But he takes the biblical formulation "in her body" to imply that the woman has to have a *sensation* of the blood-flow "inside her body" in order to attribute a status of impurity to her. By reading the principle of her sensation as the decisive factor for determining a woman's status into the verse—"'in her body'—[meaning that] unless she has a sensation 'in her body' [she is not considered to be in the status of impurity]"—he introduces a principle that is so general that it could be applied to any case, regardless of where blood traces as possible evidence for the occurrence of a woman's menstrual bleeding are found.[8] That is, if a woman has a physical sensation of the beginning of her blood-flow she can be considered or can consider herself to have her menstruation.[9] If she does not have that sensation, no matter where blood is found, it would seem, she cannot.

Beyond the immediate context of the discussion, Shmu'el's reading of the biblical verse also stands in contradiction to the metaphoric constructions I have discussed so far. Those readings have used the verse to think the interior of the woman's body as architectural, and therefore as an inanimate structure, a thing about which the rabbis can have a conversation. As inanimate object with the status of object, it can be claimed discursively, and inserted into the folds of halakhic circumscriptions. Shmu'el's reading, on the other hand, reconfigures the female body as animated, as a sentient entity. All of a sudden, the "house" is no longer empty, but has a master of its own. It is already occupied, so to speak, by her "sensation," thus rendering it uninhabitable for the androcentric perspective. In fact, this reading renders the woman's body at least partially inaccessible to its androcentric objectification in halakhic discourse.

In her reflections in *The Body in Pain*, Elaine Scarry has argued that "whatever pain achieves, it achieves in part through its unsharability, and it ensures this unsharability through its resistance to language . . . [pain's] resistance to language is not simply one of its incidental or accidental attributes but is essential to what it is" (4–5). Though a "sensation" might lack the physiological intensity of pain, I nonetheless believe that Scarry's reflection can be applied to our thinking about the discursive role of the woman's sensation in the talmudic discussions of niddah. In other words, the woman's bodily sensation lies outside halakhic discourse, and even outside of language, in an extra-discursive sphere where it does not exist independently from its subject, from her who has the sensation. The introduction of the principle of sensation in a sense restores her body to the woman. Scarry suggests that "physical pain does not simply resist language but actively destroys it" (4). Figuratively thought, Shmu'el's midrash would logically do exactly that to a majority of the mishnaic and talmudic discussions on women's corporeality in Tractate Niddah,[10] if his had been the only reading of the biblical verse. The Talmud, I claim, is rather well aware of this potential force of Shmu'el's midrash.

## The Taming of Shmu'el

The hermeneutic energy invested by the subsequent sugyah to reconcile Shmu'el's reading with the mishnaic discourse is symptomatic of the "problem" that the otherness of the woman's body presents to talmudic discourse, where it attempts to force women's corporeality into avenues of discursive objectification within the rabbinic purity and impurity system. In Shmu'el's midrash the uncontainability of women's corporeality, of their embodied subjectivity, asserts itself in talmudic discourse.[11]

Before we can draw final conclusions about the implications of Shmu'el's reading and the force that it has within talmudic discourse, however, we have to consider responses to it. Can a hermeneutic investment in Shmu'el's midrash as discussed so far be justified? Is Shmu'el's reading a lone dissenting voice that drowns in the "sea of the Talmud" and thus of little consequence, or is it a symptom of a larger complex that surges against the majority of halakhic discourse? These two questions can be answered in two different ways: as to the first question, I will analyze the sugyah following Shmu'el's case, since it is the response to an argument which more often than not indicates its force. As to the second question, I will show that Shmu'el's reading is not just his "individual" problem, but that the woman's body as sentient resurfaces elsewhere in the discussions of the Babylonian Talmud, corroborating my attempt to identify it as a counterdiscourse to the dominant talmudic discourse on menstrual impurity.

In response to Shmu'el's introduction of the woman's sensation, the Talmud basically employs three taming or domesticating strategies, all three classic argumentative maneuvers in talmudic literature.

## Taming Strategy One

Both of the first two strategies respond to Shmu'el's introduction of the principle of a woman's sensation, and neither strategy is disturbed by the fact that Shmu'el's midrash does not seem well-connected to his case scenario of the woman sitting on the ground and finding some blood. The gemara's first strategy tests Shmu'el's case by raising the classic difficulty that the verse that Shmu'el uses to argue his case has already been used for different readings.[12]

> But is not [the verse] "in her body" (Lev. 15:19) required for [a different halakhic ruling, namely] that she is rendered in the status of impurity [when the blood is still] in her body just as when it is outside?[13]

This difficulty is solved by allowing for two different readings of the same verse, owing to the specific linguistic feature of the verse, such as seemingly superfluous grammatical features:

> If that were so, Scripture could have said [merely] "in *the* body." Why [does Scripture] say "in *her* body?" Learn from this [syntactic emphasis the additional principle that she is not in the status of impurity] unless she has a sensation in her body.[14]

By allowing for simultaneous halakhic readings of the biblical verse the argumentation in the text saves the legitimacy of Shmu'el's use of the verse for his argument. This is, of course, its overt purpose. But by allowing various readings of the verse to coexist, it also limits the force of Shmu'el's reading as a possible systemic contradiction to mishnaic halakhah. Now his midrash on the verse is only one among others.

**Taming Strategy Two**

As a second strategy, which deserves closer attention, the Talmud adduces different cases from the Mishnah and other tannaitic texts that do not seem to have anything to do with the principle of a woman's sensation, and actually would seem to contradict it, since in these case scenarios her status of im/purity seems to be determined by external or circumstantial criteria. The overt question of this strategy is how Shmu'el, knowing the Mishnah, could have ruled the way he did.¹⁵ Thus in each of the four cases cited the gemara tries to reconcile Shmu'el's principle of her sensation with those cases, till the argument runs aground.

Case 1 (mNid 9:1) concerns "the woman who urinates and has a blood-flow: Rabbi Meir rules that if she is standing she is in the status of impurity, and if she is sitting, she is in the status of purity."¹⁶

Case 2 (mNid 8:4)¹⁷ concerns "the testing-rag that was placed under the pillow and some blood is found on it: if [the stain] is round, it is in the status of purity, and if it is elongated, it is in the status of impurity."

Case 3 (mNid 2:2): If blood "is found on his testing-rag they [the woman and the man] are in the status of impurity, and they are obligated to bring a sacrifice. [If blood] is found on hers immediately [after sexual relations] they are in the status of impurity, and obligated to bring a sacrifice. [If blood] is found on hers after some time, they are in a status of doubtful impurity, and exempt from bringing a sacrifice."

Case 4 (a baraita)¹⁸ is as follows: "You find yourself saying that there are three situations of doubt that apply to the woman:

a) [concerning the stain] *on her body* where there is a doubt whether it is pure or impure [or whether it establishes the status if im/purity], it is [to be considered as indicating a status of] impurity.

b) [concerning the stain] *on her shirt* where there is a doubt whether it is pure or impure, it is [considered as indicating a status of] purity.

c) [concerning the rules of transferring or contracting a status of im-purity via] touch or shaking¹⁹ go after the majority."²⁰

In each of these four tannaitic cases the criterion for determining the woman's status of im/purity is clearly an external or circumstantial one,²¹ certainly not her sensation, a point that the gemara raises repetitively in its discussion of each of the four cases. In Case 1 the criterion is her standing or sitting, in Case 2 the criterion is the shape of the stain, in Case 3 the criterion is the length of time after sexual relations before the blood is found, and in Case 4 it is the location where the blood is found, or the ambiguous princi-ple of majority of her days (see note 20).

The initial question, which the medieval commentaries such as both the Tosafists and Tosfei Rosh raise, is why the gemara uses exactly these four cases of the many possible cases in the Mishnah to think with against

Shmu'el's midrash, and whether the sugyah has a reason to choose these and no others.[22] What these commentaries recognize, and what I want to emphasize more in terms of our discussion, is that Shmu'el's principle actually would undermine the entire mishnaic and tannaitic discourse of menstruation, and not just individual cases. If all those cases cited in our sugyah claim to describe circumstantial, objective evidence by which the rabbis evaluate a woman to be menstruous or not, Shmu'el's principle relies on the woman herself, the subjective evidence of her sensation.

Beyond the question of the medieval commentaries, however, the choice of cases is not arbitrary. Another angle in the plan of the sugyah's construction eludes the Tosafot: that the unifying principle of the selection of these specific cases is not borne out by the cases themselves, but by the "solutions" that the gemara provides for each contradiction to Shmu'el raised by these cases. That unifying principle, which forms the basis for the literary structure of the sugyah, is the sensation of the woman. The gemara—carefully, one might say—selects those cases that allow for a discussion of the woman's sensation of a blood-flow, and which allow the gemara to consider a sequence of what might be called "mistaken sensations."

The reconciliation between Shmu'el and Case 1 is as follows:

לעולם דארגשה ואימור הרגשת מי רגלים הואי

Indeed, [the Mishnah assumes] that she [the woman in the mishnaic case] did have a sensation, but one may say that [the reason that in spite of her sensation she remains in the status of purity in the case of sitting while urinating with the evidence of blood spotting is that here her sensation was not one of her blood-flow but] it was a *sensation of the flow of urine* only [הרגשת מי רגלים].[23]

Here is the reconciliation between Shmu'el and Case 2:

לעולם דארגישה ואימור הרגשת עד הואי

Indeed, [the Mishnah assumes] that she did have a sensation, but one may say that [the reason that she remains in the status of purity in the case of the round stain, indicating a louse only, is that here her sensation was not one of her blood-flow but] it was a *sensation of the testing-rag* [הרגשת עד].[24]

The third reconciliation, that between Shmu'el and Case 3, states:

לעולם דארגישה ואימא הרגשת שמש הוה

Indeed, [the Mishnah assumes] that she did have a sensation, but one may say that [the reason that husband and wife are only in a doubtful status of impurity if the blood was found after a longer period of time had passed between sexual intercourse and her self-examination, is that her sensation was not one of her blood-flow but] it was *a sensation of the penis* [הרגשת שמש].[25]

The first three solutions to the problem posed by these cases to Shmu'el's midrash raise the possibility of a woman's mistaken or misidentified sensation. The gemara argues that Shmu'el's midrashic exegesis could still be upheld regarding even those mishnaic cases that seem to determine a woman's status of im/purity by other, circumstantial criteria. Thus the argument regarding the first three cases is that the Mishnah could be read as assuming the principle of her sensation: when the mishnaic cases describe the circumstances when a woman remains in the status of purity in spite of evidence of blood,[26] a woman may actually be considered/consider herself to be in a status of purity *even if she had a sensation*, because this sensation may be classified as mistaken. When those same mishnaic cases rule a woman to be in the status of impurity based on certain circumstances, the principle of her sensation is considered not applicable or to be overridden.[27] In those circumstances she would be in the status of impurity no matter whether she had a sensation of anything or not.

For those who read talmudic argumentation halakhically from a woman's perspective,[28] it could perhaps be argued that this argumentation actually has a positive effect for women, since in some cases—against the evidence (her sensation and evidence of blood)—a woman still does not have to consider herself/to be considered to be in a status of impurity. However, if we analyze this argumentation in terms of its discursive effects with respect to gender, the result is a different one: the argumentation tries to contain the potentially radical effect of Shmu'el's midrash. Shmu'el potentially opens up the discourse for women's interpretation of their own sensations. By definition, sensation is a matter of radical subjectivity, women's subjectivity no less. Analyzing women's sensation in the terms of the sugyah here, that is, by suggesting that women can be mistaken in their sensation, even if the text does so for the good of the women themselves, it discursively takes the power of interpreting this sensation out of the hands of women. Women may have felt something, but "here are the possibilities of their misinterpretation." Thus the text attempts to take control again of what otherwise would allow for women's hermeneutic sovereignty.

This dynamic is led to its logical conclusion in the discussion of the fourth and final case, the reconciliation between Shmu'el and Case 4:

ימיה בהרגשה חזיא טמאה דאימור ארגשה ולאו אדעתה אם רוב

[The principle of 'the majority of her days' implies that] if for the majority of her days she had a blood-flow accompanied by a sensation she is in the status of impurity [even in the present doubtful situation in which she presumably did not have a sensation], because you can say that she had *an unconscious sensation* [ארגשה ולאו אדעתה].[29]

With this explanation of how to reconcile Shmu'el's criterion of the woman's sensation as the determinant for the woman's status with a tannaitic case the gemara argues the following, now the other way around: even if a woman in the current doubtful case had no sensation, which by Shmu'el's standard would mean that she is not in the status of impurity, she can still be determined to be exactly that, because—the gemara suggests—the overriding principle now is "statistics": since usually, in all other cases, she does feel something, it may be assumed that in the present situation she did also, only she did not know it. With this notion of the possibly unconscious sensation, obviously, the implied subjectivity of Shmu'el's suggestion is reduced ad absurdum. Again, from a benevolent hermeneutic perspective this last argument can be read to take into consideration an individual woman's physiology ("if a woman in the majority of her days has a blood-flow accompanied by a sensation, then . . ."). But at the same time, discursively, the subjectivity inherent to the concept of sensation is drained out of it. By moving from a list of mistaken sensations to unconscious sensation the gemara attempts to turn the concept of sensation into a describable, definable, and (discursively and halakhically) controllable object. In an oxymoronic way the gemara has completely desubjectified the principle of a woman's sensation. This desubjectification is what characterizes this second taming strategy.

In the end the sugyah upholds the contradiction between the mishnaic discourse and Shmu'el's midrash. After a brief side discussion weighing the baraita (Case 4) against the mishnah serving as the anchor of our sugyah, the problem with Shmu'el is reiterated, now based on the first part of the baraita (Case 4, a) and the mishnah itself:

> It [the anonymous voice of the baraita] still states that "[concerning the stain] *on her body* where there is a doubt whether it is pure or impure [or whether it establishes the status if im/purity], it is [to be considered as indicating a status of] impurity"—*even though she did not have a sensation*, and furthermore our Mishnah itself [at the beginning of this chapter] teaches "[concerning the woman who] observes a bloodstain on her body close to her genitals, that she is in a status of impurity"—*even though she did not have a sensation*. (bNid 57b, bottom; emphasis added to indicate the problem with Shmu'el)

After all this discussion that could explain how the four cited cases could be reconciled with Shmu'el (and vice versa), the sugyah points out that there are yet more cases that raise problems. Shmu'el's midrash seems untenable against the force of the majority of the mishnaic literature. Realizing that this second strategy has reached such a strange impasse, we have to conclude that it presents itself as an exercise of thinking through Shmu'el's midrash, rather than as suggesting that "real women really" might misidentify their sensations in such a way, or a "real woman" might "really" have an unperceived sensation. The suggested mistaken sensations are compromises between two fundamentally opposed approaches to involving the woman's subjectivity in determining her status of im/purity. Since Shmu'el's midrash, which splits open the discourse to allow for the total involvement of a woman's subjectivity, and the mishnaic cases brought up against him contradict each other in such a fundamental way, the second strategy logically had to reach such an impasse.[30]

### Taming Strategy Three

In its third strategy, then, the gemara turns away from Shmu'el's midrash altogether, and offers the two readings of the last generations of Babylonian rabbis, of which only the latter is relevant to my discussion.[31]

רב אשי אמר שמואל הוא דאמר כר׳ נחמיה דתנן ר׳ נחמיה אומר כל דבר
שאינו מקבל טומאה אינו מקבל כתמים

Rav Ashi interpreted: Shmu'el ruled in accordance with Rabbi Nehemiah, because we learn in our Mishnah: "Rabbi Nehemia holds: Anything which cannot contract a status of impurity, does not contract [the impurity] of blood stains either" (mNid 9:3; par. tNid 7:4).

According to Rav Ashi, a leading Babylonian rabbi among the last generations of amoraim of the Talmud,[32] the decisive factor in Shmu'el's case is not his controversial midrashic reading of Lev. 15:19, but the fact that in Shmu'el's case-scenario the woman sat on the ground. Rav Ashi turns the conversation in a completely different direction. He argues that since the ground cannot contract a status of impurity Shmu'el declares the woman to remain in a status of purity, in accordance with Rabbi Nehemiah's principle, which we learn in the Mishnah in the next chapter. The specific context of Rabbi Nehemiah's principle is the discussion of a case-scenario in which three women sit together on a bench and blood is found on it. The anonymous voice of the Mishnah rules all of them to be in the status of impurity, whereas Rabbi Nehemiah declares them to be in the status of purity if the bench is made of stone, a material that does not receive the status of impurity.

Rav Ashi's explanation, however, harbors an extreme difficulty. This difficulty lies already in Rabbi Nehemiah's principle in the Mishnah. Thus, the Tosafot (bNid 58a, ד״ה כרבי נחמיה) attempt to clarify: "Rabbi Nehemiah's reason is that in a case where the bloodstain is found on material which is in the status of purity [and cannot receive the status of impurity], they did not decree a status of impurity on the woman herself either." If the three women of mNid 9:3 sit on a stone bench, which cannot contract a status of impurity, according to Rabbi Nehemiah all three women remain in the status of purity when a bloodstain is found on the bench. This is formulated in distinction to the anonymous majority ruling in mNid 9:3 that "if three women sat on one bench, and blood is found on it, they are all in the status of impurity." This latter ruling makes logical sense, in that we assume that the blood must have derived from one of them, but since we do not know from which one, all three of them are declared to be in the status of impurity. The material of the bench would not seem to matter. Rabbi Nehemiah's principle, however, makes their status of im/purity dependent on the material of the bench.

Does he mean to say that the stone bench cannot receive a status of impurity in general, and certainly not that of the bloodstain, so that the stone cannot serve as a medium through which the impurity of one woman's bleeding passes on to the other?[33] Applied to Shmu'el's case: Does Rav Ashi's interpretation intend to explain that since the ground cannot receive the status of impurity it cannot serve as a medium through which the woman's own impurity passes back to herself?

Rabbi Nehemiah declares all three of the women to be in the status of purity, that is, not only the two "others" to whom the impurity would have been transferred, but also the one—unknown and unrecognized—from whom the blood had originated. The blood must have originated from one of them, and yet Rabbi Nehemiah declares all three of them to remain in a status of purity. This realization would seem to indicate that the transferral of impurity to the others is not the only concern. Here, then, lies the point in which Rav Ashi sees Shmu'el's case intersecting with Rabbi Nehemiah's ruling. For just like Rabbi Nehemiah in the Mishnah holds the opinion that all three women on the bench of stone (a material that does not receive impurity), including the one from whom the bleeding must have originated, remain in the status of purity, so does Shmu'el declare the woman who sits on the ground (which does not receive impurity) and finds blood upon getting up to remain in the status of purity. As Rav Ashi points out, Shmu'el would thus agree with Rabbi Nehemiah.[34]

At the same time, Rav Ashi's interpretation either completely disregards the midrashic introduction of the woman's sensation into our sugyah, or it assumes that the midrash was actually not connected to Shmu'el's case but was a subsequent attempt to explain Shmu'el's ruling. His interpretation thus dismisses the previous two strategies, which both assumed that the midrash belonged inherently to Shmu'el's reasoning in his ruling.[35] In either case, Rav Ashi's interpretation as the concluding moment of this discussion circumvents the midrashic substantiation of Shmu'el's ruling altogether, as well as the subsequent attempt to uphold hermeneutically the principle of the woman's sensation. Thus, the third strategy in this sugyah presents itself as the ultimate rhetorical taming of Shmu'el and attempts to pour oil on troubled waters, without quite smoothing the waves. It attempts to provide closure for the coherence of the mishnaic discourse which is so disturbed by Shmu'el's reading of Lev. 15:19, but only with an extreme effort.[36]

What is the result of this discussion? Why this exercise? If Shmu'el's reading is indeed so disturbing, could the gemara not have directly presented Rav Ashi's interpretation instead of making the long detour through the discussion of the woman's possible mistaken or misidentified sensations? Could it be plausible to assume that ultimately the gemara makes this detour to force its students to come to the same conclusion as the sugyah, that is, that Shmu'el's reading leads us to an oxymoron, and that therefore Rav Ashi's conclusion, which ignores the discussion of a woman's sensation, seems to be the only possible hermeneutic solution, albeit a rather difficult one? In other words, could it be that the interest of the sugyah is to provide closure at the end, a closure that is doubly corroborated by having ruled out alternative hermeneutic possibilities? But if that were the case, would it not have been easier to go the straight way instead of through the logical and hermeneutic detour?

These are general questions about how to read talmudic literature, but they are all the more important for my current attempt to assess the force of Shmu'el's alternative reading of Lev. 15:19 and its alternative construction of women's corporeality, and what are genuine disturbances in the multiplicity of opinions in talmudic discourse. Some of the questions might be answered if we follow David Kraemer's formulation on the pedagogical nature of talmudic literature:

> [The Babylonian Talmud] concerns itself and its students with multiple interpretations of Scripture, with multiple opinions in the law, that is, with multiple approaches (but only approaches) to the truth. Even when it renders decisions or favors particular interpretations, the [Babylonian Talmud] makes it clear that the process, and not the conclusion, is its utmost concern. It makes a mitzvah out of studying study (*talmud torah*). (*Mind of the Talmud*, 190)[37]

The point of following the labyrinth of the discussion is not primarily to arrive at Rav Ashi's interpretation of Shmu'el's case; this clearly cannot be the point for the current project. Though it is presented as the final answer to the problem which the second taming strategy of our sugyah was not able to solve, it does not cancel out the second strategy's approach, since for that matter Rav Ashi's interpretation does not answer the whole problem. The sugyah, therefore, does not follow a dialectics of closure in which the problem is solved and laid to rest, even though it may follow that direction. Rather, it allows the student of talmudic literature to think through all the various hermeneutic options considered in its process. "The process, and not the conclusion, is its utmost concern." But the question remains: in what way does Shmu'el's midrash present a true disturbance, and not just serve as one of the multiple interpretations of Scripture, or multiple opinions in the law?

This question can be answered if we consider that the multiplicity of opinions is not a comprehensive or inclusive multiplicity. Rather, it is determined by its fundamental androcentric perspective. Obviously, the exclusiveness is explicit, since women are not participants in the discussions. However, beyond this obvious exclusion we have to analyze which kind of discursive mechanisms enable this exclusion, especially in a tractate that deals so exclusively with women, with women's bodies, with women's physiology. Hence, in spite of its fundamental multivocality of hermeneutics, talmudic literature has a center in its androcentric perspective and evolves from that center. Nowhere more than in its concern with women's bodies is this androcentric perspective played out more clearly, as we have discovered in its signification of women's bodies as the interior, and as the architecture of the interior. And it is to this center that Shmu'el's introduction of the woman's sensation as the decisive criterion in the discussion of her status of im/purity appears as the alternative from within. His reading is genuinely marginal, in that it lies on the margins of the androcentric signification of women's bodies. On the margins it opens a rupture in the fabric of the androcentric fabric/massekhet of the rabbinic discussions on menstruation. This rupture allows an alternative discourse to be imagined, or at least it causes enough disturbance to preclude closure, in which the androcentric imagination holds a firm grasp on women's bodies as its object, as if the subject of those bodies were nonexistent. A small rupture, but a rupture indeed.

## The Resha de-Niddah: A Conceptual Framework for the Construction of Menstrual Impurity

Shmu'el's rupture might be larger than it seems. For the question of women's sensation surfaces in the opening chapter of the tractate as well as here in the gemara. In the sugyah on Shmu'el's midrash in the eighth chapter of the tractate it is discussed most thoroughly, and, significantly, is presented as a midrashic reading, that is, as rooted in Scripture. In Shmu'el's case the woman's sensation is introduced as an alternative hermeneutics of the same verse which otherwise serves as the cornerstone for the architecture of the interior of the female body and, as argued in the previous chapter, as the hermeneutic cornerstone for the entire rabbinic discourse on menstruation. The constellation of both models as possibly alternative models is best illustrated when both are based on a reading of the same verse. When the marginal model derives its legitimacy from a different reading of the same scriptural foundation, it has its greatest rhetorical force. Hence, we have observed the sugyah on Shmu'el's midrash devoting a more thorough analysis to the potential alternative model, while at the same time attempting to diffuse its force.

In the second part of this chapter I want to turn to the opening sugyah of the tractate called the Resha de-Niddah (bNid 2a–3b), which I will read as an intertext to the sugyah discussed so far. We will be able to observe discursive and rhetorical mechanisms that are quite similar to those already observed. The Resha de-Niddah outlines, in all its complexity, the conceptual framework for the talmudic discussions of menstruation in the rest of the tractate. As is the case with opening sugyot in other tractates, the Resha de-Niddah overall is rather long, and multilayered in its argumentation.[38] From the earliest beginnings of scholarship on talmudic literature, scholars have argued that the opening sugyot of tractates are the youngest with respect to the editing history of the Babylonian Talmud.[39] If sugyot in general sometimes make references to others, due to their redactional layering, it is especially these opening sugyot which are cross-referential and make allusions, if often only implicitly, to discussions later on in the tractate. Thus, when the concept of women's sensation surfaces in the discussion of the Resha de-Niddah, it may do exactly this, that is, make a textual allusion to the sugyah on Shmu'el. In terms of developing a methodology of reading gender in talmudic literature, this point is important, since in this chapter I argue that we can find a counterdiscourse in the rabbinic discussions on menstruation, as well as the mechanisms to repress or tame it. To strengthen this argument I want to read the opening sugyah as an intertext of the sugyah on Shmu'el, and not merely as a citation of it.

In the following analysis, however, we will see that even if we assume the opening sugyah is referring to Shmu'el, it is doing so only in the form of an allusion, and not explicitly. Rather, the consideration of the woman's sensation is an integral part of the argument of the opening sugyah and its attempt to frame the discussion as a whole. Thus we can read this consideration one more time as an encroachment of the "a-normal" into what the Talmud constructs as its "normal."⁴⁰ Rather than analyzing the sugyah as a whole, I want to focus on those of its structural elements that are directly relevant for my reading of it in the terms developed in my reading of the problem of Shmu'el's midrash, that is, as constructing the woman's body in terms of an edifice as the "normal" of talmudic discourse, and the woman's body as sentient as the "a-normal," the marginalized counterdiscourse.

### Hillel and Shammai: The Fathers of Niddah

The basis for the sugyah is the following mishnah, which records the disagreement between Hillel and Shammai,⁴¹ two of the legendary first-century C.E. founding fathers of rabbinic Judaism.⁴² It is this disagreement which lays out the foundational principles of the tractate:

שמאי אומר כל הנשים דיין שעתן
הלל אומר מפקידה לפקידה ואפילו לימים הרבה
וחכמים אומרים לא כדברי זה ולא כדברי זה אלא מעת לעת ממעטת על יד
מפקידה לפקידה ומפקידה לפקידה ממעטת על יד מעת לעת

*Shammai* holds the opinion: for all women it is sufficient to [be considered in the status of impurity from] the time [of their blood-flow onwards].

*Hillel* holds the opinion [that they are in the status of impurity] from [the time of their last] examination to the examination [when they found the blood].

But *the Sages* say: Neither according to the words of this one nor according to the words of that one, but a twenty-four hour period diminishes [the period of time] from [her last] check to [the current] check, and [the period of time] from [her last] check to [the current] check diminishes a twenty-four hour period.⁴³

The three opinions offer alternative opinions as to how the woman's status of impurity is determined. As mentioned above, here the question about a woman's status of impurity has relevance only to those objects related to the Temple. One medieval commentator, the Meiri, emphasizes this and expresses this very clearly: "This mishnah is taught with respect to the issue of the status of im/purity to clarify whether we declare Temple-related items (requiring of the person who handles them, such as the wife of a priest, a status of purity) which she touched to be impure from the moment of the current blood-flow retroactively, or not. But as far as matters of marital intercourse are concerned, even though she has a blood-flow now, there is no issue whatsoever with respect to the question, whether they [husband and wife] might have committed an inadvertent transgression [of the prohibition in Lev. 18:19] if they had sexual intercourse yesterday" (*Beit ha-Behira*, Massekhet Niddah, 4).[44] Hence, as to the question of actual impurity, in the absence of the historical Temple the following debate in the Talmud has to be understood to be entirely theoretical. Being theoretical only in this respect, however, does obviously not mean that the discussion is irrelevant. Rather, it again teaches us about the rabbis' thinking about women's bodies.

According to Shammai the blood-flow itself serves as the starting point. Hillel, on the other hand, requires the external evidence secured through her examination, presumably by wiping herself, the details of which are laid out subsequently in the Mishnah. According to Hillel, then, the examination that last ascertained the absence of bleeding and, therefore, her status of purity, serves as the *terminus ad quem* retroactively, presumably even if many days have passed in between. The anonymous majority opinion of the Sages finds a compromise between the two, for against Shammai's opinion it does accept a principle of retroactive impurity, but against Hillel it fixes arbitrarily the possible period of retroactive impurity at a maximum of twenty-four hours.[45]

For our understanding of this conceptual framework it is important to reiterate that the rabbinic principle of retroactive impurity is not one restricted to menstrual impurity, but is a principle that applies to various impurities in various circumstances. It is so basic, even fundamental, to the Mishnah that subsequently the Talmud is most astonished about Shammai's opinion, since it seems to completely disregard this principle.[46] Retroactivity is a halakhic or heuristic principle, which has to do with certainty and doubt concerning reality and the requirement of certainty to determine the status of a thing or person. I use the phrase *heuristic retroactivity* to describe the mishnaic principle in thinking impurity that in the absence of certainty we apply the status that is last known about an item retroactively to it and treat the item for that time period *as if* it were indeed in that status.[47] In the absence of the evidence necessary to establish certainty, retroactivity of the current status is the bridge to the last preceding point of certainty. Hence, the subsequent talmudic discussion is interested in the possible theoretical halakhic principles which might form the basis for Hillel's and Shammai's rulings.

In this context, even more than before, it becomes evident that the Talmud uses the various principles that guide the mishnaic system of im/purity as material with which it thinks menstrual impurity, embedded in women's corporeality. The retroactivity of menstrual impurity, the main topic of the opening sugyah, lies at the intersection of these principles. In its response to the vacuum underneath the mishnah, the vacuum that is created by the absence of explication behind the three alternative options attributed to Hillel, Shammai, and the Sages, the Talmud activates those theoretical principles primarily to understand Shammai's blatant disregard of the principle of retroactivity. The discussion in these terms is generated by the predominant androcentric perspective of rabbinic literature, since once again it attempts to get hold of its slippery object—that is, the woman's body—as an object.

## Is the Woman's Body Like a Leaking Miqveh?

After a brief introductory discussion, the sugyah cites three cases from elsewhere in tannaitic literature—the leaking miqveh, the barrel of wine turned to vinegar, and the alleyway in which dead impure vermin is found—which, it suggests, may be analogous to the case of the woman. Each of these cases follows a similar structure: (1) a current examination establishes a change of status; (2) it is unknown when exactly the change occurred; (3) a previous examination serves as the last preceding point of certainty as to the prior status; (4) the mishnah or baraita construct and rule on a *heuristically retroactive change of status* of the items during the period between the points of certainty. This part of the sugyah explores whether the case of the beginning of menstrual impurity is analogous to this structure: (1) a woman's current examination establishes that now she finds blood and that, therefore, her status is changed to that of ritual impurity; (2) it is unknown when exactly her bleeding began; (3) her last examination without evidence of blood serves as the last previous point of certainty as to her still having been in a status of purity; (4) our mishnah (mNid 1:1), however, does not provide a ruling, but records a disagreement between the two most mighty rabbis of the mishnaic period as to when her status of impurity heuristically begins.

The cases are, then, introduced as questions to Shammai, who seems to reject *heuristic retroactivity* (of impurity in the case of the woman), since each of these cases operates on the basis of this principle. The discussion in the sugyah of each of these cases, which explores differences and similarities between the woman and each case, teaches us about possible associations or (mishnaic and tannaitic) contextualizations for which talmudic reasoning allows, and again the conceptual framework for thinking women's bodies. The discursive strategy employed here differs from the metaphorical constructions analyzed in the previous chapter, even though, as I will argue, it has quite similar effects. Let me explain the cases first. Here is Case 1:[48]

מקוה שנמדד ונמצא חסר כל טהרות שנעשו על גביו למפרע בין בר״ה בין ברה״י טמאות

> [Concerning the case of] a miqveh which is measured and found to be lacking [in its required minimum quantity of water and thus has become invalidated] the rule is that all *taharot* [those Temple-related items that need to be handled in conditions of purity] that have been prepared on its account—are retroactively in the status of impurity, whether [the miqveh is located] in the public or in the private domain. (bNid 2b; mMikv 2:2)[49]

I will lay out here the explanation of Case 1. A problem arises if a miqveh is examined and found to lack the halakhically required amount of water to serve as a valid pool for ritual purification. The question is how long it has not had the sufficient amount of water. For example, food items dedicated to the Temple or its procedures, such as the *terumah* or food dedicated to the priests, has to be prepared in vessels or by a person in the status of purity. If for the purpose of purification they were immersed in such a miqveh, these vessels or this person would have remained in the status of impurity, since the purification in a pool without sufficient quantities of water is rendered invalid. In such a case the Temple-related food prepared in those vessels would have become useless.

The mishnah rules that since it is unknown how long the miqveh has had insufficient quantities of water, the items that were immersed in it previous to the examination of the miqveh are rendered impure retroactively [למפרע]. It does not specify how long backwards, but presumably to the last point of certainty. Clearly, retroactivity in this case poses a problem to Shammai in the case of menstruation, if the cases are considered to be analogous.

Case 2 uses a baraita:[50]

היה בודק את החבית להיות מפריש עליה תרומה והולך ואח"כ נמצא[51] חומץ כל ג' ימים {הראשונים}[52] ודאי מכאן ואילך ספק

[Concerning the case of] someone who examines a barrel [of wine] to separate the obligatory contribution to the priests [*terumah*] on its behalf, and [then] continues [to tithe from it without further examinations] and afterwards [finds out that] it is vinegar, [the ruling is that] all {first} three days [it is still wine] with certainty, and from then on it is doubtful [whether it turned into vinegar].

The scenario that is imagined in Case 2 is that a person has produced several barrels of wine. Before they become available for personal use, he is biblically obligated to set aside a contribution to the priests, called *terumah*. One barrel is, therefore, designated to serve as the barrel from which consecutively wine is to be set aside as the terumah for the entire crop of wine, enabling the owner to use the wine from the other barrels for his personal consumption. Rashi emphasizes that this case must imply that the owner designates a terumah barrel only mentally, but does not physically set it aside as required, and starts making use of his wine. The owner "relies on this barrel and goes and drinks the other barrels and intends to separate the terumah from this barrel on behalf of the other barrels *later*, so that [at the time of consumption] the terumah-portion is separated (only) in his mind" (bNid 2b, ד"ה להיות מפריש). The reasoning is that if he had already set it aside physically, it would not matter if the wine turned into vinegar, since at the time of its required setting aside it had been wine and would have been valid terumah there and then (cf. mTer 3:1; tTer 4:7).

It is unknown to the owner exactly when the designated wine turned into vinegar. The baraita rules that for "{the first} three days" from the last point of certainty, the liquid is considered to be wine "with [heuristic] certainty," since, according to Rashi, "it takes wine three days to turn sour" (bB.B. 96a).[53] But from then on we would consider the wine to have turned into vinegar, retroactively. Again, if this case and the case of mNid 1:1 are analogous, as the sugyah wants us to consider, the case of the wine barrel poses a problem to Shammai.

Finally, Case 3 draws on a mishnah:

> השרץ שנמצא במבוי מטמא למפרע עד שיאמר בדקתי את המבוי הזה ולא
> היה בו שרץ או עד שעת הכבוד

> Any [dead] kind of impure animal (Lev. 11) which is found in an alleyway causes a status of impurity [to the things requiring a status of purity, which were handled in that alleyway] *retroactively* until [the point] that a person can say: I have examined this alleyway and there was no dead creeping thing in it, or until the time of [the last] sweeping. (mNid 7:2; bNid 3a)[54]

The alleyway or gateway is considered to be a private domain.[55] The general principle, that in a private domain a doubtful situation is regarded with more stringency, applies also in this case. That is, since it is not known how long the dead vermin has been in the alleyway, this mishnah rules that anything in the alleyway that requires ritual purity is considered to be in a status of impurity *retroactively*, till the last point of certainty. Again, this case poses a difficulty to Shammai's position in our mishnah at the beginning of Tractate Niddah, if we consider this case to be analogous to the case of a woman's menstrual impurity.

∾

What do these cases have in common, and how can the sugyah suggest them to be analogous to the case of the woman's body? The commonality is not established by the issue of impurity, since the case of the wine barrel is concerned with the invalidation of the priestly share in the produce. What they do primarily share, of course, is the factor of heuristic retroactivity. The terms of connection are temporal terms of retroactivity, either למפרע in Cases 1 and 3, or the "three days and beyond" of Case 2. This is the overt reason why the Talmud chooses these cases to discuss the issue of the retroactivity of menstrual impurity and to challenge Shammai's refusal of the principle in the context of discussing menstruation. Thus, we can spell out the analogous structure of all the cases introduced above:

1. A current examination establishes a change of status:
    the miqveh now has insufficient water (has been leaking)
    the wine is now vinegar (has been souring)
    the alleyway now has dead impure vermin in it
    the woman now has evidence of a blood-flow
2. It is unknown when the change occurred:
    when did the miqveh's water level sink below minimum?
    when did the wine turn sour enough to be considered vinegar?
    when did dead impure vermin get into the alleyway?
    when did the woman's bleeding actually begin?
3. A previous examination serves as the last preceding point of certainty as to the prior status:
    the (implied) last measuring of the water level
    the examination of the wine barrel prior to designating it
    the last sweeping or examination of the alleyway
    the woman's last self-examination w̶.out evidence of blood
4. The mishnah or baraita construct and rule on a *heuristically retroactive change of status* of the items during the period between the points of certainty:
    the miqveh is retroactively lacking till 3
    the wine is considered to be vinegar after three days from 3
    dead impure vermin are retroactively considered to have been there since 3
    (according to Hillel only) the woman is retroactively considered to be in a status of impurity

This principle of *heuristic uncertainty* is only the overt reason the Talmud chooses its test cases of (halakhic) analogy, however. Again, as in my discussion of the sugyah on Shmu'el's midrash in the first part of this chapter, I want to suggest that we move beyond the rhetorical surface of the sugyah and analyze what kind of discursive effect the sugyah produces with respect to gender. Again, we have to ask what kind of gender thinking the sugyah reflects and produces. Again, we have to ask what discursive mechanisms enable the rabbis to exclude women as partners in discussion even when the discussions revolve around menstruation. What are the implied and, therefore, hidden structures of the sugyah which, by virtue of being hidden, are all the more powerful in terms of affecting our thinking?[56]

Starting with the most basic observation, the following are other, only implicit similarities, hidden in the complex rhetorical surface of the sugyah: all of the paradigmatic cases are employing three-dimensional, spatial structures, used as examples with which to think the case of menstrual impurity. It has to be emphasized that in this sugyah the relationship between the woman's body and these other cases is not a metaphoric one, but one of suggested analogy. The question the sugyah asks is how principles that apply to the case of the miqveh apply to the case of menstrual impurity, and how not? However, it is because the Talmud "thinks" in terms of the dominant mishnaic paradigm of the woman's body as the architecture of the interior that it chooses these cases. We can read the choice of analogies as another one of those discursive mechanisms that aid the objectification of women's bodies. Metaphor and analogy support each other.

A further observation can be made: The case of the miqveh and of the wine barrel deal with fluids and the nature of their "behavior" in relation to their space of origin.[57] The implied question is how water leaks, and how exactly wine turns sour, which in turn engenders the question of how the woman "leaks." Beyond merely producing halakhic logical problems, these test cases serve as imaginative illustrations for the mechanics of female physiology. They form the discursive horizon in terms of which a woman's body can become an object of halakhic discussion. As a selection of cases, they function as epistemological devices to facilitate a certain understanding of women's corporeality, which entirely separates the body from its subject, desubjectifies it.

Hence the following talmudic discussion in our sugyah about the difference and similarity between these cases and menstrual impurity. The two positions of the talmudic dialectic that discuss the similarity of the case of the miqveh and the case of menstruation can be read as challenging and defending a "Shammaite" position. To facilitate understanding of the discussion I mark the position that challenges the Shammaite position in the mNid 1:1 with C (for "challenger"). The position that defends the Shammaite position is labeled D (for "defender"). The defender's strategy is to insist on the difference between the test cases, so that Shammai's position in the mishnah seems justifiable. The challenger, on the other hand, will argue that they are similar, and that Shammai would therefore have no basis to defend his position. Case 1 (or The Miqveh, Take Two), structured dialogically, is as follows:

התם משום דאיכא למימר העמד טמא על חזקתו ואימא לא טבל
אדרבה העמד מקוה על חזקתו ואימא לא חסר
הרי חסר לפניך
הכא נמי הרי דם לפניך

[D]: There [in the case of the miqveh] the reason [that the person who has immersed in the lacking miqveh is retroactively in the status of impurity] is because it is possible to argue that the person who was in the status of impurity [prior to the invalidated immersion] remains in the status of impurity [because his immersion has been proven to be invalid], so that you could say that [the situation is as if] he had not immersed at all. [Therefore, this case cannot be compared to the menstruating woman and Shammai is justified].

[C]: But on the contrary! [If the concern is the principle of retroactivity in cases of doubt, you should focus your argument on the lacking miqveh itself, and not the person who immersed in it, and since the miqveh originally had a sufficient quantity of water] the miqveh remains in its previous status and could be considered as not lacking.

[D]: But it is lacking right in front of you.

[C]: But in that case [of the menstruous woman] blood is right in front of you also. (bNid 2b)

The question is, when did the miqveh begin to leak? Did it begin to leak right after it was measured previously, so that at the time of the subsequent immersion of a person it was already lacking the sufficient quantity of water, and thus rendered invalid? Or did it begin to leak only shortly before the current measurement when it was found lacking, so that the immersions in question could be considered valid ones? The only "fact" is that the miqveh is lacking now, in front of us. And this is where the Talmud establishes the comparison with the woman's body, because the only "fact" is that the woman—now—has a blood-flow, as becomes evident by the self-examination in which she finds the blood outside her body. The problem the Talmud attempts to tackle is how this evidence is to be evaluated. The visual evidence in and of itself is insufficient to establish facticity, since this visual evidence requires interpretation: what are the circumstances that lead up to the evidence? So the discussion continues:

השתא הוא דחזאי
הכא נמי השתא הוא דחסר
הכי השתא התם איכא למימר חסר ואתא חסר ואתא הכא מי איכא למימר
חזאי ואתא חזאי ואתא
ומאי קושיא דלמא הגס הגס חזיתיה

[D]: It is only now that she observes the blood-flow.

[C]: [If you argue like that we could apply the same point to the case of the miqveh and claim that] here also it is only now that it is lacking. [Therefore, the case of the leaking miqveh and the bleeding woman are similar and Shammai has a problem].

[D]: Is that so!? There [in the case of the miqveh] you should say that it gradually leaked [hence, was not lacking all at once]! But could you say that here [in the case of the woman's menstruation] she only gradually observed the blood-flow?

[C]: Why not? Perhaps she observed the blood-flow only when it came in large quantities [but it had gradually begun to flow previously].[58]

Where the problem is considered to be the interpretation of the visual evidence of the blood, the argument that defends Shammai's position in the mishnah [D] posits a fundamental contemporaneity between "seeing the blood" and the flow itself.[59] This is what, according to the position defending Shammai, would distinguish the case of the blood-flow from the leaking miqveh, since in the latter the leakage can be imagined as a gradual one, whereas in the former case the woman "saw" the blood only *now* and thus started bleeding only *now*. The challenging position [C], however, argues for the similarity between the two cases. The trickle of the blood-flow, therefore, is only the external evidence of that which took some time to find its way out.[60] Hence, according to the position challenging Shammai [C], the application of the principle of retroactivity to menstrual impurity is justifiable.

We can read the dialectics of these two positions in different but not necessarily contradictory ways. First, one might wonder whether behind the explanation of the disagreement between Shammai and Hillel lies a process of adapting Greek medical theories. The position that argues for the analogy of leaking miqveh and bleeding woman, therefore challenging Shammai, has an Aristotelian affinity. "Aristotle believed that the womb existed in the body as the proper receptacle for the seminal residue when it had been finally concocted and that the menses flowed into the womb naturally throughout the month without any force. . . . Menstrual blood remained in the womb until it was used in conception and reproduction or had reached such a volume that it had emptied itself" (Dean-Jones, *Women's Bodies*, 64).[61] Thus the menstrual blood is considered to exist inside the woman's body long before it appears outside, a position that could explain Hillel's ruling. The position in the talmudic dialectic that defends Shammai, thus arguing for the difference beween the leaking miqveh and the bleeding woman, could betray a Hippocratic affinity, in that according to one of the Hippocratic texts "the descent of menstrual blood from a woman's flesh to her womb happens all at once when the woman is not pregnant" (cited in Dean-Jones, *Women's Bodies*, 62). That is, the Hippocratic writers held a "view of a month's menses as a discrete quantity of blood which entered the womb only at the end of the month" (62), while during the month the blood was stored in the flesh. The parallels are too tempting not to suggest some sort of cultural absorption.

If we approach the discussion in terms internal to rabbinic culture, we can perhaps shift the hermeneutic angle somewhat. The difficulty of this discussion lies in the ambiguity of the rabbinic use of the Hebrew term ראה or its equivalent Aramaic חזי, whose meaning oscillates between seeing and experiencing the flow itself. When the position defending Shammai rejects the similarity between the leakage of the miqveh and the menstrual blood-flow, the referent of the verb for blood-flow seems to be the flow itself: "but could you say that here she only has a gradual blood-flow." On the other hand, the phrase דם לפניך—"the blood is before you"—employed by the position challenging Shammai and insisting on the analogy between the leaking miqveh and the bleeding woman, indicates the visibility of the blood. What, however, does a linguistic inscription of visibility onto the flow itself mean? On the one hand, it is of course the woman herself who "observes" the blood-flow. But at the same time, the phrase employed is "the blood is before *you*," the implied (male) subject of the discourse. The latter sees through the eye of the woman. Hence the insistence on visual perception as a marker of her bleeding enables the subject of the rabbinic discourse to think himself in the woman's place and to displace her. If the visual perception is all that matters, the bleeding does not require the woman as the embodied subject of her bleeding, for as Elizabeth Grosz points out, "the gulf between subject and object is never so distant as in vision," since "the seer sees at a distance and is unimplicated in what is seen" (*Volatile Bodies*, 101).[62]

To summarize this section of the sugyah, so far it has constructed a pattern of argumentation that confines the thinking about menstruation and by extension about women's bodies within the walls it erects around women's corporeality. The sugyah selects those cases of analogy that not only serve its halakhic reasoning, but also illustrate women's bodies and the physiological mechanics of menstruation. The selection of these cases can be judged to be quite ingenious in some respects, since the analogies appear to be quite compelling. Because of this, however, because they seem so compelling, it is important to highlight the selective principle of these cases, since it is linked with the metaphorization of women's bodies discussed in the previous chapter. It is these only implied or hidden principles that allow for the objectification of women's bodies in order to create an object of discourse. They also permit the exclusion of women as subjects, and thus as participants in the discourse.

Lest a student of the text be all too compelled by the analogy, a moment occurs in the text that allows us to link this sugyah with the one on Shmu'el's midrash, discussed in the first part of this chapter ("The Crumbling of the House"). This moment, again, almost involuntarily discloses the main conceptual framework as a constructed one, however compelling its suggested analogies may be. But it also suggests an alternative discourse altogether. The discussion of these cases and their challenge to Shammai's position in the case of women's menstruation runs its course, in the end upholding the distinction between the test cases and the woman's bleeding. This distinction is based on a formal argument applied in all three cases rather than a substantial argument,[63] so that the fundamental analogy remains unchallenged.

## The Rupture in the Massekhet/Fabric of Niddah, Take Two

The woman's body as object remains a slippery object to the rabbinic discourse, since its excess inexpressible in language (a body is always more than its representation) threatens once again to explode its objectified circumscription. As a "reluctant" object it escapes once more through the rupture that Shmu'el's midrash made in the androcentric fabric of the discourse, and reenters through a different rupture, as a return of the repressed to the dominant discourse of androcentrism. For as a second approach to Shammai's reason, an alternative to the entire discussion pursued so far, the sugyah suggests the following (bNid 3a):[64]

היינו טעמא דשמאי הואיל ואשה מרגשת בעצמה
והלל כסבורה הרגשת מי רגלים היא
ולשמאי האיכא ישנה
ישנה נמי אגב צערה מיתערא מידי דהוה אהרגשת מי רגלים

This is what Shammai's reason is: [He disregards the principle of retroactive impurity in the case of menstruation] since a woman has a *sensation* [of bleeding] inside herself.[65]

And Hillel [why would he not have considered this argument]? [He would argue against this] that she thought it to be the *sensation of urine* [הרגשת מי רגליים].

And against Shammai, is there not the case of the one [who starts to have a blood-flow while she is] sleeping?

He argues that she wakes up because of the pain, just like [she would wake up] on account of the sensation of having to urinate.

This approach to Shammai makes astonishingly strong allusions to the sugyah that discusses Shmu'el's case, in an entirely different framework. With this hermeneutic supplement to the mishnah's enigmatic disagreement, Shammai's opinion theoretically would accord with the reading of Lev. 15:19 presented by Shmu'el: " 'in her body'—[meaning she is not in the status of impurity] unless she feels it in her body," thus canceling out the notion of retroactive impurity altogether. Hillel's opinion, on the other hand, would theoretically accord with Sifra's and the Mishnah's reading of Lev. 15:19: " 'in her body'—[this formulation teaches that she is in the status of impurity [already when the blood is still] inside her body." Since it could have been there many days, Hillel allows for an even more prolonged period of retroactive impurity. Here in this sugyah, however, a woman's sensation that is presented as Shammai's possible reason is not presented as a midrashic argument, but as a factual observation of text-external reality. Shammai simply holds that women feel, hence know by sensation, when their menstrual period begins. Therefore, the heuristic principle of retroactivity that determines mishnaic cases everywhere else does not apply to the case of women. The mishnaic Shammai here is put by the sugyah in the position of considering women's embodied and subjective reality as a determinant factor for menstruation.[66] Vice versa, the sugyah argues, if Shammai argued this way, that Hillel's answer would be to dismiss the factor of women's sensation altogether, since this factor is not reliable, and—his argument would be—women cannot make careful distinctions of their sensations.

How can we understand the connection between the opening sugyah of the tractate and the sugyah on Shmu'el's midrash? Neither of the sugyot cites the other and both can be read independently from each other as sovereign, coherent arguments. There is no explicit textual relationship between the two. The most we can say is that the opening sugyah alludes to the sugyah on Shmu'el's case.[67] That this sugyah alludes to the other one seems clear, since it uses the identical phrasing: the "(mistaken) sensation of urine [הרגשת מי רגליים]" and "she has a sensation in herself [מרגשת בעצמה]."[68] If we approach this question from the perspective of redaction criticism we may recall that the opening sugyot are considered to be the youngest in many cases. Thus the anonymous editors, the *savoraim*, of the sugyah would have known the sugyah on Shmu'el's midrash and, based on their reading of it, would have integrated it into the current argument. If that were the case, my hermeneutic of reading gender in talmudic literature, particularly the discourse on niddah, would seem to be undermined, since we would not be dealing with a return of the repressed or with a trace of the reluctant, perhaps involuntary recognition of the problematic objectification of women's bodies. However, whether or not this approach is sound in terms of literary history, the case cannot be proven, and is, from a textual point of view, far from self-explanatory. We still would have to ask why the editors/savoraim integrated this alternative approach into the opening sugyah, which conceptually frames the entire fabric/massekhet of niddah as a discourse. I would argue, then, that we are dealing with a recognition of how totally alternative the concept of sensation as a determinant factor is to the discourse as a whole. Various effects are achieved by integrating it into the opening sugyah as well. First, Shammai's opinion and Shmu'el are linked. This in turn has a doubled rhetorical effect. On the one hand, Shmu'el is marginalized once again, since Shammai is, clearly, on the margins of the Mishnah.[69] At the same time, however, we can reverse this point and argue that the more alternative voices are linked, the stronger the counterdiscourse as such begins to appear.

Finally, the motif of the woman's sensation appears once more in a subsequent part of the opening sugyah, which discusses the hypothetical reason of the Sages in mNid 1:1. To express a medium between Hillel and Shammai as the two extremes they rule that a woman is considered to have been in a status of impurity retroactively for twenty-four hours at most:

אמר רבה מאי טעמייהו דרבנן אשה מרגשת בעצמה
א״ל אביי אם כן תהא דיה שעתה
ורבה לחדודי לאביי

> Rabbah said: What is the reason of the sages [in our opening mishnah that they seemingly arbitrarily determined the period of retroactivity to be a twenty-four-hour period]? A woman has a sensation [of the blood-flow] within herself!
>
> Abaye responded to him: If that were so [that this is the reason of the sages], [their ruling should have been] the time [of her blood-flow] is sufficient for her.
>
> And Rabbah? He [only meant] to sharpen Abaye's mind. (bNid 4b)

Rabbah's hypothetical answer is that the Sages also considered women's sensation of their blood-flow as the decisive factor for determining their status of im/purity, which clearly makes no sense.[70] If Rabbah holds this to be the reason for the Sages, Abaye's refutation is more than convincing. For if that were indeed the reason of the rabbis in the mishnah they should have ruled in accordance with Shammai and canceled out the principle of retroactivity of a woman's status of impurity altogether. Abaye's refutation is so convincing that the Talmud suggests that Rabbah's point was merely to sharpen Abaye's mind, since he was his student.[71]

What happened in this strange side-argument? Why did the woman's sensation resurface yet again in this context in which it seems so out of place? Again, as in the previous case, we can see a double effect at work. On the one hand, this is another strategy of marginalization: turning the concept of women's sensation into a mere pedagogical tool in a rabbinic discussion, where it can all too easily be dismissed. But at the same time, the curious repetition of the concept, exactly because of its nonsensical deployment, intensifies the hermeneutic suspicion of the reader even more.

I suggest that the repeated resurfacing of the question of a woman's own sensation of her blood-flow is not just a minor disturbance that merely appears in localized arguments, but is a conceptual threat to the primary discursive perspective of halakhic thinking on menstrual impurity. These repeated ruptures in the fabric of niddah form a counterdiscourse to the dominant androcentrism of the tractate and its instrumentalization of women's bodies. The attempt to deal with women's bodies just like any other spatial structure, which can contract a status of retroactive impurity, just like any other space that is readily available to containment and unambiguous circumscription, fails. Her body resists being forced into these avenues of objectification, because it is never only body, but always someone's body.

I have attempted to analyze the ways in which talmudic literature conceptualizes the woman's body in its discourse on the regulation of menstrual impurity. My starting point has been to redefine the systematization of the principles that guide the impurity and purity system developed in the Mishnah as the framework that talmudic literature uses to think about the particularity of the woman's body. Menstrual regulations had been one of the essential corporeal practices the rabbis inherited from biblical legislation. They strove to preserve such practices as that which constitutes the ethnos of the Jews as a distinct people in late antique cultures. The ways in which different corporeal bodies are inscribed by halakhic discourse must be seen clearly if we want to understand how gender difference is produced in rabbinic culture. This may help us to study the nature of androcentric discourses and their strategies of excluding women as subjects. But this approach also helps us to analyze the moments in which the androcentric perspective of the rabbis fails to sustain itself,[72] and to find traces of those options of thinking and seeing the world that are culturally repressed.

Thus we have seen that in its very "naming" of the woman's body, in its metaphoric construction, mishnaic literature and the Talmud(s) constitute woman's body as the interior, as inscribed by the social location of women in the household. Here the female body as object of the androcentric imagination of the rabbis serves to reinforce the social function of women within the patriarchal culture. At the same time it is important to maintain that women's bodies are not "naturally" interior. They are constituted as such in the discourse and in the language.

Within the semantic framework of im/purity regulations, men and women in their differentiated corporeality have a potentially symmetrical or complementary relationship with its sacred center, the reference point of the whole system. The tannaitic literature (Tosefta and Sifra), and specifically the mishnaic discourse, however, reconfigure this potentially symmetrical relationship in ways that strive to reinforce the androcentric perspective of the rabbinic discourse. Thus the architecture of the interior of women's bodies is constructed as a function of the male subject.

Nonetheless,[73] when the discussion of the Mishnah in the Babylonian Talmud introduces the concept of a woman's sensation of her own physiological processes, it allows for a corrosion of the "center" of androcentrism. First an alternative reading of the biblical text (through Shmu'el's midrash in bNid 57b) opens this possibility, and second, the discussion of the retroactivity of status (through Shammai's opposition in the case of the menstruating woman in bNid 2a-b) shakes the foundation of one of the fundamental principles of the mishnaic im/purity system. Here, the woman's body is no longer thing or object readily available to the androcentric imagination. It is reconstituted as the embodiment of its subject, the woman. This alternative constellation lies on the margins of the androcentric universe, but in its repeated appearance and in the hermeneutic energies that the Talmud invests to contain it—a symptom of its threatening plausibility—we can glimpse the possibility of an alternative Talmud, one in which women's corporeality is constituted and inscribed not in relation to and as a function of the androcentric imagination.

Finally, I have to ask once more the question of gender difference, this time in conversation with feminist scholars, who have claimed the heritage of de Beauvoir's history of patriarchy and who have resigned themselves to bemoaning women's status as the Other of rabbinic discourse. In my theoretical refusal to reinforce the status of women as object and victim I am now in a position to differentiate the notion of Otherness. The critique of the androcentric perspective of rabbinic literature, where it constructs women's corporeality as its "other" in terms of objectification, is only one step in the hermeneutic enterprise. However, I choose to focus on those moments in rabbinic discourse which I have called the reluctance of the object. In other words, it is those moments where the "Other" is constituted as the "Other" of the androcentric imagination altogether—and not merely as the other within androcentrism—that allow us to preserve the notion of an ontological heterogeneity. This "Other" from without is hidden in the crevices of the "Other within."

# 4 THE HERMENEUTICS OF COLORS AND STAINS

## THE RABBINIC SCIENCE OF WOMEN'S BLOOD

IN THE PREVIOUS CHAPTER I have only touched upon a phenomenon that characterizes rabbinic discussions of menstruation beginning with the Mishnah. Much of the second part of Tractate Niddah of the Mishnah focuses on what in mishnaic Hebrew is called the *ketem* or bloodstain, defined as evidence of blood whose origin is unkown. Among the questions with which the Mishnah deals are where evidence of blood is found, what the size and shape of such evidence is, and what the location and shape of the blood can tell us about its origin. The Mishnah develops a whole hermeneutics of bloodstains. Parallel to the phenomenon of the bloodstain, and often hard to distinguish from it, is the discussion of blood whose origin is known to be genital, but of which it is not clear whether it is of *uterine* origin. Here, the criteria of distinguishing types of blood as either uterine in origin or stemming from an internal wound are mostly by color. Again, the Mishnah develops a hermeneutics of blood. In this chapter I want to foreground this feature of the rabbinic discussions of menstruation, which we may call the nascent rabbinic "science" of women's blood. What I will analyze is the kinds of authority structures that this rabbinic science discursively produces, and how gender is inscribed into these structures. We can read the Mishnah, and subsequently the talmudic discussions of the Mishnah, as producing a certain kind of knowledge, an expertise, regarding women's blood. In the process of producing this knowledge, the texts produce also the knowing subject and the objects of knowledge, both visibly and invisibly gendered. Who are these experts and on what basis is their expertise founded? How is this knowledge acquired? What are the textual and discursive mechanisms that enact the relationship between expert and clients?

Let us look first at what is clearly the dominant discourse both in the Mishnah and in the subsequent talmudic discussions. Later I will present a narrative from the Babylonian Talmud that appears as a moment of disturbance in the dominant discourse, or as evidence "that 'dominance' is, although present and in many ways obnoxious, not unproblematically established" (Bal, *Lethal Love*, 3).

**Biblical Foundations**

There are basically three verses in the biblical chapter on the impurity of genital emissions (Lev. 15) that provide the foundation for the rabbinic discussion of the nature of women's bleeding. These verses define menstrual impurity or menstruation primarily by a time line. Similarly, the distinction between menstrual impurity and impurity resulting from other genital bleeding is dependent on a time line:

ואשה כי תהיה זבה דם יהיה זבה בבשרה שבעת ימים תהיה בנדתה

When a woman has a discharge, her discharge being blood from her body, she remains in her menstrual impurity *seven days*. (Lev. 15:19)[1]

ואשה כי יזוב זוב דמה ימים רבים בלא עת נדתה או כי תזוב על נדתה כל ימי זוב טומאתה

When a woman has a discharge of blood *for many days, not at the time* of her menstrual impurity, or when she has a discharge *beyond the time* of her menstrual impurity, as long as her impure discharge lasts, her impurity shall last. (Lev. 15:25)

ואם טהרה מזוב וספרה לה שבעת ימים ואחר תטהר

When she is purified from her discharge, she shall *count off seven days*, and after that she will be purified. (Lev. 15:28)

These verses assume that at some point in time the woman has a blood-flow and that she will be in the status of menstrual impurity (בנדתה, Lev. 15:19) from that point on. The biblical text, therefore, defines her impurity entirely by a simple time line. According to that time line she has a fixed menstrual period (עת נדתה, Lev. 15:25) of seven days, apparently regardless of how long the actual bleeding lasts. Any bleeding beyond this period, or outside of this period,[2] constitutes the abnormal impurity of the *zavah*.[3] Her menstrual impurity lasts seven days, counted from the first day of her bleeding. For the impurity of *zavah*, parallel to the impurity of the *zav* or man with irregular discharges (Lev. 15:13),[4] she needs to count off seven additional days once she ceases to bleed, after which she will be in the status of purity again. Leviticus somewhat unproblematically takes the blood-flow itself, whether it be menstrual or some abnormal blood-flow, as the starting point of the period of her impurity. It does not take issue with the appearance of a bloodstain whose origin we do not know, nor does it hint at any notion of different colors or types of menstrual blood.

### The Taxonomy of the Colors of Blood

Beyond the biblical text, the Mishnah introduces the idea of distinguishing between types of blood. The basic idea here is that not all blood is menstrual blood. Hence, not all blood establishes a status of impurity for the woman, the primary (theoretical) question of Tractate Niddah. Here, this can by implication be extended to indicate that not all blood would prohibit husband and wife from marital intimacy, a point that the Mishnah does not discuss.

It is important to take note of this basic idea by way of introduction to the following, since again, as in previous contexts, we may observe a double effect. Reading the Mishnah halakhically or legally, we may find it to create a positive effect for women, when compared with the biblical text. It limits the cases of menstrual impurity since it distinguishes between different kinds of genital blood.[5] However, reading the texts on a different level, that is, as to their discursive effects, and as to their construction of new kinds of (rabbinic) knowledge and authority, which in turn are gendered, the result may be a different one.[6] In the Mishnah we read the following passage:

חמישה דמים טמאים באשה האדום והשחור וככרן כרכום וכמימי אדמה
וכמזוג
בית שמאי אומרים אף כמימי תלתין וכמימי בשר צלי
ובית הלל מטהרין
הירוק עקביא בן מהללאל מטמא וחכמים מטהרין

Five [types or colors of] blood are impure in a woman: the red [color], the black [color], the [color of] saffron, the [color of] muddy water, and the [color of] diluted wine.

The school of Shammai says: also [the color of] the water of [soaked] fenugreek, and [the color of] the juice of roasted meat.

The school of Hillel declare [the latter] to be pure.

Concerning the yellow [color]—Aqavia ben Mahalalel declares it to be impure and the sages declare it to be pure. [mNid 2:6][7]

The subsequent Mishnah explicates those colorful descriptions:

איזהו האדם כדם המכה
השחור כחרת עמוק מכן טמא דהה מכן טהור
וככרן כרכום כברור שבו
וכמימי אדמה מבקעת בית כרם ומציף מים
וכמזוג שני חלקים מים ואחר יין מן היין השרוני

Which one is the red [color]? Like the blood of a wound.

The black [color]? Like the sediment of ink. If it is deeper than that—it is impure, fainter than that—pure.

And like saffron? The brightest part of it.

And like [the color of] muddy water? [Earth] from the valley of Beit Kerem, and inundate it with water.

And like [the color] of diluted wine? Two parts water and one part wine, from the wine of Sharon. [mNid 2:7; tNid 3:11]

One is prone to ask what so moved the creators of the Mishnah to establish this list of colors of impure or uterine blood or blood that establishes a status of impurity for a woman. What could it be that drives this taxonomy? If all these different shades of red to black are impure anyway, why even bother to distinguish them? These two *mishnayot* are probably the ones that read as the most grotesque and bizarre in Tractate Niddah, regardless of the fact that they rule that not all genital blood is uterine. Here the cultural context of the reader comes most into play in trying to gauge these texts. Are they self-consciously grotesque, choosing items such as the water of soaked fenugreek or the juice of roasted meat as terms of comparison? Or are these texts enacting a form of self-deconstruction by forcing the attempt to transform color into language to the limits of discourse? These questions have to be answered in the negative.

First, we have to remember that this mishnaic text continues to "be alive" in contemporary halakhic handbooks on the Laws of Niddah and is thus read by some as structuring reality and as guiding their vision.[8] Readers with a halakhic mind or a mind that accepts these texts as authoritative do not have a problem with reading them "straightforwardly," as attempting to accurately articulate even that which resists language, in this case hues of color. Most of the talmudic discussions of these *mishnayot* read in similar terms. It is the nature of mishnaic discourse to try to categorize, define, organize. Within this textual universe the color taxonomy of women's blood is not at all bizarre. This teaches us that what seems grotesque and bizarre is so primarily in our contemporary cultural context, and because such a taxonomy is applied to menstrual blood. What Foucault writes with respect to Borges's *Chinese Encyclopedia* containing a list of fantastic things that do not seem to have any connection applies to reading this Mishnah: "in the wonderment of this taxonomy, the thing we apprehend in one great leap, the thing that by means of the fable is demonstrated as the exotic charm of another system of thought, is the limitation of our own."[9] Admittedly, the mishnah may only with difficulty be read as exhibiting "exotic charm."

Thus before discarding this rabbinic menstrual science as merely some fantastic outgrowth of male ignorance or paranoia about menstrual blood, as some critics have argued too hastily,[10] I want to make an effort to understand the text. Mary Douglas's remarks about anthropological scholarship and its production of meaning also applies to the study of rabbinic texts: "We study taboo, symbolism, blessings and curses, oracles and magic come into our purview. Largely our effort is to make sense of what we find. We are not there to pour contempt or to despise. If an anthropologist can only attribute nonsense to a ritual or a text, it is a confession of defeat" ("The

Anthropologist and the Believer," 2). From an anthropological perspective this preoccupation with the various colors of women's genital blood is unique. In fact, the vast ethnographic literature on menstrual rites and rules in other cultures does not report a similar "knowledge" of different colors of menstrual blood.[11]

### The Source for the Taxonomy of Blood Colors

If we proceed on this basis we can make an interesting observation. The mishnaic list of colors seems, even according to the logics of rabbinic discourse, quite innovative, since it does not seem to have a basis in biblical law at all.[12] Hence, the Talmud attempts, after the fact, to lend biblical authority to the distinction of blood types and to the number of impure blood types through midrashic hermeneutics.[13] The specifics of this argument need not concern us here, since the midrashic acrobatics do not explain the cultural work of the mishnaic distinction between types of blood.

The latter point we can perhaps explain if we ask the simple question of how the rabbis in the Mishnah know about this distinction. The question implies questioning their authority. If there is nothing in the biblical texts or in other Jewish cultural precedents that raises the issue of types of blood, the question really is what makes this type of knowledge believable. If the invention of a new knowledge, in this case the distinction of colors of blood, brings with it a new class of experts to defer to, in this case the rabbis, what makes this new knowledge believable? We can approach the answer to this question by turning to an intertext that, so far, has escaped the attention of scholars. This intertextual relationship could explain how the attempt of the rabbis to establish themselves as new authorities of a new kind of knowledge could be so effective that even today women defer to rabbis for advice on their menstrual blood.

Let us turn to the discussion of skin diseases as a possible model for the taxonomy of the colors of women's blood.[14] The mishnaic discussions of skin diseases that are possible sources of impurity also feature a debate on colors.[15] In mNeg 1:1 and 1:2 we learn about the four different shades of white of lesions of the skin plus several reddish variegations. Mishnah Nega'im, however, has a biblical precedent, because there is a color code of skin diseases inscribed in the biblical text, which at times is quite graphic

(Lev. 13:19, 24, 42, 43, 49). Further, the biblical text explicitly requires the afflicted person to be brought to the priest for inspection, for it is the priest who has the expertise to identify the lesions. Indeed, the key word in this biblical chapter is ראה—to see or to inspect. By contrast, Leviticus 15, the chapter that deals with bodily discharges, never requires inspection by a priest or even hints at such a necessity, and it most certainly does not provide a color code for the discharge. Since with respect to menstrual impurity the mishnaic ruling does not have a biblical base, it seems that the rabbis looked at Nega'im as a model or an analogy, which is not to say that they regarded menstruation as if it were a disease. The analogy is a procedural one: just as in the case of skin diseases, which are an integral part of the priestly purity and impurity system in the Bible, the priest is installed as the inspector and, hence, the prime expert, so also they are to be experts in the case of (irregular) genital bleeding of women, which is also an integral part of the priestly purity and impurity system, biblically as well as throughout rabbinic culture. By analogy the successor of the priest, that is, the rabbi, as an expert on matters of purity and impurity, is installed as the inspector, who like the priest is trained in the differentiation of colors. These are then the steps in the invention of the rabbinic science of blood:

1. The priestly role of inspecting skin lesions was familiar from the biblical text. This would have been an uncontested role, once the biblical text became an authoritative source for the rabbinic community. By the time of the redaction of the Mishnah, more than a hundred years after the destruction of the Temple, this had become a historical role.

2. There was no equivalent biblical precedent for the impurity of genital discharges, specifically menstruation.

3. The rabbis of the Mishnah, therefore, redefined the biblical discussion of menstruation. Whereas the biblical text had discussed menstruation in temporal terms, the rabbis of the Mishnah began to discuss it in terms similar to skin lesions, that is, in terms of blood colors. By making menstruation analogous to skin lesions, their claim to expertise on menstrual impurity could become understandable and believable. This strategy may be all the more effective by virtue of remaining hidden.[16]

4. The inspection of menstrual blood did not turn into a historical issue, since the determination of blood as menstrual continues to be halakhically relevant to the prohibition of marital intimacy during the wife's period.

## Gendering the Expertise of the New Science of Blood

The gender code inscribed in the new science will become much clearer if we ask how the rabbis imagined the colors of menstrual blood to be determined? Who is imagined to be looking at the blood? How could even women themselves determine the exact color of their menstrual blood?

We did observe that what the mishnaic text primarily does is provide analogies. It describes colors of blood in terms of other objects: the shade of red like that of saffron, of ink sediment and so on. Both the Babylonian and the Palestinian gemaras, in their effort to interpret the Mishnah, provide further analogies: red like the blood of a slaughtered ox at the first stroke of the knife; like the blood of a live bird; of a head louse; of the little finger, or of bloodletting (bNid 19b, 20a), or, in the Yerushalmi, like the blood of a goat; black like a raven, like ink, like certain types of garment, or like blood of fish (yNid 2:6, 49d/50a). This interpretive effort in both Talmudim, which in Tractate Niddah share a large quantity of their interpretive material, reads like a desperate effort to culturally translate menstruation. If we were to conceive of menstrual blood as a different culture, we could read the creators of the talmudic texts as translating and explaining a culture foreign to them in the terms familiar and accessible to them. This process of translation then entails the displacement of the "native speakers," the women who menstruate. As soon as the translation claims it has grasped the native culture, redefined and displaced it, it has rendered an actual encounter with the native language as well as with its speakers superfluous. In our case, this is precisely what the menstrual taxonomy attempts to institute. Amid the accumulation of analogies the menstrual blood itself disappears, and along with it the women. The following story in the Babylonian Talmud will illustrate my point:

אמימר ומר זוטרא ורב אשי הוו יתבי קמיה שקלי ליה קרנא קמייתא לאמימר חזייה אמר להו אדום דתנן כי האי שקלי ליה אחריתי אמר להו אשתני אמר רב אשי כגון אנא דלא ידענא בין האי להאי לא מבעי לי למחזי דמא

Amemar and Mar Zutra and Rav Ashi once sat before a cupper[17] and when the first cupping-horn was taken off Amemar he saw it and said to the others: "The red of which we have learnt (in the Mishnah) is a shade like this." When the second one was taken off from him, he said to them: "This has a different shade." "One like myself," observed Rav Ashi, "who does not know the difference between the one and the other must not act as an examiner of blood." (bNid 20a top)[18]

This short narrative, involving three rabbis from the last generation of rabbis in the Babylonian Talmud,[19] shows us how the gemara envisioned the learning of blood types. The scene at the bloodletter's house (or cupping-house) is usually read with respect to the hermeneutic uncertainty it exposes. Since the men at the scene are rabbis of the last generation in the Babylonian Talmud, it has been suggested that this short narrative should be read historically and, thus, as indicating the decline of the ability to determine and distinguish different types and colors of women's bleeding.[20] This argument does not seem so strong to me, since the talmudic literature provides the basis for a long tradition of halakhic literature subsequently in Jewish culture, which guaranteed the training of rabbinic experts down to the contemporary period. If we read the narrative with respect to how it stages the learning of blood types, however, the gendering of the new rabbinic science of women's blood is highlighted. It shows men talking and debating among themselves the meaning of the (mishnaic) text on menstrual blood that they study together. This scene resembles, therefore, a rabbinic version of what John Winkler has called men's coffeehouse talk (*Constraints of Desire*, 12) to characterize much of Greek literature on women. Only the scenario is different: we are witnessing a cupping-house talk. The women are entirely displaced from the scene, as is their blood, which even though it is the subject of the debate is present only as text—"the red of which we have learnt (in the Mishnah)"—and is displaced even further by employing men's blood as the term of comparison.

Another piece of the rabbinic discussions about the taxonomy of blood colors is the case of the bloodstain. As mentioned above, what distinguishes the bloodstain from the discussions of the colors of blood is that the source of the stain is altogether unknown. The mishnaic focus on the hermeneutics of bloodstains will add another aspect of the discursive strategies which the Mishnah enacts in order to institute the rabbis as authorities over women's bodies.

## The Case of the Ketem

Like the distinction of blood colors, the bloodstain is a mishnaic invention. In fact, the term for bloodstain, *ketem*, comes to prominence only in post-biblical, tannaitic Hebrew.[21] In the second part of the tractate the Mishnah lists a phenomenal number of different case-scenarios of locations and sizes or shapes of such stains: whether it is on her body, and where on her body; on her shirt, and where on her shirt; whether it is round or drawn out; whether it is the size of a legume; what a woman might have done to precipitate stains, such as slaughtering an animal or killing a louse; whether she might have shared a shirt with another woman, and so on.

Within the larger impurity system of the rabbis the כתם is not an unusual phenomenon, since the effort is always made to protect what is in the status of purity and to strengthen the biblical rules by building "protective fences" around them, לעשות סיג לתורה. These principles apply particularly to cases of doubt. A stain found in the environs of a woman indicates that she is possibly in the status of impurity. Hence, the Temple-related items that she handles should be protected as to their required purity, even if the woman is only doubtfully impure. Thus, halakhically, in respect to the circumstances of doubt that it establishes, the bloodstain is not different from dead impure vermin whose presence was not detected in an alleyway (mNid 7:2), the model case of doubtful impurity that we have encountered in the previous chapter. Both the stain and the dead vermin establish retroactive impurity[22] until the point when certainty can be established, that is, the last sweeping of the alleyway, or the last washing of the woman's shirt on which the bloodstain was found. We have already seen in the previous chapter that the question of retroactive impurity is primarily a theoretical one. But the stain, depending on its location and size or shape, can also be read to indicate that a woman is menstruating now. Regardless of the aspect of impurity, therefore, such a woman would have to abstain from marital intimacy.[23]

Since the bloodstain is recognized as being a rabbinic enactment only, and not derived from biblical legislation (bNid 59a),[24] the halakhic tendency is to be lenient in problems and uncertainties arising from it. Thus the Mishnah reports the following case:

מעשה באשה אחת שבאת לפני רבי עקיבא, אמרה לו ראיתי כתם אמר לה שמא מכה היתה ביך אמרה לו הן וחיתה אמר לה שמא יכולה להגלע

ולהוציא דם אמרה לו הן וטהרה רבי עקיבא ראה תלמידיו מסתכלין זה
בזה אמר להם מה הדבר קשה בעיניכם שלא אמרו חכמים הדבר להחמיר
אלא להקל שנאמר ואשה כי תהיה זבה דם יהיה זבה בבשרה—דם ולא כתם.

> A case about a woman who came before Rabbi Aqiva:
>
> She said to him: "I saw a bloodstain."
>
> He said to her: "Perhaps there was a wound in you?"
>
> She said to him: "*Yes, but* it healed."
>
> He said to her: "Perhaps it is possible that it tore open and exuded blood."
>
> She said to him: "Yes," whereupon Rabbi Aqiva declared her to be in the status of purity.
>
> He saw his students glancing at each other. So he said to them: "Why is this matter difficult in your assessment?" For the sages did not lay down the rule [of the כתם] in order to be stringent but to be lenient, because it is said: "When a woman has a discharge, her discharge being blood in her body. . . ." [Lev. 15:19]—blood—and not a stain. (mNid 8:3; emphasis added)

In this tannaitic legal case story a woman comes to consult Rabbi Aqiva, one of the giants of the mishnaic universe. This case story, finally and for the first time, stages the new rabbinic science of women's blood. A woman comes to a rabbi to consult with him as to the evidence of blood she found. Reading the story with respect to the effects it is supposed to create, it is irrelevant whether this case is a historical case or not, or whether the historical Rabbi Aqiva actually did consult with women with respect to their menstruation. What is extremely relevant, however, is the fact that already in the founding rabbinic discourse on menstruation women are represented as coming to the rabbi to consult. Already in the Mishnah the rabbis are staged as "gynecologists," so to speak, as authoritative interpreters of women's bodies, as opposed to the women who are staged as the object of interpretation. This is the only such story in the Mishnah Tractate Niddah itself. The Tosefta and subsequently the Babylonian Talmud list a number of case stories in which a woman is represented as coming before a rabbi to consult with him. It is always the woman who comes before the rabbi.[25]

The mishnaic story is remarkable as to its length and as to constructing an extended conversation between the rabbinic expert and the woman. The length of the conversation is unusual also in that it grants the woman the position as speaker repeatedly. Other case stories, for instance in the Tosefta, often are structured much more simply: something happens to an anonymous woman who normally does not speak, and the rabbi is represented as pronouncing his ruling.[26] In our story we do not learn much about the particular circumstances of the woman, since obviously the Mishnah is primarily interested in Rabbi Aqiva's position and in his reasoning. It represents Rabbi Aqiva as being the one who encourages the woman to attribute the bloodstain to something other than a source of impurity, to a wound in her internal organs perhaps, which is blood that leaves her in the status of purity (and would allow her to continue to have marital intimacy with her husband).[27] But if we read "against the grain" we see more clearly how problematic the authority structure is. Reading "against the grain" here would mean to focus on the woman and apply the same interest invested in Rabbi Aqiva's position to her. Her "Yes, but . . ." reply indicates reluctance. She refuses to take Rabbi Aqiva's lead to allow her to get out of regarding herself as impure, at least initially.

There are two possibilities to interpret this reluctance. The woman might be especially meticulous as to the observance of menstrual impurity. In this case the rhetorical force of Rabbi Aqiva's advice would be to caution her not to be overly zealous. But one could read her reluctance to indicate that she did not want to be declared to be in a status of purity. In other words, she wanted to be declared as a niddah, perhaps to avoid her marital sexual duties. In this case the rhetorical force of her reluctance would be to insist that in spite of hermeneutic alternatives she wants this blood to make her impure. The first reading would make the authority structure of the rabbi as adviser and the woman as advisee appear as benevolent paternalism.[28] In the second reading that same authority structure is made to appear not quite as benevolent, in that it would align the male authority of the rabbi with the authority of the husband.[29]

Finally, the story illustrates how the bloodstain becomes the external, visible, and accessible object that is under the jurisdiction of the rabbis. The rabbis, equipped with the science that they themselves created, are now the judges to tell a woman whether she is menstruating, whether she is a *zavah* or whether she has merely an internal wound. The rabbi is the one to judge in which case to be lenient and in which to be stringent. Thus we can understand the Mishnah's focus on the types of women's genital blood and the bloodstain as *external* evidence of a woman's menstruation. My hypothesis is that the rabbis, who had no direct access to the woman's body itself,[30] focused their attention on the colors of blood and the bloodstain, because they could establish control based on external evidence more readily and more "objectively" than on the blood-flow itself. As we have seen in the previous chapter, the rabbis could not put themselves in the place of the women to grasp the sensation of a blood-flow, or put differently, the Mishnah itself did not make her sensation a criterion for defining a menstrual blood-flow. Hence, the inspection of a bloodstain or blood on a testing rag to be judged by a rabbinic expert is another way for rabbinic discourse to objectify menstrual bleeding. The emphasis on *visual* identification of blood rather than of identification via the woman's sensation or pain is a symptom of this tendency, as is the architectural conception of the woman's body. It further allows for the construction of discursive authority structures that were transformed into social reality till the modern period. What the text then attempts to project is a process of epistemologically separating menstrual blood from women. Women are disowned of their bleeding since the projected scientists of the menstrual science, scopic and theoretical (in the true, that is Greek, sense of the word) as it is, are, of course, the rabbis. The talmudic texts attempt to institute the rabbis as the menstrual experts.[31]

### Beyond the Hermeneutic Sense of Vision: Smell and Taste

Surprisingly, we have one outside source for this rabbinic science. There is rare literary evidence external to talmudic literature that attests to the expertise of certain learned men in the Jewish community to judge blood. The patristic writer Jerome mentions in his correspondence:

> praepositos habent synagogis sapientissimos quosque foedo operi delegatos, ut sanguinem virginis sive menstruatae mundum vel inmundum, si oculis discernere no potuerint, gustatu probent.

> They[32] have as heads of their synagogues certain very learned men who are assigned the disgusting task of determining by taste, if they

are unable to discern by the eyes alone, whether the blood of a virgin or a menstruant is pure or impure. [Epistle to Algasia 121.10.19 = CSEL 56:48].[33]

Jerome's remark seems to show that it was known to "outsiders" of rabbinic culture that rabbis could function as experts concerning menstrual blood and that at a certain point in time the new rabbinic science of women's blood began to be translated into social reality. At the same time, we may safely regard his statement as polemic "ethnography" since rabbinic literature never mentions taste as a hermeneutic sense. Further, it is impossible—by all halakhic standards internal to rabbinic culture—that the rabbis tasted the blood. Presumably, therefore, Jerome's statement is a polemical distortion.[34]

The one talmudic example that perhaps comes closest to Jerome's statement in terms of employing a sense different than sight for examining the blood is the quite amazing story of Rava, a fourth-century rabbi, who *smells* the blood sent to him by Ifra Hormiz, the somewhat legendary mother of Shapur II (309–379), the Sassanian king contemporary to Rava:[35]

אפרא הורמיז אמיה דשבור מלכא שדרה דמא לקמיה דרבא הוה יתיב רב
עובדיה קמיה ארחיה אמר לה האי דם חימוד הוא אמרה ליה לבריה תא
חזי כמה חכימי יהודאי
א״ל דלמא כסומא בארובה הדר שדרה ליה שתין מיני דמא וכולהו אמרינהו
ההוא בתרא דם כנים הוה ולא ידע אסתייע מילתא ושדר לה סריקותא
דמקטלא כלמי אמרה יהודאי בתווני דלבא יתביתו

Ifra Hormiz, the mother of Shapur, sent blood to Rava.[36] Rav Ovadyah sat in front of him. He *smelled* the blood and told her: This is blood of desire. Whereupon she said to her son (the king): Come and see how wise the Jews are.

He [Shapur] responded: Perhaps he was like a blind man in a window. Again she sent him sixty kinds of blood,[37] and he identified all of them, except for the last one which was the blood of lice, and he did not know it. By chance, he sent her a comb which kills lice. She said: You Jews sit in the innermost chambers of the heart. [bNid 20b]

This is the only story in which smell is employed.[38] It is דם חימוד—blood of desire,[39] that is, blood that a woman discharges prior to intercourse out of excitement and anticipation, which is inspected by smell rather than by sight.[40] "Blood of lust" is distinguishable somehow by smell from menstruous blood, but from the Talmud itself it does not emerge whether it is impure and how exactly it is related to menstrual blood.[41] Further, it is not quite clear why it is the "blood of lust" that can be identified by smell.[42]

This story has a profoundly hyperbolic tone to it, since subsequently Ifra Hormiz sends sixty different types of blood to Rava to verify "the Jews' wisdom." Rava can indeed classify them all, though he almost fails on the last sample. Curiously, just as in the case of Jerome, we are here dealing with a cross-cultural encounter concerning the rabbinic expertise in blood, though this is an insider's construction of it. Ifra Hormiz's admiration for the "Jews' wisdom" stands in stark contrast to Jerome's disgust, though one is tempted to doubt that a historical Sassanian queen mother would be all that dazzled by this particular skill.[43]

It is the miraculous element that in the end supports the rabbis' self-fashioning as experts in the science of women's blood. Beyond what is reasonable, the narrative projects an international reputation for the rabbis as blood experts.

## Women's Hermeneutic Sovereignty

Beyond the construction of authoritative expertise, there is one moment of rhetorical ambiguity built into the mishnaic discourse—or perhaps it is a moment of conceptual weakness. The Mishnah allows a woman to attribute the bloodstain to any number of reasons that she can produce: "ותולה בכל דבר שהיא יכולה לתלות—she can attribute [the bloodstain] to any reason that she can attribute it to" (mNid 8:2, tNid 6:17, tNid 7:4). It is, of course, the rabbis who halakhically define the size and the shape of the stain, by which it can be attributed to, for instance, a louse or a bedbug. In cases of doubt, a woman is still expected to consult with the rabbinic expert. But we find in the Mishnah a rhetorical opening that puts the woman in a subject position. She is to make an "informed" judgment on her status of impurity. The point of this is not so much to argue that the Mishnah can imagine a woman making her own judgments. Rather, what the rhetoric of this statement—"she can attribute [the bloodstain] to any reason she can attribute it to"—alludes to is that the whole system works only if women play along and accept the authority to define. The woman is the one who has to make the decision to seek the rabbi's advice and submit herself to his expert authority, the woman is the one who has to observe her own blood-flow, and the woman is the one who has to regard a stain as problematic or indicative of something. That this is not merely a rhetorical issue, but does indeed touch upon an issue that deeply troubles the rabbinic discourse on menstruation, will become evident as we now turn to the story of Yalta.

**Yalta's Ruse: Scene One, or the Trouble with Authority**

Amid a series of stories about the fantastic ability of certain rabbis to identify various types of blood and their origins, the Babylonian Talmud in Tractate Niddah records the following brief story:[44]

ילתא אייתא דמא לקמיה דרבה בר בר חנה וטמי לה הדר אייתא לקמיה דרב יצחק בריה דרב יהודה ודכי לה

והיכי עביד הכי והתניא חכם שטימא אין חברו רשאי לטהר אסר אין חבירו רשאי להתיר

מעיקרא טמויי הוה מטמי לה כיון דא״ל דכל יומא הוה מדכי לי כי האי גונא והאידנא הוא דחש בעיניה דכי לה

Yalta once presented some blood to Rabbah bar bar Hana who informed her that it was impure. She then took it to Rav Yizhaq the son of Rav Yehudah who told her that it was pure.

But how could *he* act in this manner, seeing that it was taught: If a sage declared anything impure his colleague may not declare it pure; if he forbade anything his colleague may not permit it?

At first he [Rav Yizhaq] informed her that it was indeed impure, but when *she told him* that "on every other occasion he [Rabbah bar bar Hana] had declared for me such blood as pure, and only on this occasion he had a pain in his eye," he [Rav Yizhaq] gave her his ruling that it was pure. (bNid 20b)

The heroine of this story is Yalta, one of the few women in the Babylonian Talmud known by name,[45] but otherwise recognizable within this literature dominated by male actors through her relationship to one of the more well-known rabbis in the Babylonian Talmud: Rav Nachman bar Ya'akov, her husband and one of the sages of the third generation of Babylonian amoraim.[46]

What is remarkable about Yalta's story in Tractate Niddah, and what sets it apart from the numerous others in which women bring blood samples to rabbinic experts, is the fact that Yalta is not satisfied with the judgment of the first rabbi, who declared the blood in question to be impure, and thus foreclosed the possibility of sexual relations with her husband. In other stories in which women consult a rabbinic expert about the status of their blood, the narrative pattern is most commonly that she shows it to him and he passes his judgment on its ritual status. According to this pattern our story could have ended after the first sentence: ילתא אייתא דמא לקמיה דרבה בר בר חנה וטמי לה—"Yalta brought the blood before Rabbah bar bar Hana and he declared it impure." Instead she follows her desire and turns around to consult a second rabbi, Rav Yizhaq, who indeed declares it to be pure.[47] The story reflects on the issue of resistance to the authority of the rabbis, and on what happens when women's desires exceed their confinement within the science of the rabbis. I want to read this story as emblematizing the trouble with rabbinic androcentrism, particularly in its discourse on menstruation.

**Yalta's Ruse: Scene Two**

Yalta's story appears in the talmudic sugyah briefly after the scene at the cupping-house. At a point where the talmudic discussions have almost completely displaced the women, as emblematized in the scene at the cupping-house, the Talmud raises through our narrative the question of how much hegemony a woman can be admitted to hold in blood matters. The narrative functions as what Mieke Bal has called a symptom, an involuntary sign, which betrays an awareness that in order for the system to work women need to play along and submit to the rabbinic readings of women's bodies.

The way this question of authority is introduced is by a ruse, Yalta's ruse. Her ruse is twofold: first, she does not rest assured with one rabbinic judgment, and takes the initiative to consult a second rabbi, thus taking her fate into her own hands and following her desire. On this narrative step in the story the anonymous narrating or editorial voice of the gemara intersperses a commentary in the narrative of the case story, asking with astonishment:

והיכי עביד הכי—but how could *he* act in such a manner? The gemara wonders not about Yalta's behavior, as we might have expected, but Rav Yizhaq's disrespect or ignorance of Rabbah bar bar Hana's preceding judgement.[48] Such disrespect or ignorance creates a halakhic incoherence that needs to be solved to explain Rav Yizhaq's behavior. The implicit assumption of the text is that he knew about the prior evaluation. Based on this assumption, the Talmud can ascribe intentionality to Rav Yizhaq and focus the discussion on him, away from Yalta. It adduces a baraita, an earlier authoritative tradition, which is cited repeatedly throughout the Talmud,[49] that if one rabbi has declared something or someone to be in the status of impurity, no colleague can reverse such a declaration. Rav Yizhaq would thus seem to contradict an authoritative tradition.

To solve this contradiction and to explain Rav Yizhaq's otherwise questionable reversal of a preceding opinion, we learn about Yalta's second ruse. She is turned into somewhat of a trickster figure.[50] The anonymous narrator of the gemara claims that originally Rav Yizhaq had indeed agreed with Rabbah bar bar Hana: "At first he informed her that it was indeed impure." Thus he is presented as originally having acted in accordance with the principle stated in the baraita. However, the gemara suggests that he reversed his assessment only because Yalta convinced him otherwise. It was Yalta who explained to him that Rabbah bar bar Hana was indisposed to do an adequate judgment: "*she told him* that on every other occasion Rabbah bar bar Hana declared such blood as pure, and only on this occasion he had a pain in his eye." At first view, Yalta seems to fabricate the story of Rabbah bar bar Hana's ailment. It would then seem puzzling that Rav Yizhaq is so foolish as to be persuaded by such a fable. Such a reading of Yalta's second ruse, indeed, strengthens her subject position in the case, since she does not even rest with the second rabbi's judgment, and continues to pursue her desire.[51] She refuses the first rabbi's judgment and she bends the second rabbi's opinion. In such a reading she appears as questioning the authority of the experts by bending it.

We can read the story from a somewhat different angle, though, which throws a different light on the character. There is more to Yalta's argument than would appear at first sight. From this angle Yalta is not represented as fabricating a story in order to circumvent the rabbi's authority. Rather, she can be read as making a coherent argument, quite acceptable within the terms of rabbinic culture. Reading the story from this angle, we see her not as circumventing the authority of the self-fashioned experts, but as competing with it.

Yalta's argument presents, I would suggest, an allusion to a mishnah from the mishnaic tractate dealing with the impurity resulting from skin lesions. We have already encountered this tractate as an intertext in the discussion of the mishnaic taxonomy of blood colors. Once again, this tractate can be read as a subtext to the discussion of menstrual impurity. Yalta's argument presents an allusion to Mishnah Nega'im 2:3, according to which "a priest who is blind in one eye or the light of whose eyes is dim may not inspect leprous lesions, for it is written 'as far as appears in the eyes of the priest'" (Lev. 13:12)."[52] With this allusion Yalta is presented as suggesting that the inspection of women's genital blood is modeled on the priestly inspection of leprous lesions. According to the *midrashic reading* of Lev. 13:12—"and if the zara'at [skin disease] breaks forth on his skin, and the zara'at covers all the skin of him that has the plague from his head to his foot, *as far as the priest can see*, then the priest shall consider . . ."—the biblical text demands that the priest have perfect eyesight in *both* eyes in order to qualify for the inspection of leprous lesions. Just as in the context of inspection of leprous lesions, so equally in the context of the inspection of women's genital blood: the inspecting rabbi should have perfect eyesight, which according to Yalta Rabbah bar bar Hana did not have on this particular occasion. The sugyah catapults Yalta rhetorically into an argumentative position in which she is familiar with mishnaic halakhah or halakhic midrash, and can replicate rabbinic knowledge. But she is presented also as making a creative halakhic argument, which is strong enough to convince Rav Yizhaq. In its desire to harmonize the baraita with Rav Yizhaq's behavior, the text ends up putting Yalta on equal footing with the rabbis and makes her a participant in talmudic discourse, instead of its mere object.

Thus we see several dynamics at work in the narrative of Yalta and its discussion in the talmudic sugyah, which identify the story as a symptom of Mieke Bal's principle that "'dominance' is, although present and in many ways obnoxious, not unproblematically established" (*Lethal Love*, 3). First, the Talmud deploys one of the few named women characters, hence rendering her recognizable and memorable. Second, in the discussion of the story Yalta is portrayed as making a halakhic argument, as encroaching into what is normally the rabbis' territory. This is characteristic of what Mieke Bal calls a *lapsus*: "There are also slips, *lapsus* in the classical sense. We can speak of a *lapsus* whenever a word is attributed to a woman that is 'normally' exclusively attributed to a man" (83), only that Yalta is represented as making a whole argument that is normally attributed to a man. Hence the story is not about the trouble with Yalta.⁵³ Rather, it is about the trouble with the rabbinic science of blood, and the power dynamics that it tries to establish.

## Containing the Power of the Ruse

The reaction of the gemara to Yalta's argument is remarkably laconic, given its humor, but it is to the point. The subsequent dialectic argumentation in the sugyah is an interesting exercise in containing the force of Yalta's ruse. We can see strategies at work that are parallel to those deployed to contain the force of Shmu'el's midrash in the previous chapter. The sugyah introduces the question of women's believability. It asks whether Yalta can be believed in such a situation. By framing the discussion of Yalta's case in this manner the sugyah clouds the force of Yalta's argument, thus countering the encroachment of the a-normal (a woman who makes a halakhic argument) into the normal. Yalta, and along with her all women, are once again pushed into the position of the other, of the "them" (women) that can be and need to be evaluated by "us" (the rabbis), especially when "they" question "us." Thus, women are strictly distinguished from the "us" of the rabbis, a distinction that the discussion of Yalta's story so far has questioned. By introducing the question of trustworthiness women are once again marked as clearly being "them":

ומי מהימני
אין והתניא נאמנת אשה לומר כזה ראיתי ואבדתיו
איבעיא להו כזה טיהר איש פלוני חכם מהו
תא שמע נאמנת אשה לומר כזה ראיתי ואבדתיו
שאני התם דליתיה לקמה
תא שמע דילתא . . .
אלמא מהימנא לה
רב יצחק בר יהודה אגמריה סמך

But is she reliable?⁵⁴

Yes, since has it not indeed been taught [in a baraita]:

[Case A] A woman is believed when she says "*I saw* a kind of blood *like this one* but I have lost it." [bNid 20b]

The sugyah sets out to argue that Yalta can indeed be believed. Its answer to the question of whether Yalta can be believed is positive, in the tone of "surely she is believed": אין. It cites an abstract case from a baraita as being parallel. According to this baraita a woman is believed when she brings a blood sample which is—according to her own judgment—similar to the one that she consults the rabbi about, but absent and not accessible to the gaze of the male scholar. This case is suggested to be analogous to Yalta's, in that Yalta can be read as comparing her current blood sample in front of Rav Yizhaq's eyes to those which Rabbah bar bar Hana had declared pure on every other occasion. Thus the question about Yalta's reliability is an amazing strategy of refocusing. The focus is on the question of whether she *sees* correctly, and moves away from whether she made a good argument. The implied assumption is that the rabbinic experts can see, are in full control of the scopic science of blood, but women themselves may not be able to see.

A question was raised:
[Case B: What is the rule concerning the case of a woman who says] "A kind of blood *like this* has been declared pure by such and such a sage?"
[The preliminary answer is:]
Come and hear: A woman is believed when she says "I saw a kind of blood like this one but I have lost it."

The sugyah continues and raises the question about another abstract case-scenario in which a woman claims that the blood currently in question is like the one that has been declared nonmenstrual by a different rabbi. This case would seem to be more analogous to what Yalta is doing. In this abstract case the woman would almost be fulfilling the function of the rabbinic expert eye. That is, in effect it is she who judges the blood in question. Such an assessment would be completely based on her own authority, even where she has to bolster that authority by her reference to a different rabbinic authority, who has declared such blood to be pure. Still, in this case she no longer consults another—male—authority about the blood in question, but in fact forms her own opinion about it, and is the one who also pronounces it to be pure. Rashi, in fact, suggests that the scenario of this case has to be imagined as one between two women: one woman comes to her woman friend to ask her about her blood type, and the first declares it to be nonmenstrual. This scenario would undermine the gemara's attempt to gender the rabbis' expertise and authority on menstrual blood as male. If a woman was believed in such a case, a rabbi's expert eye would be displaced. The woman of the case is still represented as referring to a previous rabbi's evaluation of another, similar type of blood, but it is she who is making an independent judgment on blood that a friend brings her.

As a preliminary answer the sugyah suggests that the two abstract cases are analogous and that, therefore, a woman is considered to be reliable in her own take on the science of blood. However, the sugyah continues: "But is not this case [Case B] different, since there [Case A] the blood is not in front of her?"

Thus, the sugyah rejects the suggested analogy of the cases based on the following argument. In Case A the blood in question is absent. The woman evaluates the similarity of two blood types herself and brings a different sample to the expert. The blood sample in question no longer exists, in which case the woman's vision is relied upon. The rabbinic expert has the last word. In Case B, however, the blood in question exists, in front of the woman. Rashi comments on the force of this objection in a telling rhetorical manner by spelling out the difference between the two cases: "אבל הכא דראיתיה קמן ניחזי אנן—but in this case [Case B], where the blood is in front of us, we will look at it."[55] The "we" in this case is to be understood as an exclusivist we, a self-consciously gendered "we." That is, "we, the (male) scholars" do not have to let the woman make a judgment, since the blood in question is present and "we" can judge it ourselves.

However, against such an objection the other position in the dialectical argumentation of the sugyah insists that, nonetheless, the woman in Case B is to be believed. This time it bases this assertion on the claim that this case is parallel to Yalta's case. As Rav Yizhaq did indeed believe Yalta, so the woman who pronounces a blood sample to be pure can be considered to be reliable.

Come and hear the case of Yalta: [now the whole case of Yalta from above is cited and then the gemara continues: From Yalta's case and Rav Yizhaq's acceptance of her argument] It follows that she is believed!?

The Talmud's question behind these cases is about how much hermeneutic sovereignty a woman can be granted in assessing her own and perhaps even another woman's status of purity or impurity. Discussing this question and refocusing Yalta's story in this manner is the sugyah's strategy to control the moment of crisis in the invention of the rabbinic science.

**And Her Real Question Is?**

It would be hasty to read this argumentation solely as a struggle to establish the rabbis as the expert readers of women's blood. We can add another dimension that is embedded in this argumentation. Another legal issue that plays into this discussion is the problem of biased witnesses: that is, the prohibition on testimony concerning matters pertaining to a person's own interests or to that of their relatives. The suspicion on which the abstract cases in our sugyah are predicated is that a woman may be *driven* by desire when she comes to ascertain the status of her bleeding, since her real question to the rabbi is whether she can engage in sexual intercourse with her husband. She might therefore not be truthful, or she may be biased in her judgment. This suspicion is not necessarily based on the rabbis' perception of women's trustworthiness per se, as a generic gender problem, as if on principle women were considered unreliable. Rather, it is a question of legal principle concerning testimonies in general.[56] In our context of the inspection of women's genital blood, the case of the inspection of leprous lesions might again be considered as an intertext, since here the examined person's status of purity or impurity is at stake. In mNeg 2:5 we learn: "A person may inspect any leprous lesions except his own. Rabbi Meir [adds to the exception and thus] says: Not even the leprous lesions of his relatives." We do not learn why this is so,[57] but the most obvious reason is that the examiner might easily be biased in his or her judgment. The abstract women in the cases in our sugyah are, then, analogous to the self-inspecting person in Mishnah Nega'im. Just as there a person may not evaluate him- or herself, so in the case of menstrual impurity a woman may not evaluate herself.[58]

In spite of the strong echo of the discourse of biased testimony, however, we may point out that this echo would only question a woman's self-evaluation in cases of menstruation. It does not pose an obstacle to a woman's evaluation of another woman's blood, a scenario suggested by

Case B. The dialectic flow of the argumentation in our sugyah reached a point where such a scenario of hermeneutic sovereignty of women remains a possibility. But the sugyah concludes with the following statement: "Rav Yizhaq ben Yehudah [actually] relied on his own traditions" (bNid 20b).

The final statement of this sugyah is that Rav Yizhaq, the rabbinic expert who is represented as trusting Yalta's argument in the opening of the story, really had his own traditions. He was not really convinced by Yalta's claim at all, but had his own reasons to declare her blood to be pure, over and against the previous judgment by Rabbah bar bar Hana. This last concluding suggestion would render superfluous the whole discussion of women's trustworthiness in our sugyah, which ended up granting women a certain limited amount of sovereignty with respect to evaluating their own blood.[59] It seems that even though this reading of Rav Yizhaq's evaluation has the final say in the sugyah, it appears as an afterthought, and a pretty weak one at that. If we were to dramatize the sugyah, the editorial voice that grants women hermeneutic sovereignty in the new rabbinic science of blood, to whatever limited degree that may be, has clearly dominated the discussion. The sugyah leaves us convinced that the explanation of the Yalta story is that Rav Yizhaq simply believed her.

What this episode suggests is first that the question of the (male) rabbis' control over women's menstrual blood was indeed a "problem" in the cultural conscience of those who told the story of Yalta and those who subsequently integrated it into the talmudic structure. Even where we cannot prove, owing to lack of other historical data, that historically women resisted this kind of rabbinic control, the text itself shows that it has to negotiate this tension. Furthermore, the gemara plays with the considerable differences of opinion concerning women's hermeneutic sovereignty. One voice promotes actively not only women's trustworthiness in menstrual matters, but women's (limited) autonomy of judgment. The other voice questions the former. In the end, neither cancels out the other.

It is ultimately up to the readers of rabbinic texts to highlight this difference encoded in the text, in terms of the various gender-political options. None of the options considered suggest total hermeneutic sovereignty for women. Even that position in the dialectic which is most open to the concept posits a woman's basic reliance on some rabbinic expert's prior judgment. At the very least, this sugyah brings to the fore the struggle that is involved in the creation of the new rabbinic science. The rabbis will become experts concerning menstrual bleeding in social reality.[60] The story of Yalta, however, leaves a trace of how problematic establishing structures of displacement and dominance may be.

We can read Yalta in many ways, but there seem to be two primary options. We can read her as a proto-feminist hero of protest, whose somewhat lonely voice made it into the canon of rabbinic literature. Or we can read her story as an index of a more systemic problem in the discourse of the rabbinic science of women's blood. Both readings have advantages: in the first case, we highlight an individual woman, one of the few in talmudic literature; in the second case, we make the story much more central to the discourse as a whole, as a moment of disturbance or another kind of rupture in the androcentric fabric of niddah. Both readings also have disadvantages: in the first case, the Yalta story would be marginalized discursively as the story of the token woman. In the second case, the one named woman character we find as a model of women's protest is dissolved into an abstract element of discourse, however powerful that may be. The question is, in the end, not one of truth but of strategy. In this chapter I have pursued the second strategy of reading, leaning on a similar approach in the previous chapter. This has allowed me to interrogate the issue of who has the power to see in the rabbinic science of blood in a more systemic way.

## 5 WOMEN'S MEDICINE IN RABBINIC LITERATURE

BETWEEN FEMALE AUTONOMY AND MALE CONTROL

---

IN THE PREVIOUS CHAPTER I focused exclusively on the question of how talmudic literature attempts to establish the male rabbis, the subjects of halakhic discourse, as experts on women's menstrual bleeding. As we have seen, the rabbinic discussions of the woman's status of im/purity were largely theoretical in post-Temple times. The complex system of im/purity functions primarily as the framework within which the rabbis construct the woman's body as a significant and signifying entity within their discursive universe. At the same time, the discussions attempt to endow the rabbis, as those who discursively construct the female body, with the authority over the distinction between menstrual and nonmenstrual bleeding, between a bleeding that interferes with marital intimacy and one that does not. Such authority would come into play with irregular bleeding only, since a regular cycle would not raise any question as to the menstrual nature of bleeding. Nonetheless, such authority would imply that in cases of irregular cycles a woman would (and today does)[1] surrender the "knowledge" of her own body and its physiological processes to a male authority, for better or for worse. Within this framework I have read the story of Yalta as emblematic of the nonclosure of an androcentric discourse. On one level of reading, the narrative reflects on the possibilities for women to maneuver within the web of controlling relationships they are put in and to pursue their own desires. On another level, one which we pursued, the Yalta narrative can be read symptomatically as an involuntary sign of the problem with gender domination. The rabbis do not render women's bodies culturally invisible, nor do they construct them as incomplete, unfinished, and hence inferior versions of male bodies. Culturally and historically, they had such an option at their disposal. Instead, the rabbis chose to construct women's bodies as different from men's, differently human, with differing cultural significance. As we have seen, this is not necessarily more advantageous to women than cultural invisibility, since the rabbis develop discursive strategies to contain this difference within the parameters of their discourse.

In this chapter I want to think more about the nature of gender-specific "space," and about the possibility of women's space within the discursive universe of the rabbis, particularly with reference to women's bodies. Obviously, there are multiple ways in which "women's space" in a culture with gender-segregated spaces could be described and analyzed, both anthropologically and textually.

By "women's spaces," I mean cultural spaces in which women relate directly to women and can establish relationships that are not under the immediate control of male authority, whether of father, husband, or rabbi. A qualification of immediate control here is important, since even if a culture allows for independent women's spaces, such spaces are in most cases under the indirect control of male authority. Such indirect control can function in very subtle ways. For instance, women may mediate it psychologically through their self-perception and their perception of other women as taught to them by the culture in which they are raised. In spite of the indirect male control, however, women's spaces may allow a consciousness of a collective gender identity to emerge. They may therefore turn into potential sites of resistance against gender domination, or at least allow for questioning it and for creating temporary reprieve from immediate forms of gender domination. For a concrete example, we may think about the institution of menstrual huts in some so-called tribal cultures. Thomas Buckley and Alma Gottlieb have suggested that these institutions can also be read as actually sustaining something like women's subculture, and can even provide temporary relief from the drudgery of everyday maintenance of the family (*Blood Magic*, 31–34).

I restrict myself to only one aspect of "women's space," which I consider a fundamental one for the maintenance of women's lives, and that is the care of the body, specifically of women's bodies. The question of authority of judgment over women's bleeding that I have pursued in the previous chapter deals only with one specific aspect of the "maintaining" of women's bodies. We have seen also that the rabbinic science of blood actually displaces women's bodies. The mishnaic text renders colors of blood and shapes and locations of stains visible textually, but what rabbis are imagined as looking at is samples of blood, sometimes women's blood collected on fabric. In the scene at the cupping-house, learning evolved around a combination of (mishnaic) text and men's blood. Further, mishnaic texts construct the various chambers of women's bodies, thus making women's genitalia and internal organs visible textually. But rabbinic texts, whether in halakhic-prescriptive texts or in case stories, hardly ever imagine rabbis to be looking at women's bodies directly.[2]

Talmudic literature, however, again particularly in Tractate Niddah, considers various other situations in which women's bodies are examined. These situations most commonly do not arise from an interest in women's health care, as in Greco-Roman gynecological literature, but from a halakhic problem, determined by the interest of the text. Nonetheless, even if it is primarily the halakhic interest of the text that determines when and how the question of the examination of women's bodies is raised, each of these individual cases and their inherent assumptions about accessibility of women's bodies touches upon larger questions that reach beyond those individual cases. If, indeed, one set of cultural norms, the rules of modesty, precludes the rabbis' access to women's bodies, and it is women who examine women's bodies, it is perhaps in these textual fragments that we can search for the possibility of women's spaces in rabbinic culture. Such a space will have to be carefully examined as to its possibilities as well as its limitations.

In order to develop the larger questions let us turn to the debate on Greco-Roman gynecological literature which has emerged over the last fifteen years. The discussions of the Greco-Roman literature will help us to develop methodological tools for interrogating the rabbinic texts.

## Greco-Roman Gynecology

Scholars of late antique culture have recently paid increased attention to Greco-Roman gynecological literature as a resource for writing the history of gender. Neglected for a long time, the Hippocratic writings of the Greek classical period and the works of Galen, Soranus, and Rufus of the Roman imperial period enjoy a new popularity among cultural historians of the era. The gynecological writings appeared at first to open up the lives of Greco-Roman women to contemporary scholarship. One hope was to discover an accessible dimension of women's real lives beyond their mere reflection and distortion in the philosophical and dramatic literature produced by men. Real women's lives beyond the monolithic screen of male perception and construction of such a reality could perhaps become visible in those texts. Feminist historians, however, have pointed out the limitations of these sources for the purposes of reading women's history "from the inside." First and foremost, just like rabbinic literature, most of the medical literature is indeed written by men.[3] Feminist readings of these texts have further shown the extent to which these gynecological writings actually reflect Greek philosophies and their respective gender ideologies, rather than presenting a counterliterature. As Ann Ellis Hanson writes in her discussion of the Hippocratic texts: "The medical writer is projecting upon the woman a man's experience" ("The Medical Writers' Women," 314).

The questions that have been raised in this debate relating to the gender politics pervading the gynecological literature can be divided into three fields:

First, who undertook the examinations of women, external or internal? Who deemed him-/herself authorized to heal, in whatever way that was understood, be it merely to test some new cure on the human body,[4] or to reduce the pain of the patient, or to establish the wife's body as the husband's property? That is, who considered him-/herself, or who was considered, the legitimate authority over the well-being of the woman? Was this authority gendered male or female? And if women were given this authority, can we thus automatically conclude that women were inhabiting an autonomous sphere in which they were sovereign over their own bodies?

Connected with this first field of questions is a second one, about how medicine as a practice was organized and how it was institutionalized. Who called whom what, with what kind of authoritative voice? Who was deemed to be a healer, or a charlatan, or an expert?

Last, a problem area that is often neglected concerns the text as medium of medical knowledge in general, and gynecology in particular. What are the implications of the rise of the "scientific" medical textbook as a cultural phenomenon,[5] corresponding to the rise of literacy and the production of a (mostly male) literary elite?

On the basis of these questions modern readers of the ancient texts have come to very different conclusions about the development of women's place in late antique culture and the role that the gynecological literature played in this development.

From the vantage point of women's history, Aline Rousselle regards the Hippocratic gynecological treatises as a symptom of the decline of women's autonomy and sovereignty within the general culture: "Women were no longer mistresses of their own bodies, relying on their own observations and the interpretation of these observations by a few specialists who were women" (*Porneia*, 32). Rather, the Hippocratic texts would provide the illustration of the development of "a male policy towards women, a *gyna-economy*, which required the contribution of the doctors to make it more effective and which in this case consisted of legally sanctioned domination by fathers and husbands, indeed by men in general, over women's bodies" (32).[6] Subsequently, the gynecological writings of Soranus and Rufus of Ephesus were also manuals on fertilization written primarily for husbands, or at least for the husbands' interests: "The tradition of female experience collected and passed on by women, which had been handed over to the Greek doctors and integrated into their theories, had become a tool to help men retain control over their family life" (40).[7] Rousselle also describes a pre-Hippocratic and oral medical tradition visible behind the gynecology of the corpus; she sees oral tradition as being preserved solely by women and knowledge of it as restricted to women's circles ("Observation féminine," 1091–92).[8] This tradition of women's experience, which had been handed over to the Greek doctors and integrated into their theories, becomes a tool to help men retain control over their families and fulfill their duty to beget male heirs. Rousselle traces a historical development from a preliterary period of women's sovereignty over their own bodies to the beginning of the literary phase, with the Hippocratic gynecology in which the male medical authority took over.

Rousselle's model is methodologically problematic on both ends of the historical development, however. Even if one agrees with her contention that the gynecological literature amounts to manuals of fertilization, one must still be cautious with the assumption that women in the "preliterary Greek world" were indeed sovereign over their own bodies. Thus, even though Hanson agrees with Rousselle on the existence of women's oral tradition, traces of which are preserved in the Hippocratic corpus, she contests Rousselle's hypothesis that this tradition would have existed outside of a patriarchal context.[9] She suggests, instead, that "there was . . . considerable overlap between the gynecology of Greco-Roman medical writers and the societal traditions and experiences familiar to anyone who cared to think on gynecological topics, and there was, as well, free circulation of ideas and recipes back and forth between the two traditions" ("Continuity and Change," 78). Rather than assuming an extra-patriarchal women's sphere, she proposes that Hippocratic medical theory and what remains of pre-Hippocratic (that is, pretextual) lore were both part of the same set of fundamental cultural assumptions about gender.[10]

As far as the other end of Rousselle's historical development is concerned—that the literary gynecology replaces women's medical oral traditions—it seems questionable that the male medical literature would determine all of social reality and transform actual medical practice completely. Thus Dean-Jones argues that in spite of the Hippocratic writers' claim to authority over women's health issues "the proportion of case histories (in the treatise on Epidemics, with twice as many male as female case histories) could suggest that women tended to avail themselves of traditional medicine at the hands of wise-women rather than seek the advice of (Hippocratic) physicians who were generally male" (*Women's Bodies*, 34). She suggests that women did not flock to male doctors, but that traditional medicine for women continued to exist side by side with the scientific medicine preserved in texts. Women's space may, indeed, be highly resistant to overdetermination by the androcentric male discourse: "Ancient women may have felt that men could not understand or sympathize with their exclusively female experiences, and this may have led them to rely more on the diagnoses and therapies of wise-women" (*Women's Bodies*, 35).

We can see that the question of women's space depends on how the relationship between the male-authored texts and the women's lives they attempt to circumscribe is constructed. Rousselle's critique of Greco-Roman gynecological literature is important, in that beyond stating its obvious male authorship, she points out its androcentric bias, which serves to reinforce patriarchal social arrangements. Nonetheless, we could also argue that she endows the texts with too much power over women's lives when she assumes that they historically eradicated women's space within those patriarchal social arrangements. In spite of the emergence of "scientific" literature and the nascent importance of literacy in this period, the texts are only beginning to establish a claim to control over women's bodies, fertility, and reproductive capacities. But it has to remain questionable how far the controlling force of literate sources on gynecology extends within a presumably predominantly illiterate society, a point that has also been advanced by Monica Green in her study of medieval gynecological literature ("Women's Medical Practice," 471). Further, Green argues, "it is incumbent upon us to distinguish between the purpose with which a text is written and the purpose to which it is later put. This distinction is absolutely crucial if we are to determine the relationship women—either as practitioners or patients—had to gynecological literature" (460). Only later, when the texts are used, studied, and transmitted (by and to whom?) do they come to function as a displacement of women as authoritative sources of knowledge and care of women's bodies.[11]

Particularly with respect to the care of women's bodies, the gender politics of a text and the culture in which it is embedded come to the forefront. The debate on the function of Greco-Roman gynecological literature shows clearly how important questions such as who had access to women's bodies, for what purpose, and with what claim of authority, are for the analysis of relations between men and women—whether ideal or real, fantasized or enforced relations—in a given culture. It is these questions that have to be taken into consideration when we study the rabbinic texts that pertain to the care of bodies.

### Was There a Rabbinic Gynecology?

On the basis of the methodological issues emerging from the debate on Greco-Roman gynecological literature, I turn to the analysis of the sources in the Talmud on the care of women's bodies. Some of these questions can be asked of rabbinic literature as general methodological questions in women's history. However, caution is required when asking similar questions of both Greco-Roman and rabbinic texts in order to compare both cultural worlds. It is all too easy to neglect the differences between the rhetorics of the gynecological tracts of the Greek medical writers and those passages in the Talmud that deal with the examinations of women's bodies. Julius Preuss explains in the introduction to his now classic work on biblical and talmudic medicine: "There does not exist a work from Jewish antiquity devoted exclusively to medicine; nor even a compendium of natural history, such as that of Plinius. The Torah and the Talmud are primarily law books,[12] and medical matters are chiefly discussed only as they pertain to the law. . . . There is, therefore, no 'medicine of the Talmud,' which might perhaps be compared to the medicine of Galen or of Susrutas. There is no Jewish medicine in the sense that we speak of an Egyptian or a Greek medical science" (*Biblical and Talmudic Medicine*, 4).

In contrast to the Greek medical treatises,[13] the scattered talmudic passages on what we would commonly call gynecological issues are woven into a much larger corpus, the textual accumulation of centuries of oral transmission. These passages, assembled, cannot "reconstruct" *a* talmudic gynecology. That approach would amount to superimposing Greek terminology and epistemology onto rabbinic texts, and asking them to produce something they cannot produce. Rather, the texts compiled in this chapter are primarily episodic passages. They each have to be analyzed separately to avoid drawing hasty conclusions about *a* presumably uniform rabbinic approach.[14] Rabbinic literature does not present one homogeneous "Jewish" view on concepts that we import from Greco-Roman ways to map out reality. Due to its nature, which defies the very idea of culture as a system (Hasan-Rakem, "Narratives in Dialogue," 129), it precludes such a systematic analysis.

### Description of the Textual Evidence

The following fragments dealing with women's bodies and their physical examinations present only moments of rabbinic gender politics. Most of these appear in two different contexts, in the Tosefta and as *baraitot* in the Babylonian Talmud. It is perhaps peculiar that in tannaitic literature it is the Tosefta that provides most of the evidence. The Mishnah does not elaborate on the issue of physical examinations at all. This may be due to the generally more elliptic nature of the mishnaic texts, upon which the Tosefta often expands. An additional factor points toward what Judith Hauptman suggested recently. She proposes that a careful comparison of the Mishnah and the Tosefta might enable us to characterize the Tosefta's approach as more concerned about women's issues than the Mishnah.[15] In our context, the Tosefta's consistent interest in the question of who performs certain examinations of women's bodies, and how, may be understood in similar terms.

Further, the discussion of Tractate Niddah in the Babylonian Talmud subsequently cites a large percentage of the textual material from the Tosefta. This allows for a comparative analysis in addition to that between Mishnah and Tosefta. In those cases where two versions of the same material can be compared, sometimes conspicuous textual differences come to light. Rabbinic scholarship has commonly tried to establish the historical and literary relationship between Tosefta and Talmud. Its main concern has been to establish such a relationship in order to understand the origin of a rabbinic tradition, or the genesis of a talmudic textual unit, or sugyah.[16] Such an understanding is crucial for analyzing the process of argumentation in any given sugyah. To this set of questions traditionally asked in textual scholarship of the Talmud, we can perhaps add another dimension. If we foreground the question of gender, such differences between versions of a tradition can perhaps be analyzed in light of the underlying gender politics each of the versions suggests. It reflects on the textual changes in terms of their implications for how cultural spaces of women's bodies are constructed. For instance, the following texts, as they appear in the Tosefta's version, often remain ambiguous on the question of who is performing examinations on women's bodies. The version of the same text in the Talmud often smooths over these ambiguities. In fact, in the Talmud the baraitot on women's examinations are consistently (re)phrased to the effect that it is only a woman who could possibly examine women's bodies. Looking at the texts from this angle, the analyses of Greek gynecological treatises and of rabbinic texts intersect.

Based on these reflections, I have sought to organize the relevant passages around the fields of questions outlined above. To begin with, I have tried to locate texts that raise the question of who examines and has access to women's bodies. In the next section I take up the question of whether it is possible to trace the existence of women healers. In this context I will look at the neglected passages that cite a woman's voice as authoritative in medical matters of healing. I trace how this nameless woman, known to us only as Abaye's mother, fares within the predominantly male-produced text-corpus. Her traditions, perhaps a vestige of the preliterary oral culture or even an extra-talmudic "handbook," and their incorporation into talmudic literature *simultaneously* allow me to reflect on the process of textualization and its self-representation as a gendered culture.

## The Gender Politics of Examinations of the Female Body in Rabbinic Literature

The situations when rabbinic texts imagine or theorize the examination of a woman's body might be described as forensic contexts. By and large, we do not have any texts on examinations that are rhetorically descriptive. One text in the Tosefta describes the procedure of a gynecological examination designed to establish whether a certain kind of bleeding is uterine, and therefore menstrual, or whether it is merely vaginal:

מביא שפופרת ונותן לתוכה מכחול ומביא מוך ונתן בראש המכחול נמצא על ראשו הרי זו טמא מפני שהוא דם המקור ועל הצדדין הרי זה טהור מפני שהוא דם הקנוח

Someone brings the tube and inserts into it a painting-stick and brings a cotton-pad and puts it on the tip of the painting-stick. If [after insertion into the vagina] there is [any blood] on its tip she is in the state of impurity, since it is blood from the מקור ['source' or uterus] and if on its sides, she is in the state of purity since it is blood from the wiping. (Tosefta 8:2; cp. bNid 65b–66a)

Generally, however, the texts discussed in the following sections are all prescriptive texts. As with most rabbinic texts, we have no way of telling whether the prescribed and theorized examinations were historically implemented or not.[17] What the texts do tell us is how the rabbis imagine such examinations should be performed. We can then read these texts on the construction of gender control and autonomy.

Halakhically, a woman's body requires examination when a change of her legal status occurs, such as when she passes from minority to adulthood. In certain cases similar requirements apply to male bodies. Rabbinic legal texts of the talmudic period make this change dependent not only on abstract categories such as age, but on physiological changes as well. Just as in all kinds of other contexts, here also early rabbinic legal discourse devotes attention particularly to periods of transition, to liminal status, and to limit cases. Since a different legal status entails different rights and privileges, such texts attempt carefully to fix change and to limit epistemological ambiguity. Hence, rabbinic texts suggest that a woman's new halakhic status needs to be attested in some cases by a physical examination, before the specific halakhic rules, rights, and obligations are considered to be applicable to her.

In the following case we find discussions of women's physical examinations for such a purpose. The general framework is once again the question of the woman's status of ritual im/purity. As dicussed above in Chapter 1, this question is primarily a theoretical or historical one to the compilers of the Tosefta and certainly to those of the Babylonian Talmud.

בנות ישראל קטנות עד שלא הגיעו לפירקן הרי הן בחזקת טהרה ואין הנשים בודקות אותן וכשהגיעו לפירקן הרי הן בחזקת טמאה[18] והנשים בודקות אותן ר׳ יהודה אומר אף משהגיעו לפירקן אין הנשים בודקות אותן שמא יקלקלוהו בידיהן אלא סכות ומקנחות מבחוץ והן נבדקות מאליהן

> Legally minor Israelite women are definitely in the status of *presumptive purity* as long as they have not reached their "season,"[19] and [other] women do not [need to] examine them. But once they reach their "season" they are in the status of *presumptive impurity*,[20] and other women [need to] examine them.
>
> Rabbi Yehuda objects: even from the time they have reached their "season," other women do not examine them, so that they do not hurt them [the girls] with their hands.[21] Rather, they oil and wipe externally and [thus] they are self-examined. (Tosefta Niddah 5:4; cp. bNid 10b; my translation)

The context in which this baraita appears in the Tosefta does not help in understanding this text.[22] The Babylonian Talmud, on the other hand, cites our baraita in a completely different context at the beginning of the tractate. Here, this baraita appears in the context of case stories of young girls "whose time to have a flow of blood had not yet arrived" [תינוקת שלא הגיע זמנה לראות] (bNid 9b, 10b). The issue under debate is, therefore, a girl's potential menarche. In this context, the text is clearly made to deal with the question of from what point on a girl has to be careful in handling items related to the Temple requiring a status of ritual purity. Physical maturity that allows for the possibility of menarche is read as a ritual dividing point in the girl's life as to her potential status of im/purity.

The larger context in the Babylonian Talmud also clarifies what is meant by the heuristic category of a "presumptive status of purity." Essentially, those types of women who cannot and do not menstruate are presumed to be in a status of purity. Examples discussed in the early rabbinic texts are a girl before her menarche, a pregnant or nursing woman, or a woman after her menopause (mNid 1:3 ff; tNid 1:5 ff). If a woman is incapable of menstruating, or in rabbinic terms, in a "presumptive status of purity," she cannot render Temple-related food and other objects *retroactively* impure. In other words, when such a woman begins to menstruate her blood-flow is presumed to have started only at that point. It is not regarded to have begun at some earlier time without having come out. A "presumptive status of purity" as a halakhic or legal term, therefore, has relevance only for the (theoretical) issue of potential *retroactive impurity*, discussed above in Chapter 3.

Similarly, it may have relevance for the identification of a bloodstain as possibly deriving from menstrual blood, discussed above in Chapter 4. A stain of blood that is found in the vicinity of a woman in a "presumptive status of purity" does not establish a status of impurity or classify her as a menstruating woman, nor does it evoke a *retroactive status of impurity*.

In this context, the first part of the baraita suggests in the anonymous voice of the editor, an examination may be required. Upon reaching their "season," girls change their "presumptive status" regarding ritual purity. Having reached her "season," a girl is now considered to be in a "presumptive" status of *impurity*.[23] In other words, whereas before there would have been no concern about the girl's handling of Temple-related items, now there would be. The text, however, remains quite enigmatic as to the function of physical examination. The only aspect which the text is unambiguous about, both in its first anonymous part and in the second part attributed to Rabbi Yehudah, is that such a physical examination would be performed by "other women." This is an unquestioned assumption, mentioned almost in passing, without being discussed or questioned any further.

What, however, would the imagined function of the physical examination be? The connection between a girl's change of presumptive status and the requirement of examinations when she has reached menarche remains unclear. Rashi comments, in the Babylonian Talmud, on this baraita and on the reason why the girl's status is considered to change: "the assumption is that blood is likely to be in them" (bNid 10b, ד״ה בחזקת טומאה). Does he mean to say that we ought to think of girls once they have reached menarche as containers with a permanent presence of menstrual blood in their body, which is waiting to burst forth any minute?[24] How often then should girls be examined once they have reached menarche? These questions remain unanswered. The Meiri (1249–1306), a few generations after Rashi, deals with some of these questions. In his paraphrase of the baraita he smooths out some of its difficulties while adopting Rashi's commentary:

חזקת בנות ישראל עד שלא הגיעו לפרקן הרי אלו בחזקת טהרה ואין הנשים בודקות אותן אבל אם הגיעו לפרקן הרי אלו בחזקת דמים מצויים ונשים חוששות בהן לטהרות ובודקות אותן

Concerning the *presumptive status* of Israelite women—as long as they have not reached their "season" they are in the presumptive status of purity, and [other] women do not [need to] examine them. But when they [the girls] have reached their "season" *it is assumed that blood is likely to be in them* and [other] women are apprehensive with respect to the girl's [status] vis-à-vis the *taharot* [the food and objects related to the Temple service]. Therefore, they examine them. (*Beit ha-Behirah*, 38; emphasis added)

This comment circumvents the question of the girl's change of presumptive status of im/purity. He merely states that girls, from the time that they are physically capable of menarche onward, are considered to have some amount of menstrual blood in their bodies. Once a girl reaches such maturity, "[other] women" are concerned about her turning into a potential source of impurity with respect to Temple-related items. With this, the Meiri achieves two things: he clarifies the reference point of the discussion (that is, the Temple-related items) and, at the same time, in his rhetoric it is the other women who are apprehensive that the young girl might render the Temple-related items impure and therefore useless. This might be explained in that he imagines the women, priestly or not, to prepare the food-items for the Temple or the priests. Therefore, the women would be concerned about having the food-items being rendered useless. In the end the Meiri adds that "even if they [the girls] are not examined, the *taharot* are not rendered impure on their account based on [mere] doubt" [על ידן מספק אלא שאם לא נבדקו אין מטמאין טהרות] (ibid.). This statement appears as the Meiri's own attempt to relativize the significance of the examinations, against the text of the *baraita* in either the Talmud's or the Tosefta's versions. Based on this apprehension, women perform examinations. What kind of women?

Mothers? Experts? What kind of examinations? The projection of apprehension onto women is important when we think about the possibility of women's "spaces," since in the Meiri's formulation the women examiners are represented as the agents of rabbinic concerns. Women examiners of women's bodies do not automatically create a sovereign space for women, since the examination envisioned in this text has one specific purpose.

Let us turn to Rabbi Yehuda's objection in the last part of the baraita and to the description of the examination. Rabbi Yehuda refers only to the question of whether or not other women examine a girl once she has reached menarche. According to Rabbi Yehuda's opinion, other women do not examine the girl even once she has reached menarche. Instead, the girl performs a sort of self-examination by applying oil and wiping herself externally.

The version of the baraita offered by the Babylonian Talmud is somewhat different from the one cited above. One can only speculate whether it interprets or has a different tradition:

רבי יהודה אומר אין בודקין אותן ביד מפני שמעוותות אותן אלא סכות אותן בשמן מבפנים ומקנחות אותן מבחוץ והן נבדקות מאיליהן

Rabbi Yehuda objects: They must not examine them with their *hands*, because they might corrupt them. Rather, they oil them internally and wipe them externally, and (thus) they are examined by themselves.[25] (bNid 10b; emphasis added)

Here Rabbi Yehuda agrees that other women need to examine the girl once she has reached her menarche. His disagreement lies in the procedure of the examination. Thus, Rabbi Yehuda emphasizes that women may not examine the girls with their hands, since—as Rashi comments—"they might scratch them with their fingernail and cause them to bleed" (bNid 10b, ד"ה שמעוותות), either from a premature menstrual flow or the internal wound. The internal application of oil is supposed to be some kind of proof of the existence of menstrual blood, for if she had menstrual blood stored in her internal organs, the oil, according to Rashi, would cause the flow to start.[26] Thus, according to Rabbi Yehuda the procedure of oiling and wiping is a subset of such a "gynecological" examination.

Ultimately, what we can conclude here is that the baraita's assumption is that women execute these examinations of women's bodies, whether it is other women or whether it is the girls who are taught how to examine themselves. There is no question of presupposition here. Women's bodies are women's territory. This territory is not necessarily "sovereign" territory, since the girls are submitted to a potentially invasive procedure, and the women examiners in this case are envisioned as pursuing a very specific primary purpose: to protect Temple-related items from ritual impurity.

Another slight change in rhetoric in this version of the baraita in the Babylonian Talmud teaches us something else about a consciousness in the text about this potentially sovereign women's territory, in which women could relate to women, unmediated by male relationships. As to the reason women may not examine girls with their hands, the Talmud formulates: "because they might corrupt them." Against Rashi's reading of the verb as doing merely physical damage, this verb in most other biblical and tannaitic contexts connotes "moral" corruption.[27] Is the anxiety behind the choice of this verb about women's self-gratification, that is, about older women possibly teaching younger girls about masturbatory pleasures? This reading would remind us of the Greek anxiety about women doctors, for Ann Ellis Hanson mentions that "many ancient writers outside medicine disparage the women's tradition and what 'woman say to each other' (witness Semonides' poem on women and the tirades Euripides put in the mouth of Hermione in his play *Andromakhe*), implying that an older woman destroys a younger's sexual innocence and recalling the common male assumption that the subject matter of γυναικεῖα (*gynaeikeia*, 'women's things') is sex" ("The Medical Writers' Women," 309). Women may teach women about women's desires, and thus "corrupt" them.[28] The Babylonian Talmud does imagine the requirement of examination as a potential site of the emergence of some form of subversive collective gender identity. Thus, the baraita formulates rules designed to undermine such a possibility, and to restrain women (examiners) strictly to their roles as agents of rabbinic concerns.

### A Rabbinic Indagatio Corporis (Physical Inspection)

Another baraita, which deserves to be quoted in full, will lead us one step further. The context of this text is not the question of ritual impurity, but marital law. In distinction to the previous text this discussion would have had practical applicability for the rabbis of the second century C.E., and would not merely present an exercise in legal theory. The baraita requires physical examinations in cases when a young woman is to be married off and it is doubtful whether she is halakhically a minor or an adult. Again, the פרק or "season" is the dividing line between the two stages. In this case, however, the referent of "season" is not a girl's menarche, as in the previous text, but her twelfth year of age.[29] Here the rabbis devise an "objective," or static category. During her twelfth year a girl is in a liminal stage between legal minority and adulthood.

Strangely, however, the Mishnah also devises another category for the determination of adulthood. The rabbis discuss the physical symptoms of puberty as indications of physiological transition. The two indicators, the first of which applies to both boys and girls (mNid 6:11), whereas the second is gender-specific, are the appearance of pubic hair (mNid 5:9, 6:1, 6:11–12; tNid 6:2–7) and the growth of a girl's breasts (mNid 5:8; tNid 6:4). The pubic hair is referred to as the "lower sign," whereas breasts are referred to as the "upper sign." From a certain angle, the introduction of these signs can be read as a symptom of the rabbis' recognition that chronological age does not exhaustively define adulthood. Rather, what the signs try to address is the fact that the growth of human bodies does not follow a mechanism of chronology, but obeys individualized codes of nature not easily captured in legal discourse.[30] Thus the two categories of determining adulthood—factual, chronological age and the signs of puberty—are in conflict with each other while the rabbis attempt to superimpose the systems.[31] Again, the language of bodies is not easily translated into the language of law, and the rabbis develop a complex hermeneutics of the former in order to make it accessible to the latter.

At the same time, the rabbis of the Mishnah do not invent the signs of human maturation. In their cultural environment, Roman law similarly attempted to describe and categorize physical signs of puberty as an indicator of legal adulthood. Roman law knew an examination of children's bodies for signs of physical maturity as *indagatio corporis*, which was legally abrogated by Justinian around 530 C.E. (Preuss, *Biblical and Talmudic Medicine*, 128).Whether the rabbis knew specific Roman laws can perhaps not be proven, but we do see the rabbis participating in a legal discourse on human bodies shared by other cultures in the world of late antiquity.

We find in the third century collection of the Tosefta a text that presents a theoretical discussion as to the potential examination of a girl's body:

כל הנבדקות אינן נבדקות אלא בנשים
וכך היה ר׳ אליעזר מוסר לאשתו ור׳ ישמעאל מוסר לאמו
ר׳ יהודה אומר לפני הפרק ולאחר הפרק נשים בודקות אותן תוך הפרק אין
הנשים בודקות אותן שאין משיאין ספיקות על פי נשים
ר׳ שמעון אומר אף תוך הפרק נאמנת אשה להחמיר אבל לא להקל נאמנת
אשה לומר קטנה היא שלא תחלוץ וגדולה היא שלא תמאן אבל אין נאמנת
לומר קטנה היא שתמאן וגדולה היא שתחלוץ
אמר ר׳ אלעזר בר׳ צדוק כשהיו בית דין בודקין ביבנה כיון שמוציאין בעליון
אין משגיחין על התחתון

All those women that are to be examined are only examined by women.

Thus Rabbi Eliezer used to transfer [physical examinations] to his wife and Rabbi Ishma'el transferred [them] to his mother.

Rabbi Yehuda[32] says: before the "season" [the girl's twelfth year] and after the "season" women examine them, during the "season" women do not examine them, because "they" do not let girls who are in doubtful status, marry on account of [the testimony of] women.

[Spelled out, this means] the woman is believed to say that she [the girl examined] is [still] a minor and thus cannot perform *halitzah*.[33] [She is also believed to testify that the girl is already an] adult, so that she cannot protest, but she is not believed [if she] says that she [the girl examined] is a [still a] minor so that she can [still] protest,[34] or [already] an adult so that she can perform *halitzah*.

Said Rabbi El'azar the son of Zaddoq: When the court of Yavneh [!] used to perform examinations—they would not look for the lower sign once they found the upper one. (Tosefta 6:8–9, cp. bNid 48b)

The baraita on the examinations of women for corporeal signs of puberty opens with the general principle that all women are to be examined by women. When a girl's legal status as an adult is in doubt, the determination of her status depends on such an examination or *indagatio corporis*, as to the signs of physical maturity. There is no parallel or equivalent articulation of a principle for the examination of boys, here or anywhere else.[35] Apparently, the rabbis did not see the need to verbalize such a principle. The examination of boys did not raise a question, whereas the case of women did raise such a question. Is that self-evident? If it is considered to be self-evident it does tell us something about the gendered self-awareness of the editor. The very articulation of a principle in the case of women reveals the rhetorical gendering of the editor as male.

The text continues with citing the practice of two famous rabbis, seemingly as a corroboration of the general principle indicated by the copula: "*Thus* (וכך) Rabbi Eliezer used to transfer [physical examinations] to his wife and Rabbi Ishma'el transferred [them] to his mother."[36] A closer reading shows that in the process of the discussion the general principle is gradually restricted. The citation of Rabbi Eliezer's and Rabbi Ishma'el's practice of delegating examinations presents a first step. We learn that Rabbi Eliezer and Rabbi Ishma'el entrust these examinations to a wife and a mother. In rabbinic tradition both are known as particularly virtuous women.[37] Rabbi Eliezer's wife is Imma Shalom, one of the few women mentioned by name in the Talmud (for example, in bB.M.59b and bNed 20 a–b). She is praised both by the rabbis of the Talmud themselves and contemporary Jewish feminists. The implicit rhetorical force of this statement is that these examinations are not entrusted to just any women, but only to particularly praiseworthy and therefore reliable women. The significance becomes obvious if we consider the halakhic trajectory. According to Maimonides, for instance, בודקין על פי נשים כשרות ונאמנות—"they (the rabbis) examine them (the girls) on the authority of proper and reliable women" (Mishneh Torah, Hilkhot 'Ishut 2:20).[38] As soon as the general category "woman" is restricted by such qualifiers, more control is given into the hands of the legislators to be selective about the kind of women they can choose to entrust with the examinations. Decoding the implied gender, we can interpret the text in the following manner: "We (the male experts) have to rely on women's examinations of girls. Therefore, we will not trust just any women, but women who are trained (by us) and women who are trustworthy (to us)."

A further step in the baraita is to restrict the actual legal relevance of the examination by women. According to Rabbi Yehuda women examine girls both before and after the "season"—the year during which signs of puberty are expected and can legally render the girl an adult. It is not quite clear, however, why women would have to examine the girls before and after the year. In fact, Rashi comments that "even if [the girl's body before the פרק] has produced [the two pubic hairs] they are considered to be a mole, and she is a minor, nonetheless" (bNid 48b, ad loc.), and, Rashi continues: "[lemma:]

'women examine them'—for whether *they* (the examining women) say that *they* (the girls) have (grown pubic hairs) or whether *they* say that *they* have not—*we* assume *her* (the examinee) to be in the status of minority, and do not rely on *them* [that is, the women's testimony]." The pronouns are confusing, and Rashi's comments could also be read as referring to the girls: "for whether the girls say that they have grown the hairs or whether they say they have not—we assume *her* to be in the status of minority and do not rely on the girls' testimony." Though this might seem to make more sense of Rashi's reasoning, it does not entirely explain the change of pronouns within his comment. The same applies to the time after the girl's twelfth year: whether she has grown pubic hair or not, she would legally be considered an adult. Again, Rashi comments that "if they [the examining women] say that two pubic hairs exist, they are believed [ . . . ] because they are expected to be there, but if they say that the two pubic hairs do not exist [ . . . ] because we suspect that they fell off. Hence, we do not rely on the testimony of women."[39] Rashi's comment, therefore, spells out that regardless what the women's testimony as to the girl's physical signs of maturity is, the self-consciously gendered "we" of the rabbinic collectivity ultimately interpret the evidence. Women's testimony in these cases, even though theoretically legitimized, is practically rendered superfluous, because there are theoretical principles that override, reinterpret, or even interpret away the empirical evidence testified to by the women. If the status of the girl is determined to be that of minor or that of legal adult regardless of the signs of physical maturity, which can somewhat arbitrarily be reinterpreted, the question remains why Rabbi Yehuda would even say that women may examine them.[40]

The critical period that remains is the "season" itself, during which the appearance of the two pubic hairs would change the status of the girl from minor to fully accountable by law. According to Rabbi Yehuda, women do not examine the girls during the "season." This can be understood in two ways: it could mean that she is not examined by others at all, but performs self-examination, which is an unlikely reading. Or it could mean that those-who-are-not-women perform the physical examination, presumably male judges. The latter interpretation seems to be the stronger one, especially in view of the conclusion of Rabbi Yehuda's opinion.[41] It appears to be obvious that by raising the issue of women's testimony, Rabbi Yehuda implies that with respect to physical examinations during the period in question, he finds only men's testimony acceptable. This reading is corroborated by the end of the baraita, since here it is the court of Yavneh "who used to perform the examinations."[42]

According to the opinion of Rabbi Shim'on's opinion, cited next, women's testimony is regarded as trustworthy enough to perform an indagatio corporis even during the girl's twelfth year, her "season," when the signs of physical maturity are effective as to the determination of the status of the girl: "Rabbi Shim'on says: Even during the "season" the woman [who examines] is believed." The one rather significant restriction is, of course, that woman's testimony is only regarded as trustworthy if it induces a stricter ruling for the examinee: "[but only] to [effect] the stricter ruling, but not to [effect] the more lenient ruling." Strictness means that a girl remains bound to the obligation of levirate marriage, and is not released. A decision to enable leniency would effect her release. It seems that now we have come full circle and the initial general ruling is completely reversed and overturned.[43] What starts out as possibly suggesting an unqualified if likely reluctant reliance on women's examinations of women is brought back into the control of (male) rabbinic supervision.

One may conjecture that the discomfort of the rabbis with the general principle of women examining women, of women reading women's bodies, is that it has the potential to create a space for women that is not under rabbinic control. The subsequent restrictions of the principle, introduced as the baraita evolves, create more access for the rabbis' control into this relatively autonomous space for women.

Furthermore, it is significant to note that implied in these restrictions there is a suspicion of some form of women's solidarity. Rabbi Yehuda discounts women's testimony altogether, at least during the crucial period. Rabbi Shim'on, in spite of accepting the theoretical reliability of women's reading of women's bodies, does not allow them to give testimony for the girl to the effect that the more lenient rulings could apply to her. He rules a priori that their testimony is accepted only to induce the stricter ruling. But why are women not considered trustworthy in their testimony on behalf of other women? The issue clearly does not concern their abilities to recognize the signs of physical maturity. Rather, the suspicion appears to be that women might give a "gender-biased" testimony on behalf of the girl intended to protect her. The text then tries to rule out such a possibility.

## A Moment of Gendered Self-Criticism

Finally, the Babylonian Talmud includes a passage that reflects on the gender politics involved in the issue of physical examinations. This is one of the texts that places in the foreground some of those cultural energies spent to erect rabbinic notions of masculinity versus femininity, of male control versus female autonomy. The context is again the discussion of physical symptoms of puberty, this time much more problematically. Here, the focus is on the "upper sign" of a girl's physical maturity, the breasts. The rabbinic discussions of pubic hair may strike one as extremely invasive, as is the nature of forensic medicine in general. The impact of this language is softened by the fact that it applies, at least in theory, to both girls and boys. The rabbis do not subject only girls to their imaginary *indagatio corporis*, but boys as well. The invasiveness of a (rabbinic) court applies to both genders. In the context of the rabbinic attempt to translate the development of women's breasts into legal discourse, however, invasiveness does not adequately describe the rhetoric. The Mishnah's description of the development of women's breasts (mNid 5:9) as the sign of physical maturity is one of the more problematic texts concerning women. As with the flow of blood and women's bodies in general, the rabbis try to devise "objective" criteria to describe physical growth.

This disturbing mishnah has been read as a rabbinic form of pornography, due to its detailed fantasy of the shape of the breast and the nipple (Rachel Biale, *Women and Jewish Law*, 65). To apply a modern phenomenon to the rabbinic text of the late second century C.E. may be problematic, especially since the rabbis create a textual body only. However, imaginary or real, Biale is right in capturing the male gaze at the woman's body as object. This is again reminiscent of Boyarin's argument that "the House of Study was ... the rabbinic Jewish equivalent of the locker room" (*Unheroic Conduct*, 143). But these criteria are based on observation of the breast, and the observers are the rabbis. In this attempt the rabbis in the Mishnah make the reader or student gaze at female breasts through the implied eye of the text. The discursive objectification of women's bodies here brings the problem of the gender of the text to the foreground. In this context the Babylonian Talmud offers the following story:

ואיזהו סימנים ר' יוסי הגלילי אומר משיעלה הקמט שמואל אמר לא משיעלה
הקמט ממש אלא כדי שתחזיר ידיה לאחוריה ונראית כמי שיעלה הקמט

תחת הדד שמואל בדק באמתיה ויהב לה ד' זוזי דמי בושתה שמואל לטעמיה
דאמר שמואל לעולם בהם תעבודו לעבודה נתתים ולא לבושה

[The Mishnah asks]: What are the signs [of a *bogeret*, a legally mature woman]? R. Yossi the Galilean says: [She is a *bogeret*] from the time a wrinkle appears [under the girl's breast]. Shmu'el[44] said: Not from the time the wrinkle actually appeared, but if, when putting her hands behind it [the breast], it seems as if the wrinkle appeared. Shmu'el examined his female slave and paid her four zuz compensation for the shame. Shmu'el thereby followed his principle, for Shmu'el stated: "These [the non-Israelite slaves] you may put to work forever" (Lev. 25:46).[45] [That is] I [God] have given them to you for *work* but not [to be subjected] to shame. (bNid 47a)

Shmu'el wants to test his "theory," or perhaps more adequately put, his fantasy, on the female body directly. Here we have again an illustration of how the rabbis in the Talmud imagine the learning of the Mishnah, as in the scene at the bloodletter's house discussed in Chapter 3. In this story, two sociocultural vectors intersect. The treatment of slaves stands in the foreground of Shmu'el's examination, for the story continues with the account of how different rabbis controlled and regulated their slaves' sex lives. Shmu'el stands out as treating his slaves as his fellow human beings. The story's point is to show that according to Shmu'el the function of slaves is primarily to work, but on every other level—such as sexual morals—they are to be treated like any other human being.[46] Clearly, however, gender politics provides a second vector to the narrative. To verify his hypothesis on the development of women's breasts Shmu'el subjects the woman in her nakedness to his gaze, subjects her to "shame."[47] As in the story of the boiled prostitute, a type of woman who is socially instrumentalized is employed for the narrative. I propose to read "her shame" here not so much as the rabbis' psychocultural problem with women's naked bodies, as one might easily be tempted to do. Rather, the terminology indicates that the Babylonian Talmud regards Shmu'el's experiment as an act of improper intrusion. Thus in our narrative "her shame" is really his act of shaming her, for which he has to pay his due. In this sense then the story is not really an example showing how the Mishnah is learned but rather a reprimand, telling how it should *not* be learned. Whether Shmu'el ever really used his female slave as a guinea pig or not is immaterial. The rhetorical effect of the story is to suggest that in spite of the passage in this Mishnah which attempts to turn women's breast development into halakhic data, the Talmud indicates a recognition of the problematic mishnaic text. Shmu'el, after all, does not refrain from performing his experiment, but this is not evaluated as a good or even acceptable way of "learning Mishnah." In this case the object of mishnaic fantasy cannot be translated onto women's bodies external to the text.

**Women's Somatic Sovereignty?**

Shmu'el's act of shaming is a crucial one in the analysis of the rabbinic attempt to extend the control of the legal discourse onto women's bodies and into potential women's space. We have seen throughout this chapter examples of the Talmud's tendency to exclude the possibility of men examining women's bodies. Where the Tosefta's textual version is sometimes ambiguous, the talmudic editors emend the text on women's examination to clarify their own position that examinations, where required, are always performed by women. With the narrative of Shmu'el's experiment the Babylonian Talmud critiques the violation of this implicit cultural assumption.

The primary cultural factor influencing the imagining of women as the readers of women's bodies and men as the interpreters of such readings is the rabbbinic notion of "modesty." Throughout the Talmud we find texts that uphold modesty or abstention from potential sources of sexual arousal for men.[48] Based on this cultural notion, the Talmud *can* imagine only women as readers of women's bodies. At the same time, it creates the theoretical possibility of women's space that is not under the male gaze. The texts we have analyzed indicate an awareness of this possibility and the implications thereof. The imperative of "modesty" conflicts with the desire to control, discursively and institutionally, women's bodies.

We did observe how rabbinic legal culture tries to control discursively that which it maintains as a separate space. In some of the texts we have seen how the opinions of individual rabbis differed as to when other women should examine women and when they should not. In the context of determining whether women had reached the age of legal adulthood we could detect discomfort concerning the fact that women should be relied on as readers of women's bodies. Other halakhic principles come into play, such as the trustworthiness of witnesses. Finally, legal standards are offered that attempt to curb the relevance of physical examinations altogether. Testimonies have to support a preset standard of judgment, or an absolute age of legal maturity is determined. If we read the rabbinic text symptomatically we may observe a considerable degree of discomfort with women's reading of women's bodies in legally crucial contexts. We may argue that this discomfort betrays a rabbinic recognition of the potential power of conceptual spaces which are in the control of women. The discursive process of delegitimizing and displacing women's reading of women's bodies is part of the process of establishing the rabbis as experts on women's bodies and the ultimate authorities for women to consult.[49]

## A Woman's Voice in the Talmud? The Case of Abaye's Mother

Having dealt with texts that discuss who is imagined to perform physical examinations on the female body, I turn now to the second kind of question introduced at the beginning of this chapter—whether it is possible to trace the existence of women healers. To this purpose, I have selected a set of texts in which a woman's voice is cited as an *authoritative* voice in matters of healing, general medical advice, and, specifically, midwifery. Throughout the Babylonian Talmud we repeatedly find statements in which Abaye, one of the leading rabbis in Babylon during the early fourth century, quotes his mother. All of these statements are introduced with the formulaic אמר אביי אמרה לי אם—"Abaye said: My mother told me...."

In bKid 31b we read the following: "Rabbi Yohanan said: Happy is he who has not seen them [his parents, because] Rabbi Yohanan's father died when his mother was pregnant with him, and his mother died when she bore him. And similarly Abaye. But is that so? Did not Abaye say: 'Mother told me'? That was his foster-mother."[50] In the context of the sugyah the hyperbolic statement of the first part of this text is to indicate how difficult it is to carry out the commandment to honor one's parents. Therefore Rabbi Yohanan can find good in his tragedy. This text is important, however, because it shows that at a certain point in the editorial evolution of the talmudic text the collection of Abaye's mother's medical advice stood out to the later talmudic editors in a significant enough way to serve as a text-immanent corrective. The text in bKid 31b reports the death of Abaye's mother at his birth. An anonymous editorial voice questions this report and refers to the literary formula put into Abaye's mouth elsewhere in the Talmud: "Mother told me. . . ." The answer to this difficulty is that this oft-cited statement should be understood figuratively, and that Abaye really refers to the woman who raised him, and who educated him in these matters.

This repeated citation of a woman's voice is unique within rabbinic literature. Naturally, one of the building blocks of rabbinic literature is the citation of an earlier authority, sometimes in the form of tracing a long line of teachers who pass on a tradition. However, the form of citation in our case is somewhat unique, since the common form of citation in the Babylonian Talmud is אמר . . . אמר . . . ( . . . אמר), "Rabbi X said in the name of Rabbi Y (who said in the name of Rabbi Z)," rather than אמר. . . אמר ה לי/, "Rabbi X said: Rabbi Y told *me*." From a literary point of view Abaye's citation of his "mother" as an authority is an exceptional phenomenon in the Talmud, not necessarily in a positive sense, since the two formulas each have a different authoritative weight. The former contributes to the collective [male] character of rabbinic literature. A tradition or a specific interpretation of a biblical or mishnaic text is passed on from teacher to student and again to the student of the subsequent generation. This chain of tradition, therefore, establishes the collective community of interpretation. Against this, the individualized form of the latter formula—"Abaye said: My mother told *me*"—interrupts the collective form. The text could have said אמר אביי אמרה אמו—"Abaye said *in the name of* his mother," which might have established her as a regular member of the interpretive collective. In not doing so the text may attempt to circumscribe the authority of Abaye's mother to a more personalized "family" tradition.

This marginalization of the woman's voice is continued and even intensified in modern critical scholarship; it has been largely disregarded by scholars. For instance, Julius Preuss treats it somewhat casually as a representative of "popular" or "folk" medicine, or as the generic *vox populi*: "However, the majority of medical statements in the Talmud belong to folk medicine. The most prominent representative thereof is Abaye with his innumerable prescriptions that he had heard from his nursemaid or mother" (*Biblical and Talmudic Medicine*, 21). For Preuss this folk tradition is but a step in the cultural evolution, as he constructs it, from faith via superstition to knowledge. Thus, in his monumental attempt to show the distinction that the Talmud makes between what Preuss himself deems to be either scientific or superstitious therapies, he does indeed deal with the therapies that

Abaye's mother suggests, but mostly only in order to cite the *vox populi*. It is then interesting, though typical for his generation of scholars, to see how differently he treats similarly "superstitious" therapies when they are suggested by a rabbi with halakhic authority, rather than by Abaye's mother.[51] His distinction between folk tradition and high culture is a product of nineteenth-century positivist science. It is unwarranted when applied to talmudic literature, and only serves to doubly silence women's voices.[52]

Because of its singularity, this little corpus within the Babylonian Talmud can be taken more seriously as a uniquely authoritative woman's voice. Although already the talmudic text circumscribes the authority of Abaye's mother, it is possible to reverse the continuous process of her marginalization. On the one hand, the rabbinic strategies of marginalizing women's voices are present here; on the other hand, Abaye's mother does speak and is identified as a woman speaker. The goal of foregrounding the corpus of Abaye's mother is to preserve and even strengthen the heterogeneity of talmudic literature and culture. I can, however, admittedly not claim, in the following pages, that among the rabbis of the fourth century Abaye's mother had more importance than has hitherto been acknowledged. This we cannot know.

Abaye's mother is cited only in the Babylonian Talmud.[53] Sometimes we find only one single short phrase in her name within a larger text unit, sometimes we find a small anthology of statements on one page. Within the framework of this chapter, I discuss the collection of her wisdom on infant care, which at the same time presents the largest collection of her remedies in one place.

## A Woman's Manual of Infant Care

In the context of the following anthology the Mishnah deals with the halakhic problem of circumcision that falls on Shabbat. It prescribes that עושין כל צרכי מילה בשבת—one is allowed to perform all those actions connected with circumcision on Shabbat, such as excision, tearing, and sucking (the wound) which would normally be prohibited (mShab 19:2). The Mishnah tries to distinguish between those actions which are strictly related to matters of the physical well-being of the child and would therefore override the prohibition of labor, including certain kinds of healing, on

Shabbat and those actions which are *not* directly related to matters of health and could therefore be postponed. In its commentary on this issue in the Mishnah, the Babylonian Talmud presents very detailed material on medical questions—material that is unique to the Babylonian Talmud:

> We place a compress[54] on it [the wound of the circumcision]:
> Abaye said: Mother told me: a compress for all [kinds of] pain [is made of] seven parts of fat and one of wax.[55] Rava said: wax and resin.... (bShab 133b)

[Mishnah-lemma]: One may not make a חלוק [a shirt-shaped bandage pulled over the circumcised penis like a sheath] for him [the baby boy, if he is circumcised on Shabbat] from scratch, but instead one wraps a rag around it [the penis].

[Gemara:]

1. Abaye said: Mother told me: The חלוק for a baby should be turned outwards lest one of its threads might stick and the baby might be mutilated in its urinary canal.[56] Abaye's mother used to make a lining for half [of the חלוק]....

2. Abaye also said: Mother told me: A baby whose anus is not visible should be rubbed with oil and sit for one day; then, where it appears transparent it should be torn crosswise with a barley grain, but not with a metal instrument, because that causes inflammation.

3. Abaye also said: Mother told me: A baby who cannot suck, his lips are cold. What is the remedy? A vessel with glowing coals should be brought and held near his mouth, for this will warm his mouth and he will suck.

4. Abaye also said: Mother told me: A baby who does not breathe,[57] should be fanned with a fan, and he will breathe.

5. Abaye also said: Mother told me: A baby who cannot breathe easily,[58] his mother's placenta should be brought and rubbed over him, and he will breathe easily.

6. Abaye also said: Mother told me: A baby who is too thin, his mother's placenta should be brought and rubbed over him from its narrow end to its wide end; and if he is too fat, from the wide end to the narrow end.

7. Abaye also said: Mother told me: If a baby is too red, so that the

blood is not yet absorbed in him, we must wait until his blood is absorbed and then circumcise him. If a baby is green, so that he is deficient in blood, we must wait until he is full-blooded and then circumcise him. (bShabbat 134a)

This anthology on infant care stands out in the Babylonian Talmud. The discussions leave behind the original mishnaic context, for we are no longer dealing with the question of permissible actions on Shabbat but with infant care in and of itself. This anthology reads like a collection of recipes and remedies, in a pedagogical style reminiscent of the Greco-Roman gynecologists.[59] However, upon comparing the instructive styles some significant differences emerge. Soranus, for example, remains hidden as the author of his treatise. He erects his medical instruction on the anonymous and therefore absolutizing truth of his authority: " . . . one *must* swaddle the newborn . . . one *must* mould every part according to its natural shape . . . *the midwife should* put the newborn down gently in her lap" (Temkin, *Soranus' Gynecology*, 84). This is apodictic instruction: disembodied instruction that seeks to establish itself as nonderivative authority. On this authority Soranus, or rather the omniscient, paternal voice of science, displaces the authority of the women whose instructor he seeks to become:

the majority of the women practising midwifery approve of the section [of the umbilical cord] by means of glass, a reed, a potsherd, or the thin crust of bread; or by forcefully squeezing it apart with a cord, since during the earliest period, cutting with iron is deemed of ill omen. *This is absolutely ridiculous.* (Temkin, *Soranus' Gynecology*, 81; emphasis added)[60]

In our talmudic passage, on the other hand, Abaye declares the source of his knowledge on midwifery. His is a derivative knowledge that does not conceal its maternal origin. This maternal knowledge finds its place as such in talmudic literature.

Nonetheless, I think it is possible to observe how even in rabbinic culture the authority of Abaye's mother's wisdom is impinged upon, albeit by employing entirely different textual strategies. Even among the numerous other traditions of Abaye's mother preserved in the Babylonian Talmud, the manual on infant care displays unparalleled traits. This is the most extensive anthology of her recipes. But also she is quoted here as an authority, without being preceded or followed by the citation of a parallel remedy or incantation by one of the rabbis.[61]

It is also important to note that the Talmud does not simply evoke her as a spokesperson on women's issues or midwifery, but notes that she has competence in other areas as well. Had she been cited only in matters of infant care we could have read this as indicating that for the rabbis midwifery is merely a woman's field of expertise, an inferior one, that is, and that only because of this a woman is permitted to speak in the chorus of the collective literature. However, this is not the case. The Babylonian Talmud does not regard these instructions as an inferior field of knowledge. Obviously, it does not have the same status as halakhic discussions. Nonetheless, these instructions do not belong to an inferior ontological realm, as Preuss's epistemology would have us believe. The talmudic text itself betrays its desire to incorporate this woman's wisdom as (male) rabbinic expertise, beyond mere citation. For our manual continues by "citing" a baraita, a "rabbinic" type of text with more weight of authority than the recipes of Abaye's mother or any of her contemporaries by mere generational precedence.

> A. Rabbi Nathan[62] said: I once went to the sea-towns, and a woman came before me who had circumcised her first son[63] and he had died, and her second son and he had died; the third she brought before me. Seeing that he was red I said to her: Wait until his blood is absorbed. So she waited until his blood was absorbed and then circumcised him and he lived; and they used to call him Nathan the Babylonian after my name.
> B. On another occasion I visited the province of Cappadocia, and a woman came before me who had circumcised her first son and he had died, and her second son and he had died; the third she brought before me. Seeing that he was green, I examined him and saw no covenant blood in him. I said to her, Wait until he is full-blooded; she waited and then circumcised him and he lived, and they called him Nathan the Babylonian, after my name. (bShab134a; cp. tShab 15:8)[64]

Normally, the literary structure of the connection between the list of Abaye's mother and the baraita would indicate that at least the last remedy in the list merely represents a condensation of the earlier tannaitic story. The woman's voice would then merely announce and formulate as a general rule that which the tannaitic rabbi has already performed authoritatively. In this case, however, I think that this common reading of the literary structure can be turned on its head. That is, in all the extant textual parallels we can only find the second part of the baraita, the case of the green baby.[65] Therefore, one can argue that here actually the first part of the baraita is a later, perhaps amoraic, composition, following the narrative pattern of the second part, in response to the recipe of Abaye's mother regarding the red and green babies.

The point of this is not to make a claim about which of the textual elements precedes the other diachronically, but rather to lay bare the gender politics that are involved on the level of the composition of the text. If the first part of the baraita can be read as the secondary text, then the male hero merely institutes what the maternal voice has just offered as remedy. In simplified terms, the editorial process could be imagined to be somewhat like the following: Since the second part of the baraita is indeed an earlier authoritative text, the editors know the earlier story of Rabbi Nathan and the green baby. But they also know the list of remedies of Abaye's mother. They put together the earlier text and the amoraic discussions since the green baby links the two of them. In addition, they compose the first part of our baraita: the case of Rabbi Nathan and the red baby. They may have stylistic reasons for this. They want to compose a parallel of the red and the green baby in both textual elements. But from the vantage point of gender politics this reconstructed editorial process assumes an additional dimension. It suggests that the editors may have wanted to diminish the maternal authority of Abaye's mother. By composing the first part of the baraita, her voice seems to turn into that of Rabbi Nathan's "apprentice" rather than that of an autonomous instructor.

Again, we can briefly follow the trajectory of these text-internal dynamics of displacement. In the major medieval commentaries and halakhic codices, such as the Tosafists, this manual is passed over in silence, primarily because it does not present a halakhic controversy. Isaac ben Jacob Alfasi (1013–1103) whose digest of talmudic law became a classic of early post-talmudic scholarship, as well as Rabeinu Asher and the Meiri (1249–1306), quote the baraita of Rabbi Nathan but never mention Abaye's mother. That is not to say that the medieval halakhic literature necessarily excluded Abaye's mother because she is merely a woman. But even if the primary purpose of the codifiers was to condense the talmudic discussions, the discursive effect of their selectiveness is still the exclusion of the medical woman's voice from the stage of debate. Thus we can observe a process of progressive marginalization of Abaye's mother in rabbinic discourse.

∽

Let me take issue one last time with that which the nineteenth-century *Science of Judaism* regarded as diminishing the status of the Babylonian Talmud. These scholars considered it to be a weakness of the Babylonian rabbis to have come so intensely under the spell of popular or folk culture. In the spirit of their time the scholars of the nineteenth century made the fundamental distinction between high and low culture, where high culture is that which transcends low culture, and low culture is that which aspires to high culture. That the later halakhic literature silences Abaye's mother and preserves Rabbi Nathan as the authority can be regarded as a process of cultural rationalization.

From a feminist perspective, however, this process reads more like a process of disembodiment. The later halakhic process of codification and systematization, by purging itself from the materiality of talmudic discourse, suppresses the many embodied voices that gave birth to it. We could ascribe this desire for "cultural disembodiment" just as appropriately to nineteenth-century Jewish scholarship, manifesting itself in different ways. These scholars inscribe their scheme of high and low culture into the talmudic discourse and then regard the survival of the "lore of the masses" as more or less an accident of the discourse, but not as part of its essence.[66]

A strategy of cultural reembodiment of the Talmud, then, is to give loudspeakers to those suppressed or marginalized voices, of which Abaye's mother is one. I read her texts as a woman's voice, and I would challenge a notion of a monolithically male-authored culture in the case of rabbinic literature. Against such a view one could argue, as David Halperin did for the figure of Diotima in Plato's Symposium, that since Abaye's mother is not a woman but a "woman," a literary construction rather than a representation of a woman, it would no longer make any sense to insist on her gender. In Halperin's words: "For 'woman,' too, turns out to be a trope: in the representational economy of Plato's text (as elsewhere), 'woman' is always a sign of something else—of a spurious sexual 'difference' that men (as they see themselves) at once lack and possess. Nothing in herself, 'woman' is that pseudo-Other who both makes good what men want and exempts men from wanting anything at all; she is an alternate made identity whose constant accessibility to men lends men a fullness and totality that enables them to dispense (supposedly) with otherness altogether. ... from the perspective of the male world, at least, there is no such thing as authentic femininity. 'Woman,' and 'man' are figures of male speech" ("Why Is Diotima a Woman," 296). Against the application of this argument to the case of Abaye's mother, I would uphold the difference between Plato and the Talmud, between Diotima and Abaye's mother: on the one hand, the individual male author creates the woman of his desire. On the other hand, the Talmud as collective literature is primarily a citational literature. It quotes the traditions of the many who participate in it. Even though the overwhelming majority of speaking participants are men, we should not single out the one woman's voice as the only one not "quoted" but the mere product of male speech.

Nonetheless, what the survival of the wisdom of Abaye's mother comes to demonstrate is not so much the inclusiveness of talmudic discourse, which could sound ironic in view of the fact that even Abaye's mother's voice is mediated through her son's voice. Rather, it is a symptom of the tension within the androcentric universe of rabbinic culture. In the first part of the chapter we have traced those incidents in which women's bodies are examined in various forensic contexts. What has emerged is that it is indeed primarily women who examine women's bodies and who have access to women's bodies. This does not mean that women necessarily were in solidarity with each other against the male elite. But we have seen that at times the texts betray a discomfort with the fact that this creates a discursive and cultural space to which men have no access. The texts then attempt to project indirect means of control over that space, though it has to remain entirely uncertain how far this projection reflected back into practical life. At the same time Abaye's mother may be just one among many women who were considered health-care experts, especially that of infants. The citation of her medicinal recipes may be merely a fragment of her knowledge, and her voice mediated through her son may be merely a fragment of the voice of that wisdom that resounded through the oral culture from which rabbinic literature emerged. On this we can only speculate. But where we stand to trace and rebuild the various gendered spaces within the androcentric world of rabbinic texts that attempt to talk and write about women's bodies, she becomes an important foundation on which to imagine such spaces.

## 6 MENSTRUAL POLITICS IN EARLY CHRISTIAN LITERATURE

IN THIS FINAL CHAPTER I will turn to the Christian discourse on menstrual practices and its implication for women as embodied subjects in early Christianity. My interest in Christian menstrual politics is largely a comparative interest; the emerging cultures of rabbinic Judaism and Christianity define themselves in relation to the same collection of sacred texts, though Christian discourse often does so with greater incertitude and ambiguity. As historical, cultural, and textual foundation of both rabbinic Judaism and Christianity, those sacred texts require continuing interpretation. Both cultures produce interpretations of the same texts, largely independently, while laying a claim to revealing the texts' inherent significance, what they really are about.

At the same time these cultures differed tremendously in their hermeneutic appropriation of the sacred texts. The Christian discourse built its communal self-understanding in part from a source of hermeneutic authority separate from the texts: the Christ-event. The Christ-event in itself, however, required interpretation, which, as we shall see, produced rather different understandings of the implication of this added source of hermeneutic authority.

My interest in the relevance of (some) rabbinic texts for Jewish women's lives in late antiquity derives partly from a conversation with similar work on early Christian literature. More often than not, recent feminist readings of early Christian texts have implications for our understanding of women's lives within a Jewish cultural framework, and as such do comparative work by implication. Comparative work is performed automatically where a cultural background or context is needed in order to identify Christian conceptions of women's lives. Unfortunately, comparison with the cultural world of rabbinic Judaism often means to point out the "more" or the "better" of Christian women's lives under the reign of Christian discourse. Nobody has made the methodological and cultural blindness of this comparative approach clearer than Katharina von Kellenbach in her critical reflection, *Anti-Judaism in Feminist Religious Writings*, a work that will become relevant later on in this chapter.[1]

The inability to see diversity is a methodological and cultural blindness. It spurs the conflict and struggle over meaningfulness within the cultural discourse of the "other," a struggle that I have attempted to convey in the previous chapters for one of the most problematic "others" of early Christianity. As we shall see in the following pages, however, the discourse of the other cannot always clearly be identified as such, especially where "Judaism" and "Christianity" intersect in what has come to be called *Jewish-Christianity*, a category whose dubiousness will appear later in this chapter. Methodological blindness, then, is also the inability to recognize that the need to present one's own cultural history as redeemable for women today is based on the production of a negatively contrasting background. Such an argument stripped bare would sound something like this: if ours was not as bad as theirs for women, then the not-so-good-for-women in ours appears in a much better light and is therefore justified. This blindness then does not see that women's lives are reflected mostly through an androcentric lens in Jewish and Christian as well as Greco-Roman literatures, that women in any culture in late antiquity lived under patriarchal conditions, and that women were victims of these conditions in any cultural context, while simultaneously struggling within and against these conditions.

The following pages are conceived in conversation with that line of feminist scholarship on early Christian literature which struggles with the predominance of virginity in Christian discourse and the implications for reading women's corporeality. This analysis begins with Paul, and especially his first letter to the Corinthians, who as a Christian first had elevated a celibate life over married life.[2] Concerning Paul the historical theologian Schüssler Fiorenza argues that "the Christian missionary movement was a conflict movement which stood in tension with the institutions of slavery and the patriarchal family" (*In Memory of Her*, 216), that is, both the Roman and Jewish patriarchal family. Hence, she sees Paul's advice in 1 Cor. 7 to remain free from the bond of marriage, especially where it is given to women, as a frontal assault "on the intentions of existing law and the general cultural ethos" and as a "severe infringement on the right of the pater familias" (215). The negative definition of virginity as *freedom from* the burden of marriage was afforded great prominence in patristic literature.[3] An argument such as Schüssler Fiorenza's sets the stage for what has been called "virginal feminism" (Ruether, "Misogynism and Virginal Feminism") or "feminine advancement" (E. Clark, *Ascetic Piety and Women's Faith*). That is, feminist scholars have focused on the various degrees of autonomy and self-determination created for women by the Christian campaign for virginity, even though some of the underlying assumptions of this approach have been criticized more recently.[4] These degrees of autonomy find expression in the formation of women's communities, especially within the later monastic movement,[5] but also within the households, whether the parental one, or that of the husband (Castelli, "Virginity," 79; Brown, *The Body and Society*; Faivre, *Emergence of the Laity*, 199). The point is, of course, that women could form communities because of the ideal of virginity and sexual renunciation, whereas marital obligation prevented them from doing so.

The advantages of a virginal life for women are undeniable, since "the decision to remain a virgin and to renounce marriage and the world did provide some virgins with an opportunity to pursue intellectual and spiritual activities which would otherwise have been unavailable to them. Especially among educated aristocratic women who wished to pursue a life of study, the life of ascetic renunciation was the only institutionally established means of pursuing intellectual work" (Castelli, "Virginity," 82). There are other advantages. Thus Joyce Salisbury, in *Churchfathers, Independent Virgins*, has arranged the legends of holy women, again mostly of aristocratic background, who had vowed chastity during the fourth and fifth centuries under the rubrics of freedom of thought,[6] freedom from social expectations,[7] and freedom of movement, since some of these women, not bound by family obligations, had the opportunity to go on pilgrimages. However, she also points out that this latter freedom was quite contested among patristic writers and that "women were told to seek holiness by staying inside their homes and not traveling at all. The principle of enclosure, which was in fact what the Fathers were advocating, suggested that for women sanctity was to be found within—both within bodies that were to remain closed sexually and within rooms that were closed to the world" (84).

In spite of these advantages, however, Castelli has noted the price that women had to pay in order to fulfill the virginal ideal. Whereas the majority of the argumentation so far focused on women's sociohistorical option to walk away from the burdens of marital life and to choose the alternative of a life devoted to either study or community service, Castelli poses the question about the *meaning* of virginity and sexual renunciation for women as women. She suggests that "it is not at all clear that the ideology of virginity was not as domesticating and circumscribing of women's sexuality as the ideology of marriage" ("Virginity," 85). This contention is based on her premise that for women in a culture in which their sexuality is synonymous with their identity the ideal of sexual and bodily renunciation has much greater implications for women than for men. Since women are conceived of as bodies to begin with, and men are in their bodies only when their sexual desire for women begins to stir,[8] women have to deny their bodies altogether, whereas men only have to separate themselves from women in order to suppress and fight their desire.[9] Thus to demand sexual renunciation "is to make a far more profound demand for alienation and renunciation of self than any demand for continence on the part of men" (86). Cloke points out that it is not only that men have to separate themselves from women to transcend their bodies, but that this becomes part of women's responsibility: "On women is particularly laid the burden of avoiding being the occasion of leading others to sin. The Fathers were empathetic that if a man lusted, the woman at the very least shared the blame for his lust" (*"This Female Man of God,"* 28). This is perhaps most clearly emblematized in the reproach of a devout virgin in the fourth century who sought out the eremitic Abba Arsenius, by the archbishop Theophilus: "Do you not realise that you are a woman and it is through women that the enemy wars against the saints?" (Cloke, *"This Female Man of God,"* 29).

What concerns me here is that the virginal ideal was from its beginning in Paul's correspondence inscribed with the rhetoric of hierarchy—that is, as the ideal state Paul preferred it over marriage. Even Schüssler Fiorenza, as somebody who emphasizes the liberatory aspect of Paul's preference of celibacy, observes that already Paul "disqualified married people theologically as less engaged missionaries and less dedicated Christians." His division "posited a rift between the married woman, concerned about her husband

and her family, and the unmarried virgin who was pure and sacred and therefore would receive the pneumatic privileges of virginity" (226). Or, as Peter Brown writes, "the married person, whose heart was inevitably divided, was almost of necessity a half-Christian. . . . The apostolic gift of celibacy was too precious a thing to extend to the Church as a whole" (*The Body and Society*, 56).[10] That is to say, the argument that compliance with the patristic campaign for virginity represented an alternative to or a way out of patriarchal relations can only be advanced *at the expense of* the *hoi polloi* who were married, as well as at the expense of women in rabbinic culture, in which neither men nor women were offered a legitimate alternative to family life.[11] I use the formulation of "at the expense of" because we have to ask whether, in a discourse which builds up an elite of sexual renunciation, in which women are allowed or even encouraged to participate, married women might perhaps fare worse than in a culture in which everybody is required to marry. That is, there might then emerge an inverse relationship: the more virginity is the ideal of Christian womanhood, the more the status and options of married women decrease.

What then about those whose only merit was the production of virgins for the church, as Jerome would have it? Jerome can say "I praise wedlock, but because they produce me virgins" (Letter to Eustochium 22.20), just as Ambrose admits that "virginity itself cannot exist unless it has some means of coming into existence" (On Virginity 1.35). Jerome himself, of course, has no problem with condemning the mothers of "his" virgins to discursive oblivion, for in his argument with Jovinian he writes: "But you [Jovinian] will say 'If everybody were a virgin, what would become of the human race?' . . . Be not afraid that all will become virgins: virginity is a hard matter, and therefore rare, because it is hard: 'Many are called but few are chosen'" (Ide, *Woman as Priest*, 86; Cloke, "*This Female Man of God*," 39). He is then primarily concerned with the few, whereas the many become irrelevant to his musings about what it means to be a Christian.

What about those who opted for a life of marriage, family, and childrearing, who were to become the laity in the Christian communities, in a culture whose campaign for virginity and sexual renunciation increasingly came to focus on church leadership?[12] What about the Christianity of those who did not or could not achieve a life of virginity as the pinnacle of Christian achievement (Brown 1988, 254) and who instead relied on monks and nuns as mediators with the divine? Does not the feminist argument about "virginal feminism" repeat the argument of the patristic writers themselves? That is, if to the "fathers" the married *hoi polloi* were ultimately only half-Christian, are not the married women only half-feminists to the feminist argument, with no options left open to them to be recognized as leading a meaningful life as married women?[13]

While I am in agreement with Castelli's argument about the sexual politics of virginity, I want to look at the debate from a different angle, taking menstruation as one of my building blocks. As might be expected, the evidence is rather scarce. Giving birth, or rather the danger of giving birth and the subsequent burden of motherhood, occupies much of the patristic argumentation against marriage; menstruation and rituals concerning menstruation are almost invisible. But the general patristic silence on menstrual matters should not come as a surprise, for two reasons. The first one is the general devaluation of marriage. In rabbinic Judaism menstrual practices primarily come to concern marital relations rather than relations to the public. There exists, then, a structural parallel between virginal practices in the Christian context and menstrual practices in the rabbinic context, because both give women a tool for control over their sexual lives. Second, the discursive annihilation of the female body of difference[14] within the patristic campaign for virginity would seem to foreclose any particular interest in menstruation. Menstrual bleeding represents a marker of a gender difference that is incongruent with a world constructed from the perspective of male church authorities. By looking at the various ways in which practices or texts related to menstrual regulations are dealt with, we can study one aspect of the gendering of Christian culture in its beginning stages, an aspect that has been neglected in the recent scholarship on women's roles in early Christianity.[15]

What will become obvious is that the discussion of practices and texts related to menstruation is not merely an issue of gender politics within early Christian life, but is often located within and determined by the polemics of Christian writers against Jewish practices. Until fairly late there was no universal or "orthodox" uniformity as to what was to determine Christian life, in terms of Christian practice and rituals, since the majority of the debates centered on questions of theological doctrine. In a certain sense a uniformity of practice and rituals never really existed, since the adaptation of Christianity into different cultural contexts has created a tremendous diversity of rituals throughout its history, often against the intent of European missionaries. What remained undetermined was the *practice* of Christian life, such as, for instance, the liturgical calendar, or questions of what constituted a Christian education, what a person should know in order to become a Christian.[16] Such practical aspects of Christian life were bound to move to the foreground in local conflicts over practice. These conflicts often arose in the continuing confrontation with Jewish culture as a culture that had infused everyday aspects of marriage and family life with ritualized practices, besides having established the study of Torah as a central activity. We find early Christian literature taking pains to distinguish its community life from Jewish customary practices. It is because of its focus on doctrinal questions, on the one hand, and on sexual *askesis*, primarily for the Christian leadership, on the other, that early Christian discourse often neglected to consider the everyday lives of those who failed to rise to prominence as ascetics. I find support for this argument in Kate Cooper's study of idealized womanhood in early Christian literature. She makes exactly the same point when she writes: "Although the ascetic movement had initially served to supplement Christianity's narrow spectrum of sacred roles and priesthoods, it resulted in a further diminution of religious identity for the women and men who could claim neither clerical status nor ascetic stature. For married women the problem was particularly acute, since women's symbolic position as representatives of the household left them especially vulnerable to the erosion of the *domus* as the central icon of the social imagination" (*Virgin and the Bride*, 115).[17]

This, then, is the context for analyzing more closely a text from the margins of early Christian literature that deals with the problem of women who endow their female bodies with religious significance.

### A Third-Century Christian Community in Menstrual Conflict

In the third century C.E.,[18] during the decades succeeding the formation of the Mishnah and approximately contemporary with the collation and editing of the Tosefta, an anonymous Christian authority in Syria exclaims somewhat abusively, in his guidelines for church discipline and personal conduct[19] called the Didascalia:[20] "O foolish women, these mischances happen to you because of your opinions, and because of *these observances* you keep and because of your imaginings, you are emptied of the Holy Spirit and filled with unclean spirits, and you are thrown out from life into the burning of the fire everlasting" (Vööbus, *Didascalia*, 241). The observance referred to in this threat is the women's observance of certain restrictions during their menstrual periods.

These women are part of the group which the author addresses as those who "have been converted from the (Jewish) people to believe in God our Savior Jesus Christ" (223). The adjective "Jewish" is not included in the Syriac or Latin text: דאתפינו מן עמא למהימנו באלהא פרוקן ישוח משיחא—qui autem convertentur de populo, ut credant deo et salvatori nostro Iesu Christo. From the context of the chapter, however, it is obvious that the author refers to Jewish converts. Thus, he interprets one of Jesus' sayings (Matthew 11:28) as addressed not "to the gentiles, but he said it to us his disciples from among the Jews" [לא הוא לעממא אמר אלא לן לתלמידוהי דמן בית יהודיא אמר הוא; non gentibus sed nobis qui ex Hebreis discipuli eius fuimus] (230; Tidner, *Didascaliae*, 84). Interestingly enough, the author of the Didascalia ranks himself among those "disciples from among the Jews."[21] Further, he beseeches the Jewish converts to not "remain in your former conversation, brethren, that you should keep vain bonds" [לא מכיל תקוון תוב בדוברכון קדמיא אחין דתהוון נטרין אסורא סריקא; iam priorem conversationem non teneant observantes vincula vana] (Vööbus, 223, 225).

As we shall see, the Didascalia addresses from a unique angle the conflict between those who uphold practices signified as Jewish within the Christian community, and between those who want to distinguish Christian community life from those practices. The author of the Didascalia argues extensively with the women in his community about women's practices. The Didascalia has been widely studied for the analysis of the conflict between Jews and Christians in the early centuries.[22] It has separately been studied for its allowance for women's leadership as deaconesses and widows. According to Faivre the Didascalia is "the first document in which the function of the deaconess is presented" (*Emergence of the Laity*, 100), an office that remained virtually unknown in Western Christianity (Laporte, *Role of Women*, 111).[23] Along with others, Faivre argues convincingly that in fact the office of the deaconess was instituted as a means of control of women in a community in which widows had a highly visible and authoritative function (Thurston, *The Widows*, 96–105; Methuen, "Widows, Bishops," 197–213).

In the study of Christianity's conflict with Judaism, the role of women has been largely neglected.[24] The extensive scholarly literature on the sometimes vicious debates of early Christian writers over the significance of Jewish practices for members of Christian communities has focused primarily on what could be considered the polemic triad—circumcision, food laws or *kashrut*, and the celebration of the Sabbath and holidays—as the main issues of the conflict. In this they are justified by the predominant concerns of our sources on this conflict. For this reason the Didascalia stands out, not only as an indicator of the specific historical situation of conflict in its community, but also as an indicator of how the larger conflict over the role of Jewish customs within the Christian communities takes form when women's practices, and those practices that determine women's religious lives and identities, are located at its center, rather than circumcision. Further, I want to argue that the significance of the Didascalia lies in the observation that this is the only document in premodern history of Judaism and Christianity in which we find women developing an argument for why they wish to practice menstrual separation.

The question that has to open the following analysis is whether it is possible to perceive women's practice through the Didascalia, since again we are dealing with a presumably male-authored source. At the very least, we can say that the writer addresses himself directly to the women in the community, indicating that he expects women as well as men to be the readers of his guidelines for Christian life (or listeners, if the guidelines were read in community assemblies). This is corroborated by the fact that the Didascalia's author does not merely address women in his debate against those women who maintain the observance of menstrual rituals. Rather, women seem to play a significant role as leaders in the community, since the text develops extensive regulations for the appropriate behavior of widows, and deals with the leadership function of deaconesses within the community (Torjesen, *When Women Were Priests*; Methuen, "Widows, Bishops").[25] The text, then, can be read as an indicator of women's behavior within the community, because the author of the Didascalia reacts to, interprets, and ultimately rejects their practice in the community he addresses. I insist on this formulation to emphasize the local character and situation of the document, in spite of the anonymous author's claim to apostolic authority and representation of the "catholic church" universal, as we shall see. Even though these women's behavior is reflected only through the injunctions of the male authority, and even though we do not have the voices of the women themselves in the form of independent texts, we can catch a glimpse of women's behavior in the community if we use the Didascalia's arguments as a mirror.

My attempt to understand the practice of the women who are addressed in the Didascalia, and the gender politics which the writer of the document attempts to promote, is informed by Antoinette Clark Wire's work on the women prophets in the first-century Corinthian community whom Paul addresses in his first letter to the Corinthians. Beyond understanding Paul himself as the author of the letter, Wire attempts to "reconstruct as accurate a picture as possible of the women prophets in the church of first-century Corinth" (*Corinthian Women Prophets*, 1). Such a reconstruction is possible, Wire claims, by focusing on the "rhetorical situation" of the letter, which "includes both the goals of the speaker and the counter-arguments that are anticipated as the speaking progresses," because "to argue is to gauge your audience as accurately as you can at every point, to use their language, to work from where they are in order to move them toward where you want them to be" (3). The important definition of the starting point of Wire's analysis of Paul's letter is the contention that "what we have is not just one individual's viewpoint [Paul's] but a window into a volatile situation" (3). The volatility of the situation only disappears in hindsight, when via the history of tradition an author such as Paul is established as the primary authority for the definition of the life of the early Christian community at large.

The rhetorical situations of Paul's letter to the Corinthians and of the Didascalia Apostolorum can be compared. We have the document by the male writer laying a claim to authority within the community that he addresses. The writer reacts negatively to the behavior of the women in that community. Since their practice disagrees with his definition of what Christian life, and specifically Christian women's life, ought to be, he summons his argumentative energies to dissuade these women from continuing their practice. The two works are further comparable in that for the Didascalia, just as for Paul, it was not yet self-evident and an undebatable "fact" that Scripture for Christians had become the "Old Testament," the Vetus Testamentum, for, as we shall see, he had to argue with the women about why biblical legislations should be abrogated.

The location in time of the rhetorical situation also clearly establishes some fundamental differences, for in the third century the author of the

Didascalia could look back on a tradition of Christian literature,[26] and on a repertoire of themes for Christian polemics against the preservation of the *practical* relevance of biblical legislation within Christian communities. Before we can deal with the author's argument against the women in his community as addressing an actual conflict rather than a merely literary theme, I want to reflect briefly on the literary location he constructs for his document.

**The Claim for Apostolic Authorship**

The proem to the Didascalia makes the claim for apostolic authorship, which gives the document its name:

> We begin the book Didascalia, as the holy apostles of our Lord offered unto us, with regard to the superintendents of the holy church and the canons and the laws for believers as they commanded in it. We, however, the twelve apostles of the only Son, the eternal Word of God, our Lord and our God and our Savior Jesus Christ, as we were assembled with one accord in Jerusalem, the city of the great king, and with us our brother Paul, the apostle of the Gentiles, and James the bishop of above-mentioned city, have ratified this Didascalia. (Vööbus, *Didascalia*, 7–8)

The assembly that the proem refers to has its literary roots in the alleged apostolic council in Jerusalem described in Acts 15, which is also referred to by Paul in his letter to the Galatians (Gal. 2, 1–10).[27] Vööbus points out that the proem appears to be an addition of the secondary recension of the earlier Syriac version (37). But even so, chapter 24 of the Didascalia retells the entire event of the apostolic council of the first century, largely by citing and slightly rearranging the report of Acts 15 in its entirety, with some embellishments. The significant addition to the retelling of the apostolic council is, of course, the fact that the author puts into the mouths of the apostles that " 'it seemed to us in one mind' (Acts 15:25) *to write this catholic Didascalia for the confirmation of you all*" (214; emphasis added).[28] Strecker writes that "the author supports the 'catholic doctrine' which he represents through the apostolic claim made by his work in its title and in the fiction of apostolic authorship that it maintains throughout. Thereby he gains a legitimation that could not be achieved on the basis of his own authority, and at the same time his work acquires a universality corresponding to the presupposed missionary activity of the apostles" ("Problem of Jewish Christianity," 245). Strecker also points out that the Didascalia's claim to catholicity cannot be read as descriptive but is just that, a claim, for in fact "considering the forms in which the 'catholic doctrine' of the Didascalia appears, it is striking that it diverges significantly from the character of 'orthodoxy' with which we are familiar" (246). The claim for catholicity is repeated at the end of the report on the apostolic council, where the author adds the claim, lacking in the report of Acts for good reasons, that the apostles Peter and James remained in Jerusalem "many days": "and we were consulting and arranging together those things which are helpful for all the people and again we were writing also this catholic Didascalia" (219; see also 222).

Literarily, therefore, the Didascalia locates itself in the conflict of the mid-first century. It reinscribes that earlier conflict into its own contemporary conflict. According to Acts 15 the mid-first century conflict had broken out in Antioch, the capital of the Roman province of Syria and the third largest city in the Roman Empire. Paul was residing there at the time when certain men from Judaea came to the community in Antioch and claimed that non-Jews who joined the apostolic communities had to be circumcised "according to the custom of Moses" (Acts 15:1).[29] As a consequence Paul is sent with others to Jerusalem "to discuss this question with the apostles and elders" (Acts 15:2), meaning that the council was called together in response to the conflict in Antioch.[30]

According to the Didascalia, however, the twelve apostles assembled in Jerusalem because they found that the various churches to which they came "were observing holiness, and some abstained from meat and from wine, and some from swine [קדישותא נטרין הוו ומנהון מרחקין הוו מן בשרא ומן חמרא ומנהון מן דחזירא]" (214),[31] as well as observing various other unspecified biblical regulations. The conflict in Antioch, which in the Didascalia's retelling was similarly not merely about circumcision but about food regulations (215), is one among those others which in the Didascalia's retelling triggers the necessity for the apostolic council, and the composition of the Didascalia itself. In the Didascalia, then, the community in Antioch "knew that we [the apostles] were assembled and (that) we had all come to inquire about these things" (216). Consequently, the Antiochene community sent delegates to the apostolic council in Jerusalem, whom the Didascalia defines as "certain believers who were acquainted with the Scriptures" (216), eliding the role of Paul in the whole event.[32]

At the center of the conflict in New Testament literature stood the question of circumcision as a rite of initiation for non-Jewish converts, as well as the laws of *kashrut* as "divisive food practices" (Boyarin, *Carnal Israel*, 113; see also Dunn, *Jesus, Paul, and the Law*, 137). The Didascalia thus reinscribes the conflict of the mid-first century into its own contemporary conflict, which is also located in Syria and which also involves those who insist on the observance of practices based on biblical legislation within the Christian community. The same conflict or a similar one seems to repeat itself in the same geocultural environment.

The differences between the two events, then, are telling as to the situation of conflict in the Didascalia. Whereas in Acts 15 the conflict evolved around the question of circumcision (Acts 15:5), in addition to the question of food laws according to Paul, the Didascalia only mentions circumcision in its retelling of Acts 15 (Vööbus, *Didascalia*, 216). From then on circumcision retires to the background. Similarly, he only mentions "the distinction of meats" (223) and the impurity of the dead (242), neither of which he dignifies with a discussion. What does seem to be central to the conflict in the Didascalia among those in the community who "have been converted from the (Jewish) people to believe in God our Savior Jesus Christ" (223) are two issues. It is the argument over the keeping of the Sabbath as a rival of the "first day," that is, the Sunday as a Christian replacement of the Sabbath; the other issue is the rules of menstrual separation. The argument over the Sabbath I will leave aside. Suffice it to say that the writer calls on the "beloved brethren, you who from the (Jewish) people have believed" (233) to cease the observance of the Sabbath. He enters an elaborate discussion of biblical exegesis, to "prove" that the first day of the week is indeed more important than the Sabbath.[33] Against the women he employs a different strategy.

### Menstrual Separation in the Didascalia

From the preceding discussion we have learned more about the background of the women against whom the author of the Didascalia argues. He locates them among those in the community who "have been converted from among the (Jewish) people to believe in God our Savior Jesus Christ" (223), who are "his disciples from among the Jews" (230). The passage that introduces the argument against the observation of menstrual separation characterizes those who perform it as those "who are scrupulous and desire ... to keep the habits of nature and fluxes and intercourse [אנדין אית אנשין] [דמזדהרין וצבין למטר איך דבתנין נמוסא עידא דכינא ודובא ושותפותא]" (238).³⁴ Whereas this phrase addresses the group as a whole, the writer proceeds to enter the debate primarily with the women.

What we learn from the text is that during the "seven days of their menstrual period" these women refrain "from prayer, and from [studying] Scripture and from [participating] in the eucharist." In the formulation of the writer, they keep themselves from the fruits of the Holy Spirit, "so as not to approach to them" (329). It seems reasonable, then, to conjecture that what we do know for sure about the women is what they do. That is, they themselves have chosen to keep themselves separate from activities that are central to the religious life of the Christian community. In his argument against the women the author polemicizes against this withdrawal.

For this controversy an important intertext may be found in a rabbinic text from approximately the same time, and perhaps even from approximately the same cultural geographical space.³⁵ The Tosefta presents the following anonymous ruling:

> Men and women with irregular genital emissions, women who menstruate and parturients [all of whom are in a status of ritual impurity] are permitted to read in the Torah, and to study Mishnah, midrash, religious law and aggadah, but men who had a regular ejaculation are prohibited to do so. (tBer 2:13)³⁶

The rabbis in the Tosefta explicitly permit women who menstruate to study, among other categories of people. The same issue is discussed both in the Tosefta and in Didascalia in different contexts. Both authors rule that the women can, and in the case of the Didascalia even should, study Scripture, for different reasons. The Tosefta allows menstruating women to study Scripture in spite of their ritual status of impurity, since according to rabbinic law the text of the Torah as ritual sacred object cannot receive a status of impurity. But it certainly does not want women to otherwise abandon biblical regulations concerning menstruation. The Didascalia, on the other hand, attempts to persuade women to continue studying during their menstrual period in order to transcend their Jewish past. This convergence between the rabbinic and the Christian text is evidence for the fact that each of the two communities struggled, sharing the same textual reference in Scripture, to define the role and identity of women as part of establishing its own collective identity.

Beyond the women's behavior in the Didascalia, we may even glean the women's reasons for refraining from participation in community life during their menstrual period from the polemic reaction of the author. Here we have to proceed with caution, since a hermeneutics of suspicion is called for. There is no way of being certain whether the women really made the argument that the Didascalia strives to dismantle. In other words, what the Didascalia presents as the women's argument may be overdetermined by its own theological interests. The author may be creating a straw-woman to strengthen his own theology. What might the women of the Didascalia have argued, as the only group of women in late antique culture, Jewish or Christian, who insist on the significance of their menstrual periods for their religious lives?

### We Practice Menstrual Separation Because the Indwelling of the Holy Spirit Corresponds to Our Cycles

The Didascalia argues against two different conceptualizations. First, the women present an argument about the relationship of their bodies and "its habits" (238)[37] to the Holy Spirit.

אנגיר סבר אנתי או' אנתתא דבשבעא יומין דמדריתכי ספיקא אנתי מן רוחא
קדישא אן תמותין בהנון יומתא ספיקאית ודלא סברא תאזלין
אנדין אית בכי רוחא קדישא בכלזובן מן צלותא ומן כתבא ומן אוכריסטיא
דלא כליא נטר אנתי נפשכי אתחשבי גיר וחזי דאף צלותא ביד רוחא קדישא
משתמעא ואוכריסטיא ביד רוחא קדישא מתקבלא ומתקדשא וכתבא פתגמא
אנון דרוחא קדישא וקדישין אנון אנגיר איתוהי בכי רוחא קדישא למנא
נטרא אנתי נפשכי דלא תתקרבין לעבדוהי דרוחא קדישא

For if you think,[38] O woman, that in the seven days of your flux you are void of the Holy Spirit, if you die in those days, you will depart empty-handed and without hope.

But if the Holy Spirit is always in you, without (any real) hindrance you keep yourself from prayer and from the Scriptures and the eucharist. Indeed, think and see that prayer also is heard through the Holy Spirit, and the eucharist is accepted and sanctified through the Holy Spirit. And the Scriptures are the utterances of the Holy Spirit, and are holy. For if the Holy Spirit is in you, why do you keep yourself from approaching the works of the Holy Spirit? (239)

The women seem to keep a seven-day period of menstrual separation. The fixed number of seven days indicates the connection with the biblical regulations in Lev. 15:19ff. But the reasoning that the writer attributes to the women is a pneumatological reasoning. According to him, they "think" [סבר, speras te] that during the (presumably fixed) period of seven days, they are void of the Holy Spirit. At the end of his argument against this contention he even attributes his knowledge of it to direct communication: "You then, O woman, *according to what you say*, if in the days of your flux you are void . . ." (241; emphasis added).[39] It seems likely that this reasoning is not merely thought up by the author, but is indeed one that the women put forward. Since they consider themselves void of the Holy Spirit during their menstrual period, they refrain from the three central works (or the "fruits") of the Holy Spirit. Against this, however, the Didascalia proceeds to argue that the Holy Spirit is always in them, which eliminates the reason of their separation and turns their actions into "empty observances" (240).[40]

In its argument with the women on this point the Didascalia lays out its doctrine of baptism. Throughout the document the author elaborates on the centrality of the rite of baptism. Baptism is the rite of entry into the discipleship of Christ and into the "catholic church which is the receptacle of the Holy Spirit [עדתא קתוליקא הי דאיתיה מקבלניתא דרוחא קדישא; catholicam ecclesiam quae est susceptorium sancti spiritus]," (221).[41] Baptism signifies filiation with God and the bishop as God's servant and mediator:[42] "[The bishop] is a servant of the word and mediator, but to you a teacher, and your father after God, who has begotten you through the water" (100). But above and beyond everything else, the "unbreakable seal of baptism"

(113, 157) signifies the forgiveness of all previous sins: "to everyone who believes and is baptized, his former sins have been forgiven" (183).[43] In spite of this tenet, however, the text often appears to be preoccupied with the problem of misconduct after baptism, and especially misconduct that revokes the forgiveness in baptism. Such misconduct can be described as doing "again the abominable and defiled works of the wicked heathens" (51), meaning that the new converts do not sufficiently distinguish themselves in behavior from the pagans. But blasphemy weighs even graver, and blasphemy against the Holy Spirit, against God, against Scripture, or against the Church remains unforgivable.[44] The Didascalia demands that "when a woman who is being baptized has come up from the water, let the deaconness receive her, and teach and educate her in order that the unbreakable seal of baptism shall be (kept) in chastity and holiness" (157), in contrast to the widows who are explicitly prohibited to teach and instead are requested to send converts "who desire to be instructed to the leader."[45] The paradox is, of course, that the "seal"—חתמא—is not unbreakable, and this is what the Didascalia mobilizes against the women's pneumatological argument.

Against the women's claim that they are void and empty of the Holy Spirit during the seven-day period of their menstrual separation he expounds:

מהימנא מלא רוחא קדישא ואינא דלא הימן רוחא טנפתא . . . אינא הכיל
דאתפרק ואתרחק ושני מן רוחא טנפתא ביד מעמודיתא מתמלא רוחא
קדישא ואנהו דנעבד עבדא טבא מכתר לותה רוחא קדישא ומקוא כד מלא
ורוחא טנפתא לא משכחא לה אתרא לותה . . . אפלא גיר אית שולטנא אחרנא
דתשנא באידוהי רוחא טנפתא אלא אן ביד רוחא דאלהא דכיתא וקדישתא

Quoniam omnis homo repletus est, fidelis quidem de sancto spiritu, infidelis autem de inmundo, . . . qui vero per baptismum reiecit et deposuit et liberatus est ab inmundo spiritu, sancto repletur. Si itaq(ue) bonum operatus fuerit, permanet in illum spiritus sanctus et manet repletus, et inmundus locum non invenit. . . . nulla est alia curatio, ut abscedat ab eo spiritus inmundus, nisi per sacram purgationem et sanctum baptismum. (Tidner, *Didascaliae*, 94)

A believer is filled with the Holy Spirit, and he [sic] who does not believe, with an unclean spirit. . . . He therefore who has departed and abides afar and has departed from the unclean spirit by baptism, he is filled with the Holy Spirit. And if he does good works, the Holy Spirit stays with him, and he remains fulfilled, and the unclean spirit finds no place in him.... Indeed, there is also no other power whereby the unclean spirit may depart except though the pure and holy Spirit of God. (241)

The Latin translation differs from the Syriac in that in the Latin version the only "cure" for the impure spirit is through the "sacred purification and the holy baptism" rather than the more abstract "pure and holy spirit of God." The Syriac version seems to be based on an exegesis of Matthew 12:43–45, from a speech of Jesus to the Scribes and Pharisees, who asked him for a sign. He rebukes them with the parable of the wandering unclean spirit (τὸ ἀκάθρτον πνεῦμα) which returns to its owner. Whatever the meaning of this parable, Jesus' speech in the context of Matthew does not mention baptism. However, Vööbus remarks that some manuscripts of the Syriac version read "through baptism and the Holy Spirit" (241 n.196).

The rite of baptism signifies the endowment of the Holy Spirit, the replacement of the pre- and extra-baptismal unclean spirit once and for all. The person can only be filled by either the Holy Spirit or an unclean spirit: "The Holy Spirit stays always with those who possess Him. But from whom He departs, to him an unclean spirit cleaves" (240). Both are exclusive of the other. The "possession" of the Holy Spirit, though received with baptism, remains contingent upon "good works" [עבדא טבא; bonum]. According to the Didascalia's explanation of the significance of baptism, therefore, the women's pneumatology is inadequate, for they will not only be void during their period of menstrual separation, as they claim, but that void will be filled with unclean spirits, which leads to a battle between spirits (240), and to the ultimate replacement of the Holy Spirit with unclean spirits, which reverses the baptismal gift. He summarizes his exhortation against the women's pneumatology:

מטל הנא סכלתא הלין נדשא גדשין לכין מטל רעניכין ומטל הלין נטורתא
דנטרן אנתין ומטל מסם ברעיניכין מן רוחא קדישא מסתפקן אנתין ומתמלין
אנתין רוחא טנפתא ומשתדין אנתין מן חיא ליקדנא דנורא דלעלם

Unde stulta quae talis est, suspicio a vobis speratur. Et ex eo, quod tales observationes custoditis, per suspicionem vacatio in vobis a sancto spiritu erit et repletio ab inmundo, et ita erit vitae reiectio et conbustio aeterna. (Tidner, *Didascaliae*, 95)

On this account, O foolish (women), these happenings happen to you because of your opinions and because of these observances you keep, and because of your imaginings, you are emptied of the Holy Spirit, and filled with unclean spirits, and you are thrown out from life into the burning of the fire everlasting. (Vööbus, *Didascalia*, 241)

If indeed the pneumatological argument is an argument conceptually independent from what follows, it would seem that the women adapted what they learned about the Holy Spirit upon being baptized in a somewhat gender-syncretic way. They considered the Holy Spirit to be subjected to the cyclical habits of their physical bodies. As their bodies bleed periodically, the Holy Spirit leaves and reenters their wombs. Instead of moving from the ontological level of the flesh where bodies are gendered to the ontological level of the spirit where gender distinction are dissolved, in which there is "neither male nor female," these women reversed the move. For them, the realm of the spirit into which they enter upon being baptized does not dis- and replace the realm of the flesh, but is inscribed by it, so much so that even in the realm of the spirit there is indeed "both male and female."

This uterine pneumatology does not suit the "opinions and imaginings" of the author of the Didascalia, nor does it conform to any other Christian source that has come down to us from those centuries. The Didascalia's refutation of the women's uterine pneumatology seems illogical and inconsistent. The author's conceptual bottom line is that the women's "imagining" of the effusion of the spirit along with their blood and the subsequent spiritual void in the uterus is an unacceptable incorporation of the spiritual into the fleshly realm. The inconsistency emerges when he argues that there can be no void, but only either the Holy Spirit or the spirit of impurity. The Didascalia here does not choose a Pauline argument claiming that κατὰ πνεῦμα, there is neither male nor female, whether you menstruate or not. Rather, he admits an evacuation of the Holy Spirit, "because of your opinions" (and the accompanying observances). Because of the women's opinions, then, the Holy Spirit leaves, but only once, just as it entered only once with baptism. In this way he attempts to confine the uterine movement of the Holy Spirit to his version of its "orthodox" movement. As we have seen above, the Holy Spirit should inhabit the baptized person always [בכלזבן], which, however, is not a given but only a status of potential permanence. If the Holy Spirit has left, it is the spirit of impurity that will dwell in the person permanently [בכלזבן]. By shifting the rift to the spiritual realm, the Didascalia attempts to keep the ontological detachment of the realm of the Spirit from the realm of the flesh intact, thus foreclosing any gender distinction in relation to the Holy Spirit. The Holy Spirit gives way only to the other spirit, but cannot be bound by blood.

## We Are in the Status of Impurity Because We Consider Scriptural Legislation to Be Valid For Us

Now the author of the Didascalia turns to the other argument that the women advance. The overarching problematic to the author is still the question of the centrality of baptism, but it is tackled from a different angle. For the second, and it would seem compelling, reason on which the women base their behavior is their reading of and adherence to the biblical legislation in Lev. 15:

תוב דין אמר לכי או אנתתא בשבעא יומין דמרדיתכי טמאתא חשבא אנתי
נפשכי איך דבתנין נמוסא⁴⁶ מן בתר שבעא יומין הכיל איכנא מתדכיא אנתי
דלא מעמודיתא ואן תעמדין בהו מדם דסברא אנתי דמתדכיא אשתי תשרין
מעמודיתא משלמניתא דאלהא הי דשבקת לכי חטהיכי גמיראית ותשתכחין
בבישתא דחטהיכי קדמיא ותשתלמין לנורא דלעלם ואן לא תעמדין איך מסם
ברעינכי דילכי טמאתא מקויא אנתי ולא מדם עדרכי נטוריא ספיקא דשבעא
יומין אלא יתיראית אף מסגפו נסגפכי מטל דברעינכי טמאתא אנתי ואיך
טמאתא תתחייבין

But again I say to you, O woman; (if) in the seven days of your flux you regard yourself impure according to the second legislation—after seven days, therefore, how can you be purified without baptism? But if you shall bathe yourself, through that which you suppose, that you are purified, you shall abrogate the perfect baptism of God which completely forgave you your sins, and you will be found in the evils of your former sins, and you shall be delivered over to the fire eternal. But if

you be not bathed, according to your own imaginings you remain
unclean, and the empty observance of the seven days has helped
you nothing, but it will rather harm you—for according to your opinion you are unclean, and as one unclean you shall be condemned.
(Vööbus, *Didascalia*, 241–42)

According to this argument, the women regard themselves as being in the status of impurity during their (regular) menstrual period because they still consider this biblical legislation to be valid. Lev. 15:19, as we have seen previously, prescribes seven days of impurity, regardless of the number of days of actual bleeding. If they are indeed "formerly" Jewish women who became members of the Christian community that the Didascalia addresses, they may simply have insisted on continuing with cycles of menstrual separation. Of course, they would be supported by the fact that "Scripture," or the biblical canon, has a fundamental role in Christianity, and particularly in the Didascalia's community setting. The detailed instruction of how to study Scripture bears this out (14–15), as does the retelling of the mid-first century conflict in Antioch from Acts 15, in which the Antiochene delegates are described as those "who were acquainted with Scriptures" (216), a characterization that the Didascalia adds to the text of Acts. Finally, this is shown by the fact that the women keep themselves from Scripture during their menstrual periods, which indicates that otherwise they would regularly study Scripture.

The language of impurity now leaves the lofty pneumatological level at which we have seen the Holy Spirit and the unclean spirits at war with each other over capturing the spirit of the baptized person. Now impurity is dealt with on a more concrete level, as a concept inherited from the priestly text, which perhaps these formerly practicing Jewish and now Christian women continue to consider as authoritative.

The point of contention to the author of the Didascalia, then, is the termination of the seven-day period of menstrual impurity. The priestly text does not explicitly prescribe immersion as a ritual of purification from the period of menstrual impurity. On these grounds the writer challenges the women. If they do consider themselves to be in the status of impurity during their menstrual period—which they would be justified to do if they argue on biblical grounds—how do they purify themselves at the end of the period?

The Didascalia considers baptism to be the only legitimate rite of purification for Christians—not in its biblical-priestly sense, but in his Christian-ethical or metaphysical sense. The author presents the notion of purification in water at the end of the menstrual period as a rival ritual to baptism, and not merely as a possibly supplemental ritual. The women might have argued that there is not necessarily a contradiction or exclusive relationship between the initiating rite of baptism as a spiritual purification, and the monthly ritual of immersion as a corporeal purification. But the Didascalia does not allow for such a complementary arrangement. It insists on the exclusively spiritual sense of purification as forgiveness of sin. That insistence on the spiritual sense of purification would turn such monthly immersion into minor baptism, and therefore counteract the one and only, perfect baptism.

Interestingly enough, the author of the Didascalia considers the alternative that the women might simply choose not to immerse to mark the end of their period of menstrual separation. Is this merely a rhetorical device? Or does he think that they might concur with his insistence on the exclusivity of baptismal purification, but then could still insist on their adherence to biblical legislation? Or does he consider this to be a possible "reading" of the biblical text, which after all does not demand immersion at the end of the period of menstrual impurity, in which case they again could still insist on their adherence to biblical legislation? In either case, he anticipates a possible concession on the ritual of immersion, but not on observing the period of menstrual separation, against which he does not employ a logical but a historical-theological argument. Might this indicate that the issue of immersion at the end of the period of menstrual separation was still in debate in the Jewish community from which these women come?

Of course, the author proceeds to delegitimize this possible alternative, arguing that if it were followed the women would never be purified, since they continue to observe menstrual separation from the works of the Holy Spirit. He constructs a no-win situation for the women: if you women consider yourselves to be in the status of impurity during your menstrual period, how is the end of this period to be marked? If you immerse, you question the validity of your baptism, which was to symbolize that purification—in the spiritual sense—has been achieved once and for all. But if you don't mark the end of your period and uphold the community's once-and-for-all understanding of the purification in baptism you will remain wedded to your status of impurity. The apparent acceptance of their impurity here seems to be only a rhetorical one in the development of his argumentative refutation. All of which is to say that you should not consider yourselves to be in a status of impurity during your menstrual period in the first place, in spite of this being based on biblical legislation.

But the Didascalia does not even allow for the validity of this latter claim. In the general scheme of the Didascalia the terminology of biblical regulations of ritualized behavior is the so-called second legislation—*secundatio* in the Latin version of the text, *deuterosis* in the Greek version—and has a clearly polemic function.[47] It is his rhetorical weapon in his dispute with those people who favor the observance of certain Jewish rituals. The terminology is not only pitched to the women, but to this collective group, who continue to consider the sabbath as the biblically ordained day of abstention from work, who continue to be concerned about food regulations, and who continue to be concerned about impurity issues in the biblical-priestly sense. The term indicates that the author partially accepts an argument from the continuing authority of biblical legislation and could be saying: "you are right, what you observe is ordained by biblical legislation, but there is biblical legislation and there is biblical legislation." That is, the term introduces a division within biblical legal heritage by which the overall concept of biblical authority is kept intact, while undermining the authority of particular traditions and prescriptions. For there is the "true law," and the "second legislation."[48] The true Law, or *lex*, are primarily the Ten Commandments (Vööbus, *Didascalia*, 224), to which the writer applies the saying of the Matthean Jesus that "One *Yud* letter shall not pass away from the law" (Matthew 5:18). The Didascalia offers a midrashic reading: "Indeed, (when) He (God) spoke the ten utterings [the ten commandments], He pointed out Jesus—for ten represents Yud, but Yud is the beginning of the name of Jesus" (223). The Matthean Jesus, then, according to the Didascalia, really meant to say that the ten commandments in their continuing validity will not pass away. The *deuterosis*, on the other hand, comprises the entire legislation succeeding the creation of the golden calf, the "fall" of the biblical people of Israel, because "the second legislation was imposed for the making of the calf and for idolatry [תנין נמוסא גיר מטל עבדה דעגלא ודחלת פתכרא אתתסים]" (228). As its name implies, it is secondary, superfluous and temporary, not genuine. Indeed, it is merely divine punishment for biblical Israel's idolatry.

With the gospel story of Jesus, then, the punishment is revoked and the second legislation dispensed with, for the Matthean Jesus' principle applies only to the true Law: "Indeed, in the Gospel He renewed and fulfilled and confirmed the Law, but the second legislation He abrogated and abolished" (228).[49]

To further strengthen his juxtaposition and perhaps dissuade those in his community who adhere to rites ordained by what he calls the *deuterosis*, the author of the Didascalia repeatedly insists on the lightness of the Law and the burden of the second legislation. The Law is "simple and pure and holy" (223). "This is the simple and light Law. In it there is no burden" (225), "the Law is easy and light, of no weak voice" (226). In response to the golden calf, however, "he [god] bound them [biblical Israel] with the second legislation, and laid heavy burdens upon them and a hard yoke upon their neck" (226). "For because of the multitude of sins there were laid upon them customs unspeakable" (227). The abrogation of the "bonds of the second legislation" (229) in the story of the gospel "fulfills the power of men's liberty" (228). Again, when the Matthean Jesus says "Come unto me, all you that toil and are laden with heavy burdens, and I will give you rest" (Matthew 11:28), the author of the Didascalia argues that Jesus specifically addressed the Jews, and offered them to deposit with him the heavy burdens of the second legislation, observances such as the Sabbath or menstrual separation (230). Indeed, with the destruction of the Temple and its altar the fulfillment of the second legislation has become impossible "while dispersed among the gentiles. Wherefore, everyone who approaches it falls under a curse, and binds himself" (236).[50]

Armed with this rhetorical ammunition, then, the Didascalia attempts to lead the women's concern about menstrual impurity ad absurdum:

הלין דין על כלנש אתחשבו על אילין דנטרין דובא ושותפותא דזוונא הלין גיר כלהין נטורתא סכלתא איתיהין ומסגפניתא אן גיר כד נשתותף אנש או נאתא מנש דובא נעמד אף תשויתה נשיג ונהוא לה הנא עמלא ושחקא דלא שלוא נהוא עמד ומשיג מאנוהי ותשויתה ומדם אחרין לא נשכח למעבד

Haec igitur super omnes cogitate, qui seminum cursus et adproximationes mulierum observant; nam quae tales sunt observationes omnes stultae et nocivae sunt. Si enim cursum seminis quis passus et adproximans mulieri baptizetur, et stratum suum lavet; et erit illi hoc fatigatio, numquam deficiens a baptismo et a lavatione rerum et a stratu suo, et nihil aliut poteit agere. (Tidner, *Didascaliae*, 96)

Be thus minded therefore concerning everyone, concerning those who observe issues and the intercourse of marriage; indeed, all these observances are foolish and harmful. For if, when a man shall have intercourse, or flux come out from him, he must be bathed, let him also wash his mattress—and he will have this travail and unceasing vexation: he will be bathing and he will be washing his clothes and his mattress, and he will not be able to do anything else. (Vööbus, *Didascalia*, 242)

I consider this passage to be a rhetorical gender deflection, rather than abruptly switching from the women to men who actually observe the impurity of the *zav*, an irregular emission (Lev. 15:2–12). Now it is doubtful that the women in his community, who observed a cycle of menstrual separations, espoused the author's distinction between the true law and the second(ary) legislation. While he presents their second argument as "if in the seven days of your flux you regard yourself unclean according to the *deuterosis*," they obviously would have argued that menstrual impurity was prescribed by biblical authority, by the very texts "we" study, which are supposedly sacred Scripture to "our" community. For the women the biblically ordained practice of menstrual separation was not *secundatio*, and hence merely temporary. In spite of the destruction of the Temple they consider them as continuously valid. The Didascalia, however, rather than entirely delegitimizing their scriptural source of authority, redefines and limits that authority as only secondary legislation. He had to deal with the fact that the Torah was part of the Christian canon of Scripture. The possibility of simply throwing out the secondary legislation as an irrelevant authoritative text does not seem to have occurred to the Didascalia.[51] Instead, he maintains the status of the entire Torah as part of the Christian scriptural canon, but with a careful instruction on how to read the Torah:

ואנדין שוריה דעלמא אית לך בריתא דמושא רבא ואן נמוסא ופוקדנא אית
לך נמוסא ספרא דמפקנא דמריא אלהא מן כלהין הכיל נוכריתא אילין
דסקובלא אנין מליאית אתרחם ברם דין מא דקרא אנת בנמוסא הוי זהיר

דבלחוד מקרא תהוא קרא בה פשיטאית מן פוקדא דין ומן זוהרא דאית בה
סני אתרחם דלא תטעא נפשך ובאסורא דלא משתרין דמובלא יקירתא
תאסור אנת לך

Si autem initium generationis mundi, habes Genesim; aut si leges et praecepta, habes gloriosam domini legem. Ab omnibus igitur his tam alienis et diabolicis scripturis fortiter te abstine. Tamen et cum legem legis, ab omnibus praeceptis eius et ligaturis longe te abstine, ut non te veteribus et, qui non possunt solve, laqueis conliges et honeres. (Tidner, *Didascaliae*, 6–7)

If (you wish an account about) the beginning of the world, you have the Genesis of the great Moses; and if laws and commandments, you have the Law, the Book of Exodus of the Lord God.[52] Abstain completely therefore from strange (writings), those which are contrary[53] (to these). However, when you read in the Law, be watchful regarding (the second legislation) that you do but read it simply. But extremely abstain from the commands and prohibitions that are therein so that you may not lead yourself astray and bind yourself with the bonds of heavy burdens which may not be loosed. (Vööbus, *Didascalia*, 15)

This instruction at the beginning of the Didascalia could very well be addressed to the women, who do exactly that which the author asks them to abstain from: they observe the commandment of menstrual impurity and they bind themselves to the yoke of the Torah. Admittedly the immediate addressees of this exhortation are the men, the husbands in the community who "shall not roam and go idly about in the streets," but instead "should meditate continually upon the utterings of the Lord" (Vööbus, *Didascalia*, 14). In the subsequent chapter, which addresses the women and specifically the wives, he does not include such reading instructions. However, even if this should should be intentional and not merely an avoidance of repetition, that is, even if these reading instructions were intended for the men only, we may assume that women learned the biblical text at the very least in the setting of community gathering at which it was read (Vööbus, *Didascalia*, 37–38). Be that as it may, the women from a Jewish background who continue to observe menstrual separation most likely knew the Torah already from their former cultural context.

## The Argument from Jesus' Example

The Didascalia's third and final argument against a Christianized version of the observance of niddah is based on the author's interpretation of Jesus' acts. This argument, however, is not a response to a specific claim made by the women themselves. It does not immediately follow from the situation which the Didascalia is responding to. In fact, the discussion has inadvertently shifted from the women's public withdrawal or abstention from activities in the community to the behavior in the marriage bed. The concern shifts to the other side of the biblical regulation of behavior during a woman's menstruation: from impurity to forbidden sexual relationships, the prohibition of marital intercourse during a wife's menstrual period (Lev. 20:18). This complex is introduced by the reference to an example from the gospels. From the Didascalia's rhetoric it does not appear that he still argues against the women's behavior, or with what the women have argued.

What the author does in his third argument, then, is to have recourse to a source of authority that could be shared by any Christian, the authority of Jesus, as reported in the gospels. He bases himself on the famous story of the woman with a twelve-year blood-flow, whom Jesus heals. The reference to the individual gospel story here is in line with what the Didascalia had presented at the beginning as the study program for the members of its community: בנמוסא וספר מלכא ובנביא ובאאונגליון מוליא דהלין—"the Law, and the Book of Kings and the prophets and the Gospel (which is) the fulfillment of these" (14). In our context, then, the individual story comes to exemplify how the gospel is the fulfillment, or the *plenitudo* of the Law. The healing story appears in all three of the synoptic gospels (Mark 5:25–34; Matthew 9:20–22; Luke 8:42–48), and is the only incident in New Testament literature in which the impurity of genital discharges would appear to play any role:

ואילין תוב דדעידא אנין לא תהוון מפרשין מטל דאף הי דרדא הוא דמה כד
קרבת לקרנא דמרטוטה דפרוקן לא אתרשית אלא אף לשובקנא דכלהון
חטהיה אשתוית וכד נהוין רדין אילין דדכינא אנין אתחפטו דאיך ודקא
תהוון נקפין להין מטל דידעין אנתון דהדמיכון אנין

et quod in consuetudinibus est, id nolite segregare. Nam et ea, quae fluctum patiebatur, cum tetigisset salubrem fimbriam, non est repraehensa, sed tum sanata perfectam remissionem peccatorum meruit. Itaque, cum naturalia profluunt uxoribus vestris, nolite convenire illis, sed sustinete eas. (Tidner, *Didascaliae*, 99)

And again you shall not separate those (women) who are in the habit. For she also who had the flow of blood when she touched the border of our Savior's cloak, was not censured but was even esteemed worthy for the forgiveness of all her sins. And when (your wives have) those issues which are according to nature, take care, as is right, that you cleave to them, for you know that they are your members. (244)

As appears from this text, the Didascalia's final "proof" for the abolishing of the observance of niddah rests on the authority of Jesus' acts as told in the gospel story. The Didascalia's author only hints at the story, and does not cite it. In his reference, then, the story is significantly transformed. That is, in order to avail himself of the story of the woman with a twelve-year blood-flow as supporting his argument, he has to make a significant omission and addition. Both these devices modulate the "original" gospel story from a healing story to an anti-niddah-observance story.[54]

The omission lies in the fact that in the original story in the synoptic gospels the narrative starting point is that a woman suffers from a blood-flow for twelve years, while in the Didascalia she appears as a woman with merely (any kind of) a blood-flow. At first sight this omission might appear insignificant, for presumably the narrative device in the gospel story is only a symbolic enhancement or a dramatic exaggeration. However, the twelve years in the original story emphasize the severity of the illness, of which the woman is healed by Jesus. In the gospel narrative the question is about a pathological blood-flow as opposed to niddah. The emphasis lies on the miraculous event of healing. In the summary in the Didascalia, on the other hand, the emphasis of the story shifts away from the narrative enhancement of Jesus' miraculous healing to the touching of Jesus' garment as a transgression of biblical impurity regulations. Hence, Jesus appears to take on the biblical tradition of menstrual separation, since by praising the woman he transforms her act from transgression to exemplary behavior. This then is the Didascalia's addition in its retelling: Jesus does not chastise the woman for touching him, but deems her "worthy for the forgiveness of all her sins." To which sin is the Didascalia referring? Would it be particularly the one of touching Jesus' garment? We know nothing about the woman's sins from in the gospel narrative, nor in the Didascalia's retelling.

The Didascalia's reading of the gospel story compels us to look at the narrative in the gospel again. Does this narrative indeed critique, or even abolish or renounce, the practice of niddah? In other words, does this narrative present the New Testament's answer to the biblical tradition of menstrual regulation and abolish it once and for all? Even more significantly, what does it mean that the Didascalia's reading coincides with more recent feminist interpretations of the gospel narrative?

### The Study of the Woman with a Twelve-Year Blood-Flow

The story in the synoptic gospels, Mark 5:25–34, Matthew 9:20–22, Luke 8:42–48, runs along the following narrative line.

Of the three versions of the story Mark's is the most elaborate, of which Matthew presents a radical abbreviation,[55] while Luke remains closer to the *Vorlage* of Mark. All three start out with the fact that the woman had a flow of blood for twelve years. According to Mark and some manuscripts of Luke she had spent all she had on doctors and yet none of them could heal her.[56] According to all three she comes to Jesus from behind to touch his garment, for—according to Mark and Matthew—she tells herself that if she can only touch his garment she will be made well.[57] She is instantly healed.[58] According to Mark and Luke, Jesus asks who touched him, because he feels that something has happened to him, that power has gone out from him.[59] The disciples disqualify the question, since in the midst of the crowd around them anybody might have touched him.[60] But Jesus glances over the crowd. According to Mark and Luke the woman comes forward on her own, whereas according to Matthew Jesus sees her. Both the former gospel writers emphasize her fear and trembling while she comes forward to tell her deed.[61] Jesus' answer is the same in all three gospels: θυγάτηρ, ἡ πίστις σου σέσωκέν σε—"daughter, your faith has made you well" (Mark 5:34, Luke 8:48, Matthew 9:22).

The narrative has been dealt with in two recent monographs,[62] in numerous articles,[63] and, of course, in all the major New Testament commentaries series. Most of this scholarly literature discusses the Jewish milieu of the narrative. The story of the woman with a blood-flow becomes for New

Testament scholars the occasion to reflect not just on this particular incident in which Jesus is said to heal a woman from her sickness, but on what some call "jüdische Blutriten [Jewish blood rituals]" or "jüdische Blutscheu [Jewish fear of blood]," others "jüdische Kautelen mit dem Menstruationsblut [Jewish caution about menstrual blood]," or others women's "restrictive cultic roles in society" (Selvidge, *Woman, Cult and Miracle Recital*, 83) and most often the "menstrual taboo." Such terms indicate at best the persisting lack of understanding with which New Testament scholars reconstruct the presumed Jewish milieu of the story.

For many Christian feminists it has thus become a "banner for equality of women within church and society" (Selvidge, *Woman, Cult and Miracle Recital*, 30). Selvidge herself claims in her monograph that "this story was written to free early Christian women from the social bonds of niddah, 'banishment' during a woman's menstrual period" (30). This approach falls under what Daum and McCauley have called "Jesus-was-a-feminist strategy" (quoted in von Kellenbach, *Anti-Judaism*, 30). Such a hermeneutic strategy and the implied anti-Judaism often running alongside it has been extensively criticized from a feminist critical perspective by von Kellenbach, who builds on the work of other feminist readings of New Testament literature.

My intent here is not to indict for anti-Judaism all those feminist New Testament scholars who are engaged in the work of retrieving the meaningfulness of New Testament literature or the work of Jesus for contemporary Christian women. Nonetheless, our narrative of Jesus' healing of the woman with a blood-flow turns out to be particularly difficult. Its interpretation by both feminist and non-feminist Christian New Testament scholars proves to be part of what von Kellenbach has described as "the unself-conscious, small and seemingly innocent distortions of Judaism which add up and sustain more pernicious forms of prejudice" (13). By passing a judgment on the suffering and oppression of the woman in this particular narrative and by implication on Jewish traditions surrounding menstruation, such hermeneutic approaches also pass a judgment on Jewish women who choose to observe menstrual separation as a part of living their Jewishly defined lives today. The woman in the story becomes the emblematic Jewish woman whom Jesus comes to heal and to liberate. Such approaches do the salvage work of their own religious tradition by turning Jewish women's lives in the first century (and by implication in our own century) into the negative background of this work, or as von Kellenbach describes it: "By equating the (Jewish) foes of Jesus with the (patriarchal) enemies of feminism, some scholars arrive at the conclusion that Christianity and feminism are fighting the same battle" (74).

The challenge then is to speculate how the story would be read from the position of a woman who is committed to the observance of menstrual separation as a meaningful part of her tradition, who regards this observation as part of what it means to live her life in relation to the biblical God. The challenge is to think how the women against whom the Didascalia writes would have read the story. Such a perspective would refuse to regard the traditions surrounding menstruation as an exclusively patriarchal tool, invented by men in the service of patriarchy in order to keep women in a subordinate position. This perspective could show that most New Testament critics misrepresent the complex of niddah in biblical text and rabbinic literature. It reveals that most Christian readings choose to exaggerate the conditions of Jewish women in the first century, in order to make the contrast between Jesus and his Jewish cultural environment all the more poignant. What, then, does the miracle as part of the canonical literature for Christians really achieve for Christian attitudes toward menstruation and regulation of menstruation?

This story is one among the many in which Jesus appears as a miraculous healer. It underlines the contrast between Jesus' power to heal and that of regular doctors. In a classic article of 1959 Rudolf and Martin Hengel treated this story in the context of attitudes toward medical treatment of illness in Jewish and Greco-Roman culture. They chose as the literary context or cultural intertext of this story the genre of miraculous healings,[64] which circulated in the Greco-Roman world in various cultures, and elaborate on the typical narrative elements of such stories. They note "as far as the details about the duration of the suffering and the failure of the doctors are concerned, these are typical characteristics for miraculous healing stories both within and outside the New Testament" ("Die Heilungen Jesu und medizinische Denken," 346; my translation).[65] Similarly, the instantaneous healing at the end of the story represents "an aspect characteristic of miraculous healing stories" (347). As the Hengels point out, the narrative element of touch as a means of healing does not appear only in this story, but in others in the synoptic gospels, most significantly in Mark's summary of Jesus' fame as a healer:

When [Jesus and the disciples] had crossed over, they came to land at Gennesaret and moored the boat. When they got out of the boat, people at once recognized him, and rushed about that whole region and began to bring the sick on mats to wherever they heard he was. And wherever he went, into villages or cities or farms, they laid the sick in the marketplaces, and begged him that they might touch even the fringe of his garment;[66] and all who touched it were healed. (Mark 6:53–56; cf. also Mark 3:10, Luke 6:19; see Hengel, "Die Heilungen Jesu und medizinische Denken," 347).

The semantic weight of the woman's touching of Jesus' garment lies in the healing power of his touch:[67] after the doctors have tried their medical treatments, a mere touch of Jesus suffices to heal her. The story became popular and lived on in the religious imagination in later centuries. At the beginning of the fourth century Eusebius describes in great detail in his *Ecclesiastical History* a bronze statue erected as a memorial of her "who had an issue of blood, and who, as we learn from the sacred gospels, found at the hands of our Saviour relief from her affliction [τὴν γὰρ αἱμορροοῦσαν, ἣν ἐκ τῶν ἱερῶν εὐαγγελίων πρὸς τοῦ σωτῆρος ἡμῶν τοῦ πάθους ἀπαλλαγὴν εὕρασθαι μεμαθήκαμεν]." The statue, which Eusebius claims to have seen, apparently represented the scene of the woman's healing and stood in front of a house in Caesarea Philippi (in northern Palestine), which had been identified as the woman's house. Eusebius notes that the statue itself had certain healing powers by virtue of an herb which "climbed up to the border of the double cloak of brass [μέχρι τοῦ κρασπέδου τῆς τοῦ χαλκοῦ διπλοΐδος], and acted as an antidote to all kinds of diseases."[68] Similarly, Athanasius relates in his *Vita St. Antonii*, of the latter half of the fourth century, the story of a paralyzed young girl who had "a terrible and very hideous disorder. For the runnings of her eyes, nose and ears fell to the ground and immediately became worms." Not only that, she was also "paralyzed and squinted." Her parents "having heard of monks going to Anthony, and believing in the Lord who healed the woman with the issue of blood [πιστεύσαντες τῷ Κυρίῳ τῷ τὴν αἱμορροοῦσαν θεραπεύσαντι], asked to be allowed, together, with the daughter to journey with them." They allowed her to participate in the pilgrimage and the girl is indeed healed.[69]

In spite of the context in Mark's gospel and the later wide reception of the story as a narrative of a miraculous healing that enhanced the powers of

Jesus, the story comes to be read on the background of biblical impurity regulations and by extension also on the "background" of the mishnaic discourse of impurity. Indeed, the woman's sickness is identified mostly as what could be called specifically a "Jewish sickness." It is not only a physical ailment from which she suffers, but she also suffers from the μάστιξ[70] of her own Jewish culture. Jesus then comes to heal her from both.

First she is identified unquestioningly by almost every commentator as a Jewish woman. By "Jewish" woman commentators mean a woman whose life is unquestionably defined and circumscribed by the biblical text on the one side, and the mishnaic text on the other. But even if the narrators indeed imagined her as a Jewish woman, one would still have to ask what kind of Jewish woman, since the Jewish community in first-century Palestine turns out to be so vastly diverse. The biblical text, which is prescriptive and not descriptive, requires interpretation in order to be applied to the regulation of daily life. Would she be a woman in whose community purity laws were more strictly or more leniently interpreted and observed? Be that as it may, the fact remains that none of the gospel narrators defines her as either non-Jewish or Jewish. In fact, it is this narrative ambiguity that facilitates those allegorical interpretations in early Christian literature which take this woman as a type of gentile and take her to be representative of the gentile church, such as Jerome and Augustine.[71] The narrative ambiguity keeps the possibility open that the woman's status of impurity according to the priestly regulation in Leviticus is of no interest to them, since they are primarily concerned with the healing miracle.

Second, her sickness is identified as a "Jewish sickness" by choosing Lev. 15 as Mark's (and parallels') intertext. Hence the woman is identified as a *zavah*, or a woman with an irregular or extended blood-flow. The connection with Lev. 15 is established primarily linguistically. In the Septuagint rendition of Lev. 15:25 the woman with a discharge of blood for many days is described as γυνή ἐὰν ῥέῃ ῥύσει αἵματος ἡμέρας πλείους.[72] For Lev. 15:33 the Greek term for her (regular) "menstrual separation" is τα αἱμοροούσα ἐν τῇ ἀφέδρῳ.[73] This linguistic similarity with the description of the woman's sickness in the gospels appears to identify Lev. 15 as an intertext that the narrators, or at least the writers of the gospels, had in mind. Commentators point out the suffering of the woman caused by her "Jewish illness": "In this case the sickness itself was so grave for a Jewish woman because she was in perpetual state of cultic impurity which made entering the sanctuary and participation in religious festivals such as Passover, impossible. Indeed, similar to leprosy, it excluded her from human society in general" (Hengel, "Die Heilungen Jesu und medizinische Denken," 346, 347; cited by Pesch, *Das Markusevangelium*, 301; Guehlich, *Mark 1*, 8:26, 296). But even here it is important to keep in mind that this linguistic connection is not a necessary one,[74] for as Hengel has pointed out, "the verb αἱμοῤῥεῖν is often found in Hippocrates" (346 n35) and is a component of medical vocabulary.

Most important to this reading of the story as a repudiation of Jewish traditions surrounding menstruation, however, is the narrative moment of the woman's touching of Jesus. Identified as a zavah, she is bracketed between Lev. 15 on the one hand and mishnaic law on the other. At one end of the spectrum stands Lev. 15, according to which supposedly the zavah transfers the status of impurity by touch. Surprisingly enough, however, none of the New Testament commentators take note of the fact that as far as the zavah is concerned, the masoretic text does not include an explication that she communicates impurity by *being touched*, as does the menstruating woman (Lev. 15:19). Nor is there any mention that neither she or the menstruating woman communicate impurity by touching anyone. The difference between being touched and touching someone is significant. The menstruating woman does transfer impurity by *being touched* (Lev. 15:19). Leviticus does not mention that she communicates impurity by *touching*. Milgrom comments that this "can only mean that in fact her hands do not transmit impurity. The consequence is that she is not banished but remains at home. Neither is she isolated from her family. She is free to prepare their meals and perform household chores. They, in turn, merely have to avoid lying in her bed, sitting in her chair, and touching her" (*Leviticus 1–16*, 936). This would apply all the more to the zavah, who could even be touched. The zavah, according to the masoretic text of Leviticus, communicates impurity only indirectly: if somebody touches her bedding or anything on which she sat, "whoever touches them shall be impure; he shall launder his clothes, bathe in water, and remain impure until the evening" (Lev. 15:27). Nonetheless, some manuscripts and the Septuagint's translation of Lev. 15:27 read: "whoever touches *her*, shall launder his clothes . . ." (Milgrom, *Leviticus 1–16*, 943).[75] Only if we accept, with Milgrom, the former reading, does the zavah, similar to the zav, the man with an irregular discharge, communicate impurity by being touched.

At the other end of the spectrum stands the mishnaic ruling in mZav 5:1:

"He who touches a *zav*, or he whom a *zav* touches, transfers a status of impurity to food, drink and vessels that (can be purified by immersion)."[76] MZav 5:1 extends Lev. 15, for according to the biblical text, as we have just seen, only the person who touches (somebody in the status of impurity) becomes impure, but presumably not the one who is touched (by somebody in the status of impurity). As a mishnaic zavah the woman in our story is then compared to a leprous person (Schottroff, *Befreiungserfahrung*, 113; Schmithals, *Das Evangelium nach Markus*, 293). Selvidge goes as far as to write that "the woman in the miracle story was beaten because of her physical ailment. She was taboo to all. She could have no intimate relations with men, nor could she, as a responsible Jewess, with a good conscience, be milling about among the masses" (*Woman, Cult and Miracle Recital*, 88; cf. Trummer, *Die blutende Frau*, 84).

Consequently, the presumption is often that the woman, deliberately or not, would have rendered Jesus impure (Selvidge, *Woman, Cult and Miracle Recital*, 92; Luz, *Das Evangelium nach Matthäus 8–17*, 52). Or she touched Jesus only secretly, because she knows that she really should not touch Jesus, since a status of impurity would be transferred to him: "Coming from the rear of the crowd, the appropriate place for the defiled, she risked defiling others by approaching and deliberately touching Jesus' clothes" (Guehlich, *Mark 1*, 8:26, 297; see also Witherington, *Women*, 73; Kertelge, *Das Markusevangelium*, 58).[77] Further, her fear and trembling at the end of the story is often explained as being caused by her sense of guilt about having rendered Jesus deliberately impure (Kertelge, *Das Markusevangelium*, 59) or revealing her awareness of having violated a taboo (Ruether, "Women's Body and Blood," 14).[78]

Finally, and perhaps most significantly, Jesus is regarded as having abolished the levitical impurity regulations concerning women by not only disregarding the fact that she committed the dreadful act of touching him, but by even praising her for her faith: "The fact that the woman was neither rejected nor reprimanded, but is recognized for her faith and healed, indicates that part of the Jewish fear of blood has been overcome" (Sand, *Das Evangelium nach Matthaeus*, 201).[79]

Even if we accept Lev. 15 and by extension its mishnaic elaboration as the intertext of the story, and even if we assume that the woman is Jewish, what is disregarded in all these speculations is the fact that the woman does not commit a transgression by touching Jesus, neither according to the priestly writings, nor according to mishnaic law. Thus Jacob Milgrom points out that in Lev. 15 "there is no prohibition barring the menstruant from touching anyone" (936). That is, neither Lev. 15, nor the mishnaic expansion of biblical im/purity regulations, ever prohibit touching by the woman, and thus do not treat the event of touch as a transgression, as opposed to, for example, forbidden sexual relationships. The latter, including the sexual relationship with a menstruating woman, are indeed a matter of transgression. The biblical and rabbinic discourse of im/purity is not a punitive discourse.[80] If it should so happen that someone touches a menstruating woman, and that might even be quite often, then the person who touches her simply acquires a ritual status of impurity until the evening of that day.

The woman in the gospel story commits no transgression when she touches Jesus' garment. Neither biblical nor mishnaic law consider the case of a person in a status of impurity who deliberately touches somebody else. Rabbinically speaking, the woman of our narrative would only have committed a transgression had she done anything that might lead to or initiate sexual contact, which is clearly not the point of the story.[81] Further, as far as I know, there is not a single case story in talmudic literature of someone in the status of impurity touching somebody else.[82] Thus, in spite of the halakhic theory expressed in mZav 5:1, the concern about touch remains at the very most subdued. Selvidge's contention that "a responsible Jewess with a good conscience" would not have been milling around in the masses is, therefore, unfounded, and has polemic undertones.[83] There is no indication that rabbinic literature expresses any concern about milling around in the masses, for those who are in the status of impurity because of a regular or irregular discharge, or those who are concerned about remaining in the status of purity. We might have expected such an indication had there been hermeneutic or practical concern about being touched by a person with such an invisible impurity.

The case for impurity according to either biblical or rabbinic law as a primary concern of the narrative cannot therefore be consistently argued. The attempt to read this story as an abrogation of biblical traditions concerning menstruation and irregular discharges of blood remains unsuccessful. The Jesus of this narrative appears as someone who has the power to heal a woman with a severe sickness, where others have failed. It is because of the open and unclear relationship of this narrative with the biblical text in Leviticus that from the beginning of Christian hermeneutic literature writers could use the story for whatever purpose they wanted. The Didascalia, as the only text in early Christian literature that I am aware of, uses the story in a way similar to contemporary Christian feminists. Its author is, of course, not concerned about the liberation of the women converts from a Jewish background in his community from their old oppression. Rather, he attempts to persuade them to turn away completely from that which gave them meaning in their previous lives, in order to conform to his interpretation of what it means to be Christian.

At the same time, the same story could be used to achieve the opposite ends. In the mid-third century, at approximately the same time in which the Didascalia was composed in Syria, Dionysius, the bishop of Alexandria and a student of Origen, wrote in response to the inquiry of Basilides, a colleague in rank:

> The question concerning women in the time of their [menstrual] separation, whether it is proper for them when in such a condition to enter the house of God, I consider a superfluous inquiry. For I do not think, that, if they are believing and pious women, they will themselves be rash enough in such a condition either to approach the holy table or to touch the body and blood of the Lord. Certainly the woman who had the discharge of blood of twelve years' standing did not touch (the Lord) Himself, but only the hem of His garment, with a view to her cure. (R. Kraemer, *Maenads, Martyrs, Matrons, Monastics*, 43)

Whereas the Didascalia tried to convince women in its community to partake in the Eucharist while they are menstruating, Dionysius attempts to keep them away from it, as well as from the altar and the church altogether. Again the woman with the twelve-year flow of blood is representative of any woman who has her menstruation. But now she becomes exemplary for barely having touched Jesus, since in fact she never touched Jesus' body, and her touch is not really any touch at all. The priestly terminology and regulation of Leviticus has sunk into oblivion.[84] The rhetoric is a different one, and in a way a more misogynist one, because Dionysius is no longer arguing about the validity or abolishment of a tradition, be it legal or practical. Rather, he seems to consider menstruation as essentially and inherently forbidding, so much so that the very question about it should be regarded as superfluous, so much so that "good" women, pious women, would never even get such a horrendous idea as to partake in the Eucharist "in such a condition."

It is this discourse of menstrual repugnance which subsequently predominates in Christian legal literature over against such an argument as the Didascalia had advanced.[85] At best, menstruation may be read as emblematic of the sinfulness of corporeality.[86] That might seem logical, since the Didascalia reacted and responded to a unique and local situation. Dionysius, on the other hand, responded to the question of a colleague who wanted to know the Christian principle or ruling regarding menstruous women in their relationship to the Christian public. Nonetheless, the Didascalia's argument would seem to be the more consistent one in a Christianity in which Pauline theology won the day, for if in Christ the "law," as that which set the Israelites apart from the rest of the human world, was fulfilled and no longer the basis of what made a Christian a Christian, then the regulations concerning menstruation should also have been abolished. Dionysius's opinion persisted despite its inconsistency. Why should one part of the Law be retained, but not others? Perhaps it persisted because Christian thought, by virtue of its "Westernization"—an ever-deepening permeation by Greek metaphysics and ontology and the accompanying dualistic pattern that bred contempt of the physical world, of the body, and in particular of the female body—could allow for such an "inconsistency."

In this I would argue in particular against those Christian feminist approaches that consider Dionysius's opinion to represent a revival of "Old Testament laws of purity" (Ruether, *New Women/New Earth*, 65), and hence blame the church's Jewish past for the separation of menstruous women from the Eucharist. Thus Leonard Swidler—who was one of the first scholars to write a monograph on *Women in Judaism* (1976), which unfortunately serves as one of the main sources for many Christian feminists—unfamiliar with rabbinic literature, argued that "Dionysius forbade Christian women from entering a church during their menstruation" because he held on "to the Hebraic laws of ritual impurity, which Jesus rejected" (343). Again, here I am following von Kellenbach's brilliant critique of this "Jewish-cultural-lag-theory," which contends that "Christianity is depicted as a powerless and innocent victim of a sexist Jewish past rather than active and responsible shaper of a new patriarchal tradition. The power of sexism is underestimated; Christianity's choices, mistakes and failures are glossed over" (*Anti-Judaism*, 113).

The question that remains would be about the fate of the book of Leviticus in Christianity. If it is so often assumed to stand in the background of those arguments concerning menstrual regulation, how did the book as such, and in particular those questions concerning purity, fare in early Christian literature? Or was the story of the woman with a twelve-year blood-flow indeed the only point of reference for those who even considered the (in)significance of menstruation?

## The Disappearance of the Female Body of Difference: The Case of Origen

The only other text in early Christian literature that I am aware of which deals extensively with the book of Leviticus is the collection of Origen's homilies on Leviticus. Origen roughly follows Leviticus but omits some passages. He delivered these homilies during three years sometime between 238 and 244, toward the end of his life (Barkley, *Origen's Homilies on Leviticus*, 20). Rufinus's translation of these homilies, as well as of Origen's homilies on *Genesis* and *Exodus*, stem from the early fifth century, between 403 and 405.[87] From a Christian perspective Leviticus may be the most "Jewish" of all the books of the Torah, with its holiness code, as well as being the most carnal, the most concerned with the physicality of the body. By remaining part of the Christian canon, it comes to present a continuous challenge for the church fathers at pains to distinguish Christianity from that which it inherits, biblical Israel. As part of the Christian canon, then, Leviticus continued to transmit the explicit commands of the God of biblical Israel, who became the Christian God. What were Christians to do with this divine voice, especially seeing that again and again some Christians continued to understand this text to be addressed to them also, as we have seen in the Didascalia? Hence, special hermeneutic parameters had to be set within which the book was to be read.

As we have seen, the Didascalia posed a historical-chronological division within the period of biblical Israel, affirmed by the coming of Jesus, which invalidated those laws given in the "second nomos." Similarly, Origen outlines special reading instructions in order to refute those "who force us to be subservient to the historical sense and to keep to the letter of the law" (Barkley, *Origen's Homilies on Leviticus*, 30). Like the Didascalia, Origen seems to battle those in his community who regard the biblical legislation of Israel, and especially Leviticus, as authoritative for themselves, and not just for the Israelites in the past. In reaction to those literalists he outlines how the book of Leviticus, which as a text is indeed still valid for the Christian community, has to be read in order not to be subservient to "the letter of the Law":

> As "in the last days" (Acts 2:17) the Word of God, which was clothed with the flesh of Mary, proceeded into this world. What was seen in him was one thing; what was understood was something else. For the sight of his flesh was open for all to see, but the knowledge of his divinity was given to the few, even elect. So also when the Word of God was brought to humans through the Prophets and the Lawgiver [Moses], it was not brought without proper clothing. For just as there it was covered with the veil of flesh (2 Cor. 3:14)[88] so here with the veil of the letter, so that indeed the letter is seen as flesh but the spiritual sense hiding within is perceived as divinity. Such, therefore, is what we now find as we go through the book of Leviticus. (29)

The basis for proper hermeneutics is christology. Just as Jesus, the Word of God, is only clothed with the human flesh, so the Word of God was previously given to biblical Israel only clothed with the letter. Just as a distinction is made between the flesh or humanity of Jesus, and the understanding or knowledge of the divinity hidden in the flesh, so there is a distinction between seeing the letter and perceiving the divinity behind the letter.[89] S/he who sees but fails to perceive or understand, fails to penetrate through the surface of the flesh and the letter to the divinity in hiding. As opposed to the Didascalia, therefore, that claimed what it called the "second nomos" had been invalidated in history, but which could not provide a reason why that same "second nomos" should then remain relevant at all for the Christian community, Origen operates with a christological hermeneutics, which knows how to recognize the obvious and the hidden, the veil and the essence, the fleshly clothing of the Word of God and the Word itself, the letter and the spirit. But like the Didascalia he attempts to lead *ad absurdum* those who insist on the literal meaning of the letter:

> For if I should follow the simple understanding, as certain ones among us do, without using in their terms of ridicule the stratagems of

language or the cloud of allegory, I would draw out the voice of the Lawgiver. [Then] I, myself a man of the Church, living under the faith of Christ and placed in the midst of the Church, am compelled by the authority of the divine precept to sacrifice calves and lambs and to offer fine wheat flour with incense and oil. (29, 30)

Just as the Didascalia tells the women that if you keep part of the law, you really would have to observe it all, Origen argues that if you literalists follow the simple understanding in parts of it, I, as a man of the Church, as one functioning in the role formerly carried out by the priests, should have to offer sacrifices as prescribed in Leviticus, which is clearly not the case.

Given these hermeneutic parameters what then happens to the regulations of im/purity, particularly those concerning women? Origen's eighth homily on Leviticus deals with the impurity of birth (de eo quod scriptum est: "mulier quaecumque conceperit semen et pepererit masculum, immunda erit septem diebus" [Lev. 12]) on the one hand, and the varieties of leprosy (de diversitatibus leprae (Lev. 13 and 14])[90] on the other, but it stops short of Lev. 15 and fails to preach on the impurity of genital discharges. Thus Origen's sermon on the leprous person theoretically does not have any interest for my pursuit here. However, the first part of the homily on the impurity of birth is instructive as to why he most likely could not have dealt with Lev. 15 without turning it into "an obstacle and ruin of the Christian religion" (88). Origen begins with a reflection on the opening verse of Lev. 12, the chapter on the impurity of birth, and makes an observation similar to that of the halakhic midrash:

> "If any woman conceives and bears a male child, she will be impure for seven days" (Lev. 12:2). First let us consider according to the historical sense if this does not seem to be a superfluous addition, "A woman who conceives and bears a male child." How else could she bear a male child unless she had conceived? (Barkley, *Homilies on Leviticus*, 154)

On the first hermeneutic level, which he calls here *secundum historiam*, but which really only implies a close or literary reading of the text, Origen notes the textual peculiarity of the doubled formulation "conceives and bears." In an almost midrashic attitude toward the biblical text, paying close attention to grammatical peculiarities, he emphasizes the significance with his rhetorical question. Origen's "historical" question of the text focuses on when the woman in childbirth would be considered to be impure. Surely not when she conceives, but when she gives birth. So why did the text insert "if she conceives"? The syntactic peculiarity on the surface of the text reflects onto the mystical level, which leads him to an extraordinary interpretation:

> For the Lawgiver added this word to distinguish her who "conceived and gave birth" without seed from other women so as not to designate as "unclean" every woman who had given birth but her who "had given birth by receiving seed." There can also be added to this the fact that this Law which is written concerning uncleanness pertains to women. But concerning Mary, it is said that "a virgin" conceived and gave birth. Therefore, let *women* carry the burdens of the Law, but let *virgins* be immune from them. (Barkley, *Homilies on Leviticus*, 154)

The doubled formulation in the biblical text of the woman who conceives and gives birth according to Origen's mystical reading points to the distinction between Mary and all other women on the one hand, and between virgins and women on the other. The former distinction seems to derive primarily from a theological concern. By implication she who clothed the Word of God in her flesh, to use Origen's language, would actually have been impure through giving birth according to biblical law. This seems to be an untenable position. Therefore, the doubled formulation in Lev. 12 points to the fact that the process of conception in Mary is not an ordinary conception, but a conception without seed. The impurity lies in the act of ordinary conception, and ordinary women fall victim to that, but not Mary. Virgins, then, are included in the mystical exception of Mary from the "burdens of the Law." This last phrase, however, is difficult to understand. There is nothing remarkable about virgins being excluded from the law of impurity of birth, since they are virgins by virtue of not giving birth, unless he imagines the repetition of Mary's conception. Or does he generalize and mean to say that virgins are freed from the general "burdens of the Law," by implication also from the legal tradition concerning menstrual impurity? Does this imply other (Christian) women in the community, who do not choose the heroic path of asceticism, are supposed to observe not only the period of birth impurity, but also the period of menstrual impurity, since he does not outright reject the principle of impurity due to birth? One would think that this is not Origen's intention. But he formulates that the "law pertains to women" but not to virgins, and especially not to Mary who was the virgin among virgins. "Women may carry the burden of the Law" but not virgins.

Ultimately, however, Origen does not seem much interested in these other women. The last line in this paragraph seems almost like a throwaway line, which utters a thought but does not think it through. In other words, he only needs the "other" women as a negative contrast for Mary and all the other virgins. This becomes all the more clear when he subsequently attempts to justify why nonetheless Paul calls Mary a "woman" instead of a virgin when he writes in his letter to the Galatians: "But when the fullness of time came, God sent his son, made from woman, made under the law, that he might redeem those who were under the law" [ὅτε δὲ ἦλθεν τὸ πλήρωμα τοῦ χρόνου, ἐξαπέστειλεν ὁ θεὸς τὸν υἱὸν αὐτοῦ, γενόμενον ἐκ γυναικός, γενόμενον ὑπὸ νόμον] (Gal. 4:4–5). This causes Origen to reflect on the appellation of "woman." For one, the virgin can be called "woman [γυνή, mulier]"—"not because of corruption but because of her sex [non pro corruptela, sed pro sexus indicio nominavit]" (Barkley 155, Baehrens 395). That is, the fact that Paul calls her woman does not imply that she had been stained by the *macula admixtionis*, the stain of intercourse. She has a sex, but she never had sex. On the other hand, Origen explains at length that the term "woman" can be attached to a certain age, "when the female sex proceeds from the years of puberty and passes to that time when she seems to be suitable for a man [qua feminino sexui de annis pubertatis exceditur et ad id temporis, quo habilis viro videatur esse, transitur]." A virgin who remained chaste can be called a woman "by virtue of the maturity of age alone [pro sola aetatis maturitate mulier nominetur]."

What Origen drives at in the end is that virgins are not really women. They are merely called women, because a woman (mulier) is usually defined not merely by her gender, and not merely by her age, but by her sexuality or sexual activity. Just as Mary was detached from the physicality of human intercourse, so are all virgins, who along with Mary are separated from the rest of the women (a reliquis mulieribus) (Baehrens 396). At the same time, virgins then are, of course, the true women, for virginity was to become the ideal of Christian womanhood.

What this passage comes to emblematize, then, is both a social distinction among women and an anthropological distinction in woman, both of which exactly correspond with each other. The social distinction between *hoi polloi* and *virgines* is the distinction between those who remain wedded to the physical world and their bodies and those who achieve the ideal womanhood of renunciation of sexuality. It is the distinction between physical birth and spiritual birth, between a bleeding body and the spiritual soul that inhabits it.

We needn't wonder, then, that Origen has no interest in the impurity of genital discharges. For even the most physical event, birth, can be transformed via Mary into a spiritual symbol. But with virginity as the ideal of Christian womanhood in the literature of the early church, developed at the expense of the "rest of the women," and thus with the obliteration of the physical body as bearing any postive significance, menstruation becomes a discursive nonevent. Where it became an issue, such as when Basilides inquired from Dionysius in Alexandria what to do about those bleeding bodies of women, it was banned from the space of the church. Dionysius's ruling then would seem to correspond in the sociohistorical world to that theological discourse which obliterated the female body, which is in the habit of bleeding periodically, for the sake of the world of the spirit.

In light of this direction of Christian discourse on the female body we can now once more return to the peculiar controversy enshrined in the text of the Didascalia in order to reflect on its place within the larger discourse. Here we do not deal with (male) theologians reflecting on the ideal of womanhood, or male clergy in the upper ranks of the institutional hierarchy making rulings, but with women themselves, from among those whom Origen would perhaps rank among his *reliquum mulieribus*, interpreting the significance of their bodies for their religious lives.

### In Defense of the Female Body of Difference

From the argument of the Didascalia it appears that at the beginning of the third century there were women in a certain Christian community, or in certain communities in the cultural sphere of Syria, who had come from a Jewish cultural background. These women continued to observe menstrual separation. This observance may have provided them with an important link between their old community and the new one, between their previous religious lives and their lives within the Christian community. It is not entirely clear how they would have understood this continuity between the old and the new, nor even how this continuity is to be imagined, for it is not entirely clear from what kind of Jewish background they came. As we have seen, the tannaitic literature of the rabbis of approximately the same period allows women during their menstrual periods to read the Torah or otherwise study rabbinic texts (tBer 2:13; Cohen, "Menstruants and the Sacred," 283; Boyarin, *Carnal Israel*, 180). Do these women in the community of the Didascalia come from a Jewish community which did or did not entirely base its community life on rabbinic interpretation of Jewish practice? Or if their former Jewish community was determined by a rabbinically circumscribed life, had the women already refrained from religious activities such as reciting the liturgy and reading the Torah, in spite of the rabbinic permission? Or did they change their practice when they became members of the Christian community, when they were baptized?

In spite of these questions, which cannot be answered with certainty, we see the Didascalia dealing with these formerly Jewish women as now baptized members of its own community. Upon baptism they received some instruction from women, for as the Didascalia prescribes: "and when she who is being baptized has come up from the water let the deaconess receive her, and teach and educate her" (Vööbus, *Didascalia*, 157).

Several different though not necessarily alternative scenarios can be imagined. On the one hand, they might simply have continued what they have practiced before: menstrual separation from "sacred" activities. Just as they kept away from the synagogue or from involvement in the liturgy of the synagogue during their menstrual period, they applied this to the church. In such a case these women might have come to the Christian community from a Jewish community that was not (yet?) regulated by mishnaic halakha, or from a Jewish community that was ruled by rabbinic halakhah, but by a stricter application of it. This line of reasoning would cast them as conservatives whose motivating desire was primarily to preserve their tradition.

Thus in Christian historiography the so-called Jewish-Christian heretics have often been called "conservatives." But such a categorization is possible only from a theological point of view, one that regards Christianity as that which overrides and supersedes Judaism, or at least the legal-cultural aspect of biblical Israel. Converts from Judaism then are deemed to have remained stuck in their legal mode of thinking, and thought not to have grasped the gospel message of freedom. The inadequacy of such a theological perspective, especially for understanding the situation depicted in the Didascalia, becomes apparent when we consider that the women do not merely preserve their tradition, if that is the case, but readapt it to their Christian lives. Thus they have to engage in an act of reinterpretation of their Jewish traditions as well as of the Christian teaching that they are joining.

On the other hand, the women may not have kept themselves away from the synagogue, but began to abstain from attending the church assembly when they joined the Christian community because the church assembly might have had a different symbolic signification to them than did the synagogue. That is, they regarded the church and especially the Eucharist, the "fruits of the Holy Spirit," as a substitute for the Temple and its sacrificial cult, rather than the synagogue. This scenario seems to be the more unlikely one, but needs to be considered as possible. In this case the women should be cast as innovators.

In either case, most likely they learned about the concept of the Holy Spirit and its workings within the Christian community in those instructions after their baptism and then used and reframed the pneumatology they were taught into what I have called a uterine pneumatology, to give adequate expression to their desire to maintain rituals of menstrual separation from the sacred, very much to the dislike of the author of the Didascalia. In order for us to hear the women's argument better, against the authority of the Didascalia's author and before judging them to be either conservative or innovative, we have to consider once again what Antoinette Clark Wire wrote with respect to the Corinthian women against whom Paul argued:

> Again, any independent determination of a text's authority works against hearing the arguments in the text because it sets up an alternative authority to the conviction won by the arguments given. This explanation is not a sleight of hand to cancel out the authority of the text. It is a necessary defense of authority that operates through persuasion as found in the form and functioning of Paul's letters. If we take on the role of the reader that Paul sets up and locate the Bible's authority not in given dogmas or individual authors but in the event where the persuasive word meets conviction, this event may occur where we do not expect. (Wire, *Corinthian Women Prophets*, 10–11)

The Didascalia, of course, never attained the canonical authority of Paul's letters. But the author is often read theologically as already inhabiting the space of the "catholic" church, as speaking from the perspective of orthodoxy, even where he is not quite as orthodox in some of his theological views as one would have imagined. As far as the "Jewish Christian" women are concerned, however, he certainly is higher up on the rungs of the ladders of orthodoxy. Against this theological reading I want to consider with Wire not the authoritative weight of the Didascalia's argument against the women's argument regarding a historical development of theological doctrine, but rather the argumentative weight of both parties in the situation. In this way the women are not up against Didascalia and all the rest of theological orthodoxy, but the Didascalia's author is up against the women in his local community, in which "persuasive words can meet conviction."

The question I want to consider at the end, then, is whether these women acted primarily as (former) Jews or as women? Of course, this question can only be asked on the conceptual level, for in reality they cannot be separated. But the reason the question needs to be asked this way is that historiographers of early Christianity have so far always only considered the first part, to the complete neglect of the second.

The controversy in the Didascalia has been almost exclusively treated as one between so-called Jewish-Christians,[91] on the one hand, and the perspective of Catholic Christianity on the other, which the Didascalia claims to defend, however questionable that claim to catholicity might seem. In the analysis of the women's argumentation above I have attempted to avoid the categorization of these women as Jewish-Christians in favor of the more cumbersome "those who came or were converted from a Jewish background," primarily because both the definition or meaning of the term and the representative value of the category of Jewish-Christians has become so questionable in recent years.[92] In a recent paper, "Jewish Christianity in Antioch Before the Time of Hadrian: Where Does the Identity Lie?" Jack Sanders has aptly imagined other people asking him:

> What does he mean by Jewish, and what does he mean by Christian; and given the enormous variety of both in the period under consideration, how can he possibly get beyond the task of definition—especially when so many other scholars have met defeat on the battle-

field of contention over the definition of so seemingly simple a term as "Jewish Christianity"? (346)

This is even more true concerning the term Judaizers[93] or Judaizing Christians (Connolly, *Didascalia*, lxxxiii), which has been applied to women in the Didascalia's community as well.

As far as the women in the Didascalia are concerned, we can claim with certainty that they understood themselves as Christians, and not as a separate syncretistic group of Jewish Christians. The Didascalia itself, in spite of identifying the women and those others who still prefer Shabbat over Sunday as coming "from among the people," did not regard them as such a separate group, since it addresses them as baptized members of the community. Further, we have seen it is not even unambiguously clear in how far their practice of menstrual separation can be identified as a Jewish practice, since it does not conform to tannaitic texts, and especially in view of the "Christianized" interpretation of the practice. The conflict arises precisely because they have their own interpretation of what it means to live a Christian life as a woman, which comes into conflict with the understanding of the author of the Didascalia. Their interpretation appears to be strong enough that the author of the Didascalia finds himself forced to enter into an argument with them.

But what if we turn away from the question of their "Jewish" motivation to their motivation as women? Can we even ask that question beyond the arguments that we have seen them advancing? Clearly, the women themselves have not made an explicit case for their behavior. Nonetheless, I would like to propose that if we contrast these women's behavior with Origen and the majority discourse on virginity as the ideal of Christian womanhood, it is possible to reflect on the significance of their behavior as a gender-specific behavior, for the Didascalia's women give a positive signification to their embodied lives, embodied not in a static physicality called flesh, but in a living body that undergoes cyclic changes. Instead of transcending their body in order to free themselves from the shackles of bondedness in the flesh, they affirm their embodied lives by endowing the body with significance regarding their connection with the Spirit or the presence of the Divine. In their conception of a Christian life their bodies in the here and now are not transcended and overcome in order to participate in the fruits of the Spirit. Or, in terms of their pneumatology, the Spirit that they received upon baptism remains subject to the habits of their female bodies.

The Didascalia's author, then, instead of being viewed as someone who helps the women to their own liberation from what he calls "the burden of the Law," corresponding to what Christian feminists have regarded as Jesus' liberation of (Jewish) women from the "social bonds of niddah," in the end "liberates" them from their attempt to endow their embodied lives with positive signification with the help of the symbolic terms they found in the teaching of the community they joined. What this "liberation" amounts to is revealed in the Didascalia's final point with regard to those who "keep the habits of nature and fluxes and intercourse" (Vööbus, *Didascalia*, 238), immediately after his reference to the gospel story of the woman who touched Jesus' cloak:

וכד נהוין רדין אילון דדכינא אנין אתחפטו דאיך ודקא תהוון נקפין להין מטל דידעין אנתון דהדמיכון אנין והויתון מחבין להין איך נפשיןֿ⁹⁴(262)

And when (your wives have) those issues which are according to nature, take care, as is right, that you cleave to them, for you know they are your members, and love them as your soul. (244)

Cohen has recognized the uniqueness of this passage in Christian literature, for he writes: "The Didascalia's rejection of the Levitical impurity laws is so radical that it even rejects the requirement that husband and wife separate from each other during her menstruation" (290). What Cohen does not observe is that the Didascalia has suddenly switched addressees. After the long and protracted discussion directly with the women on their menstrual separation from Christian community life, the Didascalia's author turns to address their husbands, and orders them to engage in marital intercourse. Up to this point the question of marital intercourse had not been part of the debate at all. It is doubtful that a refusal of the women to sleep with their husbands during their menstrual periods, if they indeed did refuse, would have been visible in the community and hence known to the author, unless the husbands complained to church authorities. Though that is possible, it seems more likely that the Didascalia throws into the discussion what is part of the biblical discourse. The thought process might have been that since the author started to get into a debate about regulations concerning menstruation anyway, in which he declared the invalidation of traditions based on what he calls the "second law," he decided to settle everything contained in that "second law."

He ignores the women as the ones who had initiated the occasion of his discussion; he also completely disregards them as subjects in matters of sexual intercourse. For if the women indeed did not want to sleep with their husbands during their menstrual periods, would the Didascalia's recommendation to the husbands to cleave to their wives present a liberation from their own attachment to the regulations in the "second nomos"?

My argument in the end, then, is not that the menstrual regulation and separation in and by itself is necessarily affirming of women. We have seen that in the mouth of Dionysius of Alexandria the prohibition to enter the church and partake in the Eucharist while menstruating becomes a tool of repression of women's embodied lives. Nor is the opposite position, in which the Didascalia wants to get rid of any menstrual regulation passed down from biblical tradition, since its author enacts a discursive repression of what women do with their bodies which in the end is almost equal to Dionysius's, only in the opposite direction. Hence, the position of contemporary feminists, who want to argue that Jesus liberated (Jewish) women from their rootedness in biblical culture, and that the "reintroduction" of a menstrual taboo by Dionysius in the third century represented a fall-back into patriarchy in Christianity, amounts to the same discursive repression of the life choices of women who do not follow the Christian path. In the end, the entire difference lies in what women choose to do with such traditions, what meaning they give to them, and how they view the significance of their embodiedness for their intellectual and religious life choices. A Christian discourse, which focused almost entirely on the ideal of virginity, did not provide much space for such a reflection. In that respect, then, the women in the Didascalia present a challenge to the author of the Didascalia, who entered into a discussion with them. They present an equal challenge to contemporary feminist critics of gender constructs in the literature of early Christianity.

## CONCLUSION

THE READINGS OF a wide variety of texts throughout the chapters of this book have aimed at two different purposes. On the one hand, they have investigated what the texts reveal with respect to rabbinic thinking about gender in the context of discussing the biblical laws of menstruation. The cultural and hermeneutic presuppositions of the rabbis determined and shaped their discussions of women's bodies and corporeality. On the other hand, underlying my readings has been the question of the possible implications for Jewish women's lives emerging from the rabbinic discussions and other related textual cultures.

As to the latter, we have to conclude that it is extremely difficult to extrapolate from the rabbinic discussions as to the impact they had on women's lives. It is extremely difficult to reconstruct women's voices within the rabbinic texts, even where they focus on questions that concern women, and on intimate factors such as women's bodies and women's sexual lives. Most of the discussions are of a highly theoretical nature. They are a product of the Beit Midrash, the House of Study, an almost certainly exclusively male institution. This institutional setting of their discussions provided the rabbis with the opportunity to discuss the nature of women's bodies and to textualize them without the pressure of accountability to those who inhabit those bodies. The cultural process that I have tried to trace is the following. The Beit Midrash is a cultural innovation unique to the rabbinic movement in late antiquity. Its framing as an exclusively male institution and its production of a male leadership for the Jewish community is reflected in the nature and the framing of the discussions. It is the nature and the framing of the discussions, concomitantly, that enable and stabilize the Beit Midrash as a homosocial community.

This step I have outlined in Chapter 2, which discusses the metaphorical construction of women's bodies as houses and as buildings. We have seen that this is the predominant choice of metaphors in the Mishnah, as well in a number of baraitot in the Babylonian Talmud. Further, the Talmud in its exegetical passages on the Mishnah expands on these metaphors. This construction, which rabbinic culture shares with many other androcentric cultures, for women amounts to what Hélène Cixous has diagnosed as the violence of masculine cultures: "she has been kept at a distance from herself, she has been made to see (= not-see) woman on the basis of what man wants to see of her, which is to say almost nothing" (*Newly Born Woman*, 68). The rabbis' favored choice of metaphorical construction aids them discursively in stabilizing the Beit Midrash as an exclusively male community. Whereas one might have considered women to be important references for the reflections on menstrual impurity, the mishnaic texts objectify women's bodies. The effect of this objectification is that women are not needed to contribute to the discussions and, in fact, are excluded from the discussions altogether.

At the same time we have seen in Chapter 3 that the Talmud produces a reading of the Mishnah which potentially subverts the entire mishnaic perspective. Shmu'el's midrash, introduced and discussed in the Babylonian Talmud, produces a corrosion of the mishnaic perspective in that it introduces the criteria of sensation in its thinking about the female body. Of course, the subversion of the mishnaic perspective in this particular case is part of the Babylonian Talmud's general rigorous pursuit of dialectical strategies (Hayes, *Between the Babylonian and Palestinian Talmuds*, 180), but in this case it produces a particular effect with respect to the implications for gendering rabbinic discussions. Shmu'el's midrashic reading and its various manifestations throughout Tractate Niddah represents a rupture in the mishnaic framing of women's corporeality, because the female body is no longer the object that fortifies the androcentric universe. It now gains a life of its own, which allows for an alternative reality to break into the one that the mishnaic texts construct as dominant.

What emerges from this analysis is that despite the dominant perspective of the text, the talmudic discussions do not evolve into a homogeneously gendered discourse. Within the dialectics of the Babylonian Talmud we can witness tensions and conflicts around the creation of gender. The discussions open up alternatives rather than congealing into a closed, discursive universe.

Chapters 4 and 5 pursue this path further. Chapter 4 addresses the tension inherent in the talmudic construction of the rabbi as expert on women's bleeding. Again, rather than reading these texts primarily as representing the social-historical institution of rabbinic control over women's blood, I have traced the moments within the discourse where such control reveals itself as gendered control, as control that is not self-evident but that needs to legitimize itself. Here the story of Yalta has served as the narrative focal point. We have seen that the talmudic discussion of the case of Yalta has, at least rhetorically, as its goal the establishment of rabbinic control over women's blood. I have tried to examine this overt goal by reading the narrative and its talmudic discussion symptomatically. One side of the discussion not only considers women to be competent halakhic judges in cases of having to distinguish types of genital bloods. It also catapults Yalta rhetorically into a position of sustained halakhic reasoning. The text has to struggle hard, both rhetorically and logically, to make such rabbinic expertise believable and acceptable. By focusing our reading on the difficulty of this struggle we can reveal how fragile is the construction of such authority and control.

Chapter 5 focuses on a marginal voice that the Babylonian Talmud integrates into its discussions, on the repeated citing of Abaye's mother. The goal of this chapter is to foreground this marginal voice, to highlight its presence within the talmudic discussions that again emphasize the multiplicity of gender perspectives within the Babylonian Talmud. At the same time, the goal here is to analyze the strategies by which the dominant talmudic discourse marginalizes this voice. This process of marginalization begins already within talmudic literature, but subsequently even more so with medieval halakhists and modern academic critics. Against such a progressive marginalization the focus on Abaye's mother's presence within the talmudic texts reverses the process. She is seen as someone who is rhetorically not marked as inferior, and who is a caretaker of bodies, someone whose "medical" expertise ranks with the "medical" expertise of other rabbis in the Talmud.

Finally, in Chapter 6 I have turned to the Didascalia Apostolorum as a text that is usually discussed by scholars of early Christian literature, as part of the history of the early church. The function of the third-century Didascalia in this work is to serve as a complement to the rabbinic discussions. With the Didascalia we have access to Jewish women's attitudes toward practices and rituals concerning menstruation. In his argument with the Jewish women converts in his community, the author of the Didascalia allows us a glimpse not only of women's practice but also of their arguments in advocacy of such practices. The Jewish women converts in the Didascalia move in the same cultural universe as the rabbis toward the end of the tannaitic period, geopolitically as well as textually. For both, biblical law remains the primary reference point. These women then allow us to move away from a simplistic hermeneutic model according to which the rabbis partially expand and partially rewrite the biblical laws concerning menstrual impurity, and finally superimpose them on women who remain victims of such legislations.

The overarching goal of this project of brushing androcentrism against the grain has been to move away from a model that regards the rabbinic discourse on menstrual impurity exclusively as a product of a generic form of patriarchalism and which merely considers that discourse to be born from male fear or abhorrence of women's blood. Here it has been essential to read the rabbinic discussions as born from a hermeneutic disposition toward biblical traditions. I have claimed that the gender politics of the discourse on menstrual regulations is intersected and traversed by the discourse of ethnicity. If we consider rabbinic hermeneutics as based on the desire to preserve biblical Israel as a corporeal, embodied community, the discussions of menstrual regulations have to be analyzed in relation to that desire. The preservation of the corporeal biblical Israel, consisting of men and women, male and female bodies, is obviously inscribed by gender, yet not entirely determined by it. By the same token, then, we can consider women to have an identity-establishing investment in observing biblical traditions concerning menstrual regulations. To practice forms of menstrual abstention may allow for a particular women's form of self-perception. It allowed women to engage in the continuous reproduction of biblical Israel or in the continuous observance of Torah, with and in their bodies. The converted Jewish women in the community of the Didascalia, who desired to preserve a form of menstrual separation within their new Christian environment, which supposedly "liberated" them from biblical rulings, manifest that women could have some desire attached to the observance of "women's" practice. Within these parameters, then, the practice of menstrual separation from marital intimacy in and by itself can no longer be regarded as merely an emblematic sign of women's oppression under patriarchal conditions. Rather, it may serve as a ground to rethink the relationship between the politics of gender and the politics of ethnicity, to rethink what is at stake for women in theorizing corporeality or identities of embodiment.

To allow this to happen, however, the hegemonic structuring of the rabbinic culture of interpretation needs to be turned on its head. This created discursive conditions that allowed for the displacement of women from the reading and translating of women's bodies into language. Once these conditions are recognized, we may allow for new language to be created and for the old language to be transformed. In this endeavor, we may need the help of the poets:

> What I want to say, Linda,
> is that there is nothing in your body that lies.
> All that is new is telling the truth. . . .

# NOTES

### INTRODUCTION

1. This period, therefore, stretches over a few centuries, from the second century to the sixth century C.E. Where relevant, however, I will refer to talmudic commentaries of the medieval period. As will be seen in the following studies, talmudic texts are often highly ambiguous. Medieval commentaries may help us in understanding a passage of the Talmud, without necessarily forcing us to accept their reading as the only one possible.

2. On the meaning of the Hebrew *massekhet*, or Aramaic *massekhta*, as "fabric," equivalent to the Latin *textus*, see Stemberger, *Einleitung*, 124. See also Peskowitz, *Spinning Fantasies*, 13.

3. One might object that philology or text criticism are objective ways of engaging the text. That may be accurate. However, I would argue that such a claim of objectivity can only function within a self-contained realm of discourse. That is, within Jewish Studies as a self-referential academic discipline the historical-philological study of the Talmud can be staged as a "scientific" discourse. But where the Talmud enters a field of cross-cultural interaction, for instance in more broadly defined cultural studies or in religious studies, or in feminist scholarship, and where the study of the Talmud is pursued in dialogue with other disciplines and other cultures, producing different questions to be asked of the texts, philological and text-critical approaches are limited. It goes without saying that any cultural study of talmudic texts needs to rely on the efforts of philology and text criticism to establish reliable and accurate texts.

4. I have in mind Theodor W. Adorno's famous statement, first formulated in 1949 and maintained for at least another fifteen years, that "to write a poem after

Auschwitz is barbaric." He revised this claim only in his *Negative Dialectics*, where he wrote: "Ceaseless suffering has as much right to express itself as does the victim of torture to screaming. Therefore it may have been false to say that after Auschwitz one cannot write poetry" (355).

5. During 1992–93 I was a student in the Beit Midrash program at the Shalom Hartman Institute in Jerusalem. Without the support of some of the people at the Institute, this work would have been impossible.

6. The emphasis on becoming rather than being is derived from Rosi Braidotti's reading of Luce Irigaray's work. Irigaray's concept of becoming woman is well summarized in her statement: "In order to become, it is essential to have a gender or an essence as *horizon*. Otherwise, becoming remains partial and subject to the subject. When we become parts or multiples without a future of our own this means simply that we are leaving it up to the other, or the Other of the other, to put us together. To become means fulfilling the wholeness of what we are capable of being" (cited in Braidotti, "Of Bugs and Women," 111, her emphasis).

7. Here I am referring to Simone de Beauvoir's classic study of the status of women under patriarchy, specifically in Western culture, *The Second Sex*, the foundational text for contemporary feminist theory. De Beauvoir's basic claim is that women in patriarchal cultures such as that of the West have been objectified, made into the "Other," by association with the body and its social expression of the domestic sphere, versus the association of maleness with mind and the public sphere. In de Beauvoir's existentialist terms this is the juxtaposition of "immanence" and "transcendence." In patriarchal cultures women remain chained to immanence, and de-Beauvoir's narrative of women's liberation is to achieve transcendence, "by leaving behind the unredeemed and unredeemable domestic sphere of contingency for the public sphere of economic activity, women too can achieve transcendence. Liberation for women in Beauvoir's liberationist macronarrative consists in emerging from the dark cave of immanence 'into the light of transcendence'" (Schor, "This Essentialism Which Is Not One," 63). Obviously, these terms have long since been criticized by scholars of feminist theory, as to de Beauvoir's reinscription of Western metaphysics. What I do believe, though, is that for many women, even today, the desire to commit themselves to a life of the intellect is still experienced as flight from a woman's fate, and as an attempt to succeed in a "male world" by hiding or ignoring one's womanhood.

8. See D. Goodblatt's study, *Rabbinic Instruction in Sasanian Babylonia*.

9. On the argument regarding this point, see D. Boyarin, *Carnal Israel*. However, in this study Boyarin also argues that some of the conflicted arguments regarding women's learning may indicate that there were at least some women studying Torah (see especially chapter 5).

10. The traditional numbering of the pages extends to seventy three *dappim* or

double-leaves of gemara, ending with bNid 73a. This traditional numbering always begins with 2a.

11. The category of authorship of rabbinic texts is problematic to say the least, and that not just since Foucault. For one, the problem is posed by the nature of the texts, which have their origins in an oral culture. There is no author in the sense of the person or the people who authored the texts. As opposed to literary systems that imply or construct authors for texts, all of the texts of the rabbinic period are authorless. Nor is this juxtaposition an absolute one, as Daniel Boyarin points out: "texts, even single-authored texts, are not created by their authors but produced within a heteroglottic sociolinguistic matrix that is necessarily heterogeneous, inasmuch as it is the product of social conflict and cultural contention. By definition then, a text could not reflect its 'author's' interiority. . . . This is, of course, only more to the point when the texts are not the product of a single author but of whole communities working over generations" ("On the Status of the Tannaitic Midrashim," 456). The rabbinic texts present themselves as anthologies of quotations and discussions of scholars of several generations, as if we had access to the actual material for rabbinic oral interactions (Boyarin, "Placing Reading," 26).

12. In methodological terms I am learning from Mieke Bal, who, with respect to reading biblical love stories, writes: "I do not claim the Bible to be either a feminist resource or a sexist manifesto. . . . It is the cultural function of one of the most influential mythical and literary documents of our culture that I discuss, as a strong representative instance of *what language and literature can do to a culture, specifically to its articulation of gender*" (*Lethal Love*, 1, my emphasis). This latter question is what I am interested in asking of talmudic literature. The reader will find many reminiscences of her work throughout this book.

13. Discussing a tannaitic text, Miriam Peskowitz similarly suggests that "we modern readers tend to read this [mKid 4:14, Ch.F.] and other rabbinic passages as if we were rabbis and shared their positions as men. . . . Reading with the rabbis means accepting their unspoken truisms as truths" (*Spinning Fantasies*, 53).

14. Here often terms from psychoanalysis are employed. A text may perform a certain turn "against its own desires" (ibid., 43), which in turn may be read as a symptom, defined as an "involuntary sign" (Bal, *Lethal Love*, 82).

15. Thus, Miriam Peskowitz reads mishnaic passages "to show the difficulty that rabbis encountered as they made gender" (*Spinning Fantasies*, 32). Such a reading may make "visible something embedded in the text's logic, and it shows something the text might have wished to keep under wraps" (43), in order to create stability of meaning.

16. Again, I want to call on Mieke Bal's work. She gives tremendous weight to the process of reading as performance on the text: "Texts trigger readings; that is what they are: the occasion of a reaction. The feeling that there is a text in support of one's

view makes texts such efficient ideological weapons. Every reading is different from, and in contact with, the text" (*Lethal Love*, 132). Her stated goal is to "break[ing] open the too-monolithic readings projected on the Hebrew love stories in order to make others believe that life, love, and women are what one wants them to be" (132).

17. Genres of talmudic discussions would, among others, include halakhic discussions, midrashic interpretations, and narratives, both legal case stories and pedagogical tales.

18. This term I borrow from Ilana Pardes's *Countertraditions in the Bible*.

19. In the sense in which Ouaknin has defined the historial approach: "The historical method considers the past as belonging totally to history. The past is intelligible only after the knowledgeable and critical mediation of the historian" (*The Burnt Book*, 57).

20. For my methodological assumptions I am indebted to Antoinette Clark Wire's 1990 book, *The Corinthian Women Prophets*. Through a reading of Paul's first letter to the Corinthians Wire reconstructs the picture of the women prophets in the church of first-century Corinth. As an argumentative text, the Didascalia is quite similar in structure to Paul's letter. What Wire writes about with respect to Paul can be applied to the Didascalia: a "rhetorical or argumentative situation includes both the goals of the speaker and the counterarguments that are anticipated as the speaking progresses. . . . So what we have is not just one individual's viewpoint but a window into a volatile situation" (*The Corinthian Women Prophets*, 3). From the anticipated and, in the case of the Didascalia, even cited counterarguments, we may develop a picture of the women, as will be argued in the last chapter.

21. However, in this context it should perhaps be noted that both the Babylonian and Palestinian Talmuds report that "Israelite women took upon themselves the stringency that even if they saw a drop of blood of the size of a mustard seed they waited seven clean days" (bNid 66a; bBer 31a; compare yBer 5:1, 8d). "Israelite women" (בנות ישראל) here has to be read as Jewish women as defined by rabbinic culture, as opposed to, for instance, Samaritan or Sadducean women (בנות כותים and בנות צדוקין; mNid 4:1–2; tNid 5:1–2). The talmudic text indicates that (some) women had an interest in observing the biblical commandments of Niddah, and preferred an even stricter observance than required by biblical commandments. But the Talmud does not preserve the women's argument for this change in practice. This text will be discussed in more detail in the third chapter.

22. For much of that discussion in the specific context of discussing menstruation I have gained tremendous insights from the general discussion of von Kellenbach's *Anti-Judaism in Feminist Religious Writings*.

23. See also Urbach, *The Sages* (305).

24. When referring to the Mishnah as a whole, I will consistently capitalize it, in contrast to referring to an individual mishnah, which will be lower case.

25. For an introduction to the question of the relationship between the Mishnah

and the Tosefta, and for a discussion of the scholarship on this question, see Stemberger, *Einleitung in Talmud und Midrasch*, 171.

26. The Aramaic term, meaning "outside" tradition, has a dogmatic connotation, since it implies that the Mishnah presents the canonized inside traditions, and everything aside from the Mishnah is designated as an outside tradition. A baraita cited in the Talmud does not necessarily have to be a citation of the Tosefta. The Talmud will cite a number of *baraitot* which do not appear in any other rabbinic text.

27. The rabbinic terms for interpretation of biblical verses and texts, derived from the root *d-r-sh*, "to search."

28. In his introductory notes, Ouaknin makes a similar point: "the Mishnah and the Tosefta use a simple, concise, but often elliptical style; they avoid digressions, and the rare anecdotes one encounters here and there have the purpose of shedding light on the various opinions by means of a fact" (*The Burnt Book*, 28).

29. Again, I refer the reader to the excellent introduction of Stemberger (*Einleitung in Talmud und Midrasch*). He writes "*Gemara* (*gemar* in Babylonian Aramaic means not only 'to complete' but also 'to learn') is the 'learning of tradition' or the traditional teaching itself . . . [the Geonic usage] understands *Gemara* as the rounding off of *Mishnah* by the interpretation of the amoraim. Censorship leads to the use of 'Gemara' rather than 'Talmud' in the printed Talmud" (183). The terms Talmud and gemara can often be used interchangeably. However, to be precise, the terms are technically not the same, since gemara specifically designates the later discussion of the Mishnah, whereas Talmud includes both the Mishnah and the Gemara.

30. Compare also Ouaknin, who writes: "In *Mahloket* [dispute, Ch.F.], reconciliation is not sought. If the term 'dialectic' can be used—and it is often used to describe Talmudic thinking—we would have to talk of an 'open dialectic,' since no synthesis, no third term, cancels out the contradiction" (*The Burnt Book*, 84).

**CHAPTER 1**

1. For example, R. Adler's "In Your Blood, Live: Re-Visions of a Theology of Purity" (38–41). This brief essay presents a revision of her original popular piece, which defended the practice of the laws of Niddah, and interpreted them from a woman's perspective ("Tum'ah and Taharah," 63–71). See also J. Baskin's "The Separation of Women in Rabbinic Judaism."

2. For instance, Blu Greenberg's *Women and Judaism* and, more recently, the essays and narratives anthologized in Rivkah Slonim's *Total Immersion*.

3. See, for instance, the collection of stories in *Total Immersion*. It contains a number of stories that describe women taking the greatest of risks to immerse themselves in the miqveh under various forms of oppression and persecution. Here the self-sacrifice in order to fulfill the requirement of ritual immersion at the end of

the menstrual period is raised to a great ideal. For a discussion of this contemporary orthodox women's literature, see Jody E. Myers's essay on "The Myth of Matriarchy in Recent Writings on Jewish Women's Spirituality."

4. See Judith Wegner, "Chattel or Person?" (163), Rachel Biale, "Women and Jewish Law" (147), and Rachel Adler, "In Your Blood, Live" (40). Adler claims that "the word niddah describes a state which is neither socially nor morally neutral."

5. The two most recent commentaries on Leviticus discuss the etymological options in much more detail than the current context allows for. See Milgrom's Anchor Bible volume on Leviticus 1–16 (744–45) and B. A. Levine's JPS Torah commentary volume on Leviticus (97).

6. Milgrom, *Leviticus 1–16* (744–45) and B. A. Levine, *Leviticus* (97); compare Moshe Greenberg, "Etymology" (70).

7. This priestly text about the ritual of purifying a person who has contracted ritual impurity by touching a corpse refers to the water involved in the rite as מי נדה—*the water of purification*. The use of *niddah* in this term is not really translatable, but Rashi explains it as מי הזייה—the water of sprinkling.

8. Milgrom, *Leviticus 1–16* (744–45); compare Moshe Greenberg, "Etymology" (70).

9. Greenberg seems to agree with this assessment. He writes that "its [*niddah*] basic sense will be (like its targumic equivalent) 'distancing, apartness,' specifically, the separation of women from certain social contacts during their menstrual 'impurity' " (ibid., 75). Feminist scholars who argue etymologically and cite the root n-d-h as an etymon, have also translated the term as she who is "banned" or "ostracized" (Wegner, "Chattel or Person?" 163; and R. Biale, *Women and Jewish Law*, 147). Rachel Adler explains that "Niddah, from the root NDD, connotes abhorrence and repulsion" ("In Your Blood, Live," 40).

10. Levine, *Leviticus 1–16*, 463–64; compare Moshe Greenberg, "Etymology," 70.

11. With the sole exception of mNid 7:4, which in our standard Mishnah editions seems to refer to a בית הטמאות—a house for impure women, according to some manuscripts of the Mishnah itself as well as manuscripts of the Talmud where it cites this Mishnah (Epstein, *Introduction to the Text of the Mishnah*, 124; Harrington, *The Impurity Systems of Qumran and the Rabbis*, 271). Rashi seems to have such an edition in front of him, since he explains the term as referring to "a room which women avail of during the days of their menstruation" (Dinari, "Customs Relating to the Impurity of the Menstruant," 309). Was that the practice in Rashi's environment during the eleventh century? The standard reading of the term, however, is בית הטומאות—a house of impurities, that is, a house for objects that have protracted impurities (Harrington, *The Impurity Systems of Qumran and the Rabbis*, 271). Some scholars adduce a passage from Josephus's *Antiquities* as evidence. He refers to the practice of the Israelites of removing menstruating women from the city (i.e., the realm of the

community, his rendering of the Israelite camp: Ant. 3:11, 3). But it is not clear whether he merely intends to explain the biblical text, Leviticus 15, and thinks that this is what it implies (see Albeck's Notes and Addenda on mNid 7:4), or whether he indeed has a contemporary practice in mind, as Dinari claims ("Customs Relating to the Impurity of the Menstruant," 309). Finally, Shaye Cohen discusses a section from the Temple Scroll at Qumran, which cherishes the utopian vision of a Jerusalem entirely protected from impurity, and thus also will bar women from access. But, as Cohen points out, this is a sectarian vision of what should be, and not a description of what is ("Menstruants and the Sacred," 278).

12. This shift occurs in Ezekiel: "In Ezekiel the start of a new concretization can be seen: in אשה נדה of Ezek 18:6, the word נדה, in apposition to the word אשה, denotes an embodiment of menstrual impurity—'a woman, a menstruant = a menstruous woman'" (Moshe Greenberg, "Etymology," 75). Greenberg's little essay is most helpful in thinking etymologically. He studies Targumic Aramaic and Peshitta Syriac renditions of Hebrew derivatives of the root *ndd*, which he holds to be "the most natural etymon" of *niddah*, and the Hebrew and Aramaic equivalents of Syriac *ndd*, in order to establish their semantic fields. He concludes that "the base idea of ndd is 'distancing'—physical (e.g., flight from) and moral (e.g., abhorrence of)" ("Etymology," 69). What his study shows, however, is that different texts and translators create different connotations, thus producing a basic instability in the meaning of the term *niddah* itself.

13. A possible exception is a simile attributed in the Babylonian Talmud to Rabbi El'azar (bSot 42b), discussed in note 19 below.

14. Ezekiel is the classic, but also the only, biblical text that deploys the term *niddah* as a moral category. Describing the dire future days for the Israelites, especially in Jerusalem, Ezekiel states: "They shall cast their silver in the streets, and their gold shall be *like a niddah*: their silver and their gold shall not be able to deliver them in the day of the wrath of the Lord, . . . As for the beauty of his ornament which he set in majesty: they have set up in it the images of their abominations and of their detestable things: therefore I have set it for them *like a niddah*" (Ez. 7:19–20); "And the word of the Lord came to me, saying, Son of man, when the house of Israel dwelt in their own land, they defiled it by their way and by their doings: their way was before me *as the uncleanness of a menstruous woman*" (Ez. 36:17). Given how prevalent the notion is in Ezekiel, it is important to note that the rabbis made a hermeneutic choice not to deploy the term as a moral metaphor for morally transgressive behavior.

15. "The land, into which you go to possess it, is a *land of niddah* through the *niddah of the peoples of the land*, with their abominations" (Ezra 9:11). Both texts are associated with the priestly tradition. However, the priestly portions in the Pentateuch themselves are careful not to use the term metaphorically as a moral category.

16. See Cynthia Baker's article on the figure of the woman in the *shuq* (the

marketplace), "Bodies, Boundaries, and Domestic Politics in a Late Ancient Marketplace" (1996). This figure also produces some anxiety in rabbinic circles, as Baker shows in her article.

17. See Thomas Buckley and Alma Gottlieb's revision of classic anthropological notions with respect to tribal practices of menstrual huts. In their reading, institutions such as menstrual huts may in certain contexts suggest a strengthening of women's communal life among women. It may also be considered as a break in the usual chore of everyday life (*Blood Magic*, 31).

18. In the *Encyclopedia Judaica* article on Niddah, Ta-Shma presents the two texts as rabbinic texts, which might indicate such a practice in a radically different light. He claims: "In ancient times a menstruous woman was completely segregated, particularly in Erez Israel [the Land of Israel] where the laws of purity were still in vogue from the time when the Temple existed. Excluded from her home, the menstruous woman stayed in a special house known as 'a house of uncleanness' (mNid 7:4), she was called galmudah ('segregated,' bRH 26a)" (*EJ* 7: 1145). The latter text I discuss in the next paragraph. The former text, mNid 7:4, is extremely ambiguous as to its manuscript evidence; see note 11. Given this weakness of the sources, Ta-Shma's general statement as to women's segregation seems to be unjustified.

19. The text has a parallel in bSot 42b, where the tradition is, with slight differences, transmitted in the name of Rabbi El'azar, possibly a contemporary of Rabbi Aqiva: "Rabbi El'azar said: Every community in which hypocrisy resides is rejected like a niddah, because it says (Job 15:34) 'for the community of hypocrites is *galmud*,' and thus in the coastal plains they call a niddah *galmudah*. What is a *galmudah*? She is weaned from her husband." Again the term *galmud* is not clear, since even in the Bible it is extremely rare, occurring only three times in Job and once in Isaiah (49:21). In Job the term is mostly used with the meaning of barren (3:7, 30:3). The midrash in Sotah appears in a chain of examples in which Rabbi El'azar expounds the term חנופה—hypocrisy, citing several biblical verses in which a derivative of the term is used. This is how he comes across the verse in Job, which is somewhat cryptic. This verse also provides the association with the niddah, since he apparently knows the same tradition cited above in the name of Rabbi Aqiva. He can, therefore, make the connection with the niddah through the term *galmud*, which is also used in the verse of Job. Rabbi El'azar, therefore, seems to have in mind the explanation that we learn in the passage in Rosh Hashana: a community of hypocrites will be rejected by God, Israel's husband, in the manner of separation between the menstruant wife and her husband. That is, the subject of comparison here is not the niddah and the community of hypocrites, but the manner of separation from the respective husbands. However, the text employs the term *rejection* (מאס) rather than mere separation. Thus Rabbi El'azar is presented as exposing a metaphorically more negative attitude toward the menstruating wife.

20. In his article "The Customs of Menstrual Impurity: Their Origin and De-

velopment" [Hebrew], Dinari argues that the Talmud polemicizes *against* those customs that separate the menstruous woman from the community and that later, post-talmudic, halakhic sources that incorporate such customs as halakhah not only have no foundation in the Talmud, but sometimes even contradict it. He attributes such post-talmudic customs to widespread and deeply rooted folklore about menstruation, against which halakhah as expressed in the Talmud polemicizes but which later on found their way back into halakhic discourse. Thus, when Judith Baskin claims that the rabbinic *niddah* "must be kept separate from centers of holiness and the holy books" ("Separation of Women," 14) she does not merely read selectively but is wrong.

21. The discussion of whether women should study Torah is a different issue, which does not touch upon the issue of im/purity and sanctity.

22. Shaye Cohen offers this source ("Menstruants and the Sacred," 283), but does not comment upon the fact that menstruous women are allowed to study. For a thorough discussion of this astonishing passage and its subsequent rewriting in the Babylonian Talmud, see Boyarin, "Studying Women" (*Carnal Israel*, 180). Whereas the Palestinian Talmud quotes this baraita, as it appears also in the Tosefta, the Babylonian Talmud rewrites its gendering: "*Men* with irregular genital emissions, and lepers, and *those who have had sex with menstruating women* are permitted to study Torah, but men who have had a regular ejaculation may not" (bBer 22a). Boyarin deals at length with the more general question of women and study of Torah. The varying appearances of this text fit his larger observation that in Palestine the notion of women studying has been more acceptable, whereas the Babylonian Talmud in its discussions attempts to limit and even suppress this possibility. With respect to this baraita he writes: "Menstruants can study Torah in Palestine. Thus we have once more evidence that in Palestine the notion that women might study Torah was not by any means unacceptable. Indeed, the very casualness with which the Tosefta reveals that women study Torah and with which the Palestinian Talmud cites such study . . . constitutes an index of the acceptability of that notion there" (*Carnal Israel*, 181). It is, therefore, plausible to assume that the Babylonian Talmud changed "menstruating women" to "those men who have had sex with menstruating women" not so much because it had a problem with *menstruating* women studying Torah. Rather, the problem was that *women* were studying.

23. In her discussion in *Women and Jewish Law* of the "Laws of the Menstruant" Rachel Biale has attempted to outline a historical evolution that connects both the discourse of menstrual impurity and the biblical discussion of the prohibition of sexual intercourse during the woman's menstruation. She claims that a historical shift takes place from one to the other, already in the biblical period: "After the destruction of the First Temple (586 B.C.E.), an evolution in the laws of *niddah* had already begun to take place. The justification for these laws was shifted from the realm of purity laws to the arena of sexual taboos. This transformation became even

more pronounced in the mishnaic and *talmudic* literature which developed after the destruction of the Second Temple" (148). Biale acknowledges that the historical explanation of the shift within biblical culture is only circumstantial, due to the scantiness of the texts to give a basis to such a conjecture. Her suggestion, if modified, finds support in recent biblical scholarship. Biblical scholars attribute both conceptual contexts to different sources. Lev. 15 is part of the priestly source P, whereas Lev. 18 and 20 are part of the Holiness Code H. Both sources have different ideological emphases. A few years ago, Israel Knohl suggested that contrary to traditional views, H is actually younger than P (*Sanctuary of Silence*, based on his dissertation of 1988), a view accepted by Milgrom and Levine in their commentaries on Leviticus. The textual aspects relevant for my reading of rabbinic texts will be discussed in more detail in the next chapter.

24. There is, however, a wide-ranging debate on the ideological decentralization of the Temple among the Pharisees prior to its destruction, a tendency that the rabbis, at least during the tannaitic period, supposedly latched on to. With Gedalyahu Alon as his predecessor, Jacob Neusner is the main spokesperson of this argument. According to Neusner, "the Pharisees determined to concentrate on what they believed was really important in politics, which was fulfillment of all the laws of the Torah, even ritual purity and tithing, to achieve elevation of the life of all of the people, at home and in the streets, to what the Torah had commanded: You shall be a kingdom of priests and a holy people. Such a community would live as if it were always in the Temple sanctuary of Jerusalem. Therefore the complicated and inconvenient purity laws were extended to the life of every Jew in his [sic] own home. The Temple altar in Jerusalem would be replicated at the tables of all Israel" (*The Idea of Purity*, 146). This view, however, has been more recently contested by E. P. Sanders in *Jewish Law from Jesus to the Mishnah*, who opposes the argument that the Pharisees were trying to live as priests. Even Neusner admits that "certain Mishnaic pericopae take for granted a priestly and cultic setting, while others assume the law is to be kept at home by ordinary people, not priests" (*Idea of Purity*, 72). For a discussion of this debate see H. Harrington, *The Impurity Systems*, 267–81. Further, there is also some debate on how long practices such as eating meals at home as if one were at the Temple extended beyond the destruction of the Temple. There are some texts that seem to indicate that certain groups continued to do so. However, I do not wish to enter this debate here, since I have much less confidence than Alon, Neusner, or Sanders in our ability to read the Mishnah as a document that tells us anything about the historical reality of the practice of the Pharisees, or even the rabbis subsequently. Ultimately, historicist readings of the Mishnah must remain speculative about the historical reality it supposedly represents.

25. In terms of the social construction of *women* in traditional Jewish societies, however, an insistence on making this distinction between the avoidance of women as sex objects rather than as potential sources of impurity may prove to be insignificant.

26. See, for instance, Adler's argument ("In Your Blood Live," 38).

27. There is a wide-ranging debate on the question of whether the remainder of the Palestinian gemara of niddah existed and has been lost to us or whether it never existed. Thus Albeck claims in his extensive analysis of the relationship between the Palestinian Talmud and the midrashic anthology of Bereshit Rabbah that BerR 18:1, or at least part of this paragraph, stems from the Palestinian Talmud, referenced by the editors of Bereshit Rabba. Their Palestinian Talmud included a gemara on chapter 5 of Mishnah Niddah, which we do not possess (Albeck and Theodor, *Midrash Bereshit Rabba*, vol. 3, 72). Further, the Tosafot, the medieval commentary on the Babylonian Talmud, refer to the ירושלמי בפ׳ נדה, that is, the Palestinian gemara on chapter 7 of our Mishnah, which we likewise no longer have. Bokser concludes in his survey of scholarship on the Palestinian Talmud ("An Annotated Bibliographical Guide") that the "tentative consensus" is that "the missing chapters in Makkot, Shabbat and Niddah existed" (167), hence that the missing portions were lost at the time of the production of manuscripts that we possess, during printing or at some earlier, post-talmudic time.

28. For a summary of this debate see Stemberger, *Einleitung in Talmud und Midrasch*, 186.

29. For instance, the tractates Order of Kodashim ("Holy Things") discuss the regulations concerning sacrifices. Further, certain tractates in the Order of Zeraim ("Seeds," or laws pertaining to agriculture) discuss the laws concerning the procedures and quantities of agricultural products to be given to the priests and Levites at the Temple. This observation touches upon the long discussion of the purpose of the Mishnah. The three main suggestions today are collection of sources, teaching manual, or law code. For an introductory discussion see Stemberger, *Einleitung in Talmud und Midrasch*, 151–54.

30. See also Judith Hauptman for a brief discussion of these *mishnayot*. She reconstructs a possible historical development of the laws of niddah in Mishnah and Talmud and suggests that the lack of reference to the sexual taboo in the Mishnah indicates that "the laws of Niddah, as they were observed in the early *amoraic* period, when ritual purity for the preparation of food was no longer an issue in Babylonia, were a simple matter of refraining from sexual relations for the week of the blood flow" (*Rereading the Rabbis*, 160). This is, of course, quite possible, but does not sufficiently explain the discursive silence on the sexual taboo, nor the discursive weight given to the factor of impurity.

31. Rashi interprets this to mean "handing him [the cup]" (bKet 4b).

32. The citation in bKet 61a adds a comment attributed to another rabbi of the following generation, of the first half of the fourth century, who qualifies this remark by stating: "We hold this to apply only [if she performs these labors] in front of him [that is, in front of her husband], but if [she does] not [do them] in front of him, we have no issue" (bKet 61a). The text continues here with citing the practice of the

wives of four amoraim from the first to the penultimate generations in the Talmud concerning the mixing of wine: "Shmu'el's wife changed it [the wine-glass] to her left hand [in handing it to him], [concerning] Abaye she [his wife] would leave it at the mouth of the barrel, [concerning] Rava, on the pillow, [concerning] Rav Papa, on the bench."

33. See Rashi bKet 4b and 61a, ד"ה חוץ ממזיגת כוס; see also Tosafot bKet 4b, ד"ה הצעת המטה. Compare Judith Hauptman who emphasizes that Rav Huna's rule indicates that "all other household labors, such as baking and cooking, are permitted" to the wife (*Rereading the Rabbis*, 160).

34. In the conclusion to her book, Hauptman presents a comparison between the two texts (ibid., 248–49).

35. A comparison between the Palestinian and the Babylonian Talmud is only marginally important to the argument I am trying to put forth. In the version in the Babylonian Talmud Shmu'el is represented as going to his colleague directly and asking him a "what if" question: "What if she said: I am in the status of impurity, and then she turns around and says: I am in the status of purity?" (bKet 22b, bottom). Hauptman rightly points out that "in this version of the incident, Samuel [sic] asks Rav precisely the same question that he asked in the other one, but without any reference to his personal circumstances. . . . As a result, the charm and certainly the bite of the story are lost. The issue of a wife thwarting her husband's sexual drive because she was not interested in sex at the time, although probably implied, is not brought to the surface" (ibid., 249).

36. Hauptman goes even further to suggest that the rabbis "exhibit a liveliness of outlook and an openness to self-critique. Moreover, the redactor may have deliberately injected a feminist message, namely, that clever, resourceful women may take patriarchal structures designed to subordinate women and utilize them instead for their own empowerment within rabbinic law itself" (249). To my reading eyes, this suggestion gives the redactors too much credit and puts too much weight on the potential empowerment granted by the redactors to women, even though this element should not be belittled. At the same time, while it is not entirely implausible, Hauptman's reading discounts the framework within which this story is introduced: that of women's trustworthiness or believability. The very fact that the rabbis in those cases in which women are represented as taking control of their lives evaluate their believability severely impedes the possibility of their empowerment.

37. Compare also mShev 2:4 mentioned above, where the Mishnah employs the language of impurity in a context that clearly deals with aspects of sexual prohibition. The wife is represented as saying to her husband during sexual intercourse, נטמאתי— "I became impure," here meaning that she started her menstrual period, and that she is thus sexually prohibited. This mishnah and the subsequent discussion in the Talmud focus on a definition of male pleasure and at what point male sexual pleasure

becomes transgressive. Clearly, the woman as the provider of his sexual pleasure is instrumentalized in this context. Once more, we can see that the rabbinic text inscribes the *language* of impurity into the discussion of the biblical prohibition. The sugyah which builds on this mishnah warrants a careful analysis as to how it merges and entwines the two conceptual discourses. This analysis is beyond the means of this chapter.

38. For an example, see, for instance, the popular *Halachos of Niddah* by Rabbi Shimon Eider. Note the linguistic shift in his handbook. He writes, with respect to the different colors of blood, that "if a woman discovers a red or black discharge or stain..., *she is considered a Niddah*. If a woman discovers white, blue... discharges or stains *she is not considered Niddah*" (8–9). To be considered niddah means for all practical purposes that she cannot have sexual relations with her husband.

39. This phrase is often used in popular literature on Jewish law as well as in scholarly literature. For an example of the former, see Rabbi Shimon Eider's *Halachos of Niddah*. He writes in the moralizing rhetoric typical of this literature that the sexual act, "when performed irresponsibly, with a prohibited mate, or without proper observance of *the laws of family purity*, lowers the participants to the level of animals" (xiii). Judith Hauptman also mentions the contemporary use of the phrase without further comment (*Rereading the Rabbis*, 165).

40. Perhaps it should be noted that punishment is not precise. A commandment functioning as an act of expiation, or perceived to function as such, is not so much a punishment as a sacrifice, phenomenologically. This may not make a significant difference, but the distinction is important.

41. AdRN B 9, 13a is perhaps the most extreme formulation in that here "the first 'adam'" is described as דמו של הקב"ה, "the blood of the Holy One Blessed Be He," which the first woman spilled. However, it seems to me that AdRN has a *Tendenz* in the redaction of its traditions, which makes it one of the more misogynist texts in rabbinic literature. It would be fruitful to do a comprehensive analysis of this late Babylonian text with respect to how it edits its textual traditions on women's issues.

42. On a summary of the debate, see Stemberger, *Einleitung in Talmud und Midrasch*, 215.

43. A third-generation Babylonian rabbi, that is, from approximately the latter half of the third century, or from the early fourth century C.E. The anonymous Galilean is a topos, and appears repeatedly as somebody who presents his midrashic interpretation before Rav Chisda in the Babylonian Talmud (bShab 88a; bSanh 113a; see also bHull 27a).

44. See bSotah 5a. According to Rashi this is understood to be the minimal quantity of blood in a human being to sustain life.

45. In the sense of having established a special law.

46. Boyarin comments on this text that "these commandments, according to the

Babylonian Talmud, like any others belong in principle to the whole people, male and female alike. But these are particularly given to women because they belong particularly to women's sphere as understood by the rabbinic culture, to her body, cooking, and the comfort of the house" (*Carnal Israel*, 92). It seems important to emphasize, however, that here the midrashic explanation, which the Babylonian Talmud offers as an explicit countermodel to the midrashic explanations above, insists on the commandments as incumbent upon the community. In this specific context the effect of the text, or even its intent, is to prevent the marginalization of the three commandments as merely women's commandments that serve to punish her.

47. He juxtaposes the rabbinic discourse on the transgression of the first woman with the Greek myth of Pandora, and with Philo's reading of Eve, which, according to him, all expose a systematic "discourse of misogyny" (*Carnal Israel*, 80).

48. See, however, for example, the short "side-remark" in bShab 152a: תנא אשה חמת מלא צואה ופיה מלא דם והכל רצין אחריה—"it is taught [in support of a preceding midrash]: a woman is a bag full of excrement and her mouth full of blood, but still everybody runs after her." Even if "mouth" is to be read as her "lower" mouth, this is clearly a misogynist statement, which reflects on the apparent paradox of male desire. I do, however, agree with Boyarin's overall assessment.

49. For example, Baskin, "Separation of Women," 7.

50. Dean-Jones points out that "these beliefs are echoed in such works as Columella's *De Re Rustica* and Plutarch's *Moralia*" (*Women's Bodies*, 249), both second-century works. Plutarch's text, however, does not exactly cite Pliny, but offers an additional power of menstruation by relating "the story of hail being averted by 'hail-wizards' through the use of the blood of a mole or a woman's menstrual pads" (*Table Talk*, VII 2, 700 F). The diachronic tenacity of a text such as Pliny's becomes evident if we consider that "Pliny's claims about the powers of menstruating woman were recorded by the Inquisition in their handbook for identifying witches, Malleus Maleficarum" (Dean-Jones, *Women's Bodies*, 249).

51. Galit Hasan-Rokem points out that "another aspect of the ethnographic character of Rabbinic literature is that its generic taxonomy reveals an almost full repertoire of folk literary genres as we know them from various cultures . . . Supernatural elements, such as miracles, magic, spirits, demons and angels, occur in legends as part and parcel of the current belief system" ("Narratives in Dialogue," 110).

52. For a major discussion of this approach see his *Carnal Israel* and *A Radical Jew*.

53. I am not claiming that Boyarin generally fails to see the androcentrism of the centralization of circumcision. This statement may perhaps be regarded as a Freudian slip to make a strong rhetorical point.

54. At the same time, the centrality of circumcision as a cultural issue is not surprising, since it reflects the gendered perspective of our sources, mostly composed by men.

**CHAPTER 2**

1. As we have seen in the last chapter, a large part of the talmudic discussions of menstrual impurity, as well as the entire mishnaic Order of Purities, are of an entirely theoretical nature. The usual explanation for why the only tractate of this order to be discussed and subsequently developed into a talmudic tractate is that one aspect of the legal complex of niddah is its inclusion in the list of forbidden sexual relationships, an aspect that has remained practically relevant. Commonsensical as this explanation is, it is not very strong, since the majority of the talmudic tractate is still concerned with the aspect of purity. And, in other cases where a small part of a tractate was halakhically, that is, practically relevant, it was introduced elsewhere in the Talmud. For this latter point I am grateful to Daniel Boyarin.

2. Thus Elizabeth Grosz describes her attempt to theorize sexual difference as an attempt to "problematize the universalist and universalizing assumptions of *humanism*, through which women's—and all other groups'—specificities, positions, and histories are rendered irrelevant or redundant" (*Volatile Bodies*, ix, my emphasis). Similarly, Moira Gatens who argues that "humanism by its adherence to an 'a priori' and universal conception of human nature ( . . . ) also takes no account of sexual difference" (*Feminism and Philosophy*, 152).

3. This is of course a terribly simplified description of Western intellectual or philosophical tradition and should only be understood as a rough summary. Rosi Braidotti summarizes similarly but with a different emphasis: "the masculine qua human is taken as the 'norm,' and the feminine qua other is seen as marking the 'difference.' The corollary of this definition is that the burden of sexual difference falls upon women, marking them off as the second sex, or the structural 'other,' whereas men are marked by the imperative of carrying the universal" ("Sexual Politics," 152). Nonetheless, Judith Butler notes that in a conversation with Donna Haraway on Irigaray's tendency to reinforce Plato as the origin of Western representation, the latter argued "that the 'West' and its 'origins' are constructed through a suppression of cultural heterogeneity" (Butler, *Bodies That Matter*, 257, note 44). This is a useful reminder not to use the concept of the "West" too lightly, in ways that gloss over the West's internal differences.

4. See Stiegman on "Rabbinic Anthropology" and Boyarin's " 'Behold Israel According to the Flesh': On Anthropology and Sexuality in Late-Antique Judaisms" in his *Carnal Israel*, 31–60.

5. On Aristotle's (and other Greek) notions of female corporeality see Ann Carson, "Putting Her in Her Place" and Dean-Jones, *Women's Bodies*. Thomas Laqueur has analyzed in detail "how a biology of hierarchy in which there is only one sex, a biology of incommensurability between two sexes, and the claim that there is no publicly relevant sexual difference at all, or no sex, have constrained the interpretation of bodies and the strategies of sexual politics for some two thousand years"

(*Making Sex*, 23). He explains the apparent paradox in Aristotle as the result of his deep commitment to the existence of two radically different and distinct sexes in metaphysical terms, while at the same time he promoted a one-sex model on the biological level. Accordingly, "in the flesh, the sexes were more and less perfect versions of each other. Only insofar as sex was a cipher for the nature of causality were the sexes clear, distinct, and different in kind" (29).

6. Recently, Cynthia M. Baker has promulgated a similar argument in her dissertation on *Rebuilding the House of Israel: Gendered Bodies and Domestic Politics in Roman Jewish Galilee, c. 135–300 C.E.*, Duke University. Unfortunately, her dissertation became available too late to be considered in any detail in this book. Baker kindly made available a manuscript of her presentation "Ordering the House: On the Domestication of Jewish Sexuality" at the 1994 national meeting of the SBL. As far as I can tell, our work takes somewhat different directions, since Baker not only restricts herself mainly to tannaitic literature, but also does not deal with the rabbinic complex of purity regulations. See further below, note 36 and note 49.

7. The verse can be split up differently and be read: "When any man has a discharge from his body, his discharge is in the status of impurity." The difference lies in whether we understand the man or merely his discharge to be in the status of impurity. This is the reading which the Septuagint provides: Ἀνδρι ἀνδρί, ᾧ ἐὰν γένηται ῥύσις ἐκ του σώματος αὐτοῦ, ἡ ῥύσις αὐτοῦ ἀκάρθαρτός ἐστιν. See Milgrom (*Leviticus 1–16*, 907), who states against Septuagint that "the rest of the verse can only with great difficulty be rendered 'his discharge (it) is impure'."

8. Rather than healthy and unhealthy discharges, because the notion of health is not a biblical one. Further, in view of the biblical definition of menstrual bleeding in terms of a time line, "common" and "uncommon" as temporal adjectives may be more appropriate terms to define the distinction. "Regular" and "irregular" is not quite exact either, since a seminal discharge is not necessarily regular.

9. See Milgrom (*Leviticus 1–16*, 904) for a discussion of the different ways to structure this chapter chiastically.

10. However, there is one notable difference, which is only a side issue to my discussion. That difference lies in the fact that the man is explicitly required to "launder his clothes and wash his body in living water" (Lev. 15:13) at the end of the seven days, before he brings his offering to the priests. Not so in the case of the woman, whom the text never explicitly requires to wash herself. Thus the wide-ranging debate on whether women were required to immerse biblically (Harrington, *The Impurity Systems*, 276; Milgrom, *Leviticus 1–16*, 934, 986–91), or whether this is only a rabbinic requirement by analogy (Sanders, *Jewish Law from Jesus to the Mishnah*, 214).

11. See also David Biale (*The Eros and the Jews*, 29): "The [levitical] law did not regard a menstruating woman as any more repugnant than a man who had ejaculated: both had incurred cultic impurity by loss of their respective seed, but

the woman's period of impurity was longer because the flow continued for seven days."

12. Milgrom (*Leviticus 1–16*, 939) merely states that this can be explained by the fact that "semen impurity is less severe than blood impurity," without explaining why this would be so.

13. Similarly Baruch Levine, in his commentary on the book of Leviticus, upholds the gender-symmetric structure by stating that "the categorical difference between abnormal and normal conditions is that abnormalities ultimately require ritual expiation as part of the purification process, whereas normal conditions, though inducing impurity, require only bathing and laundering of clothing and observance of the proper period of waiting" (Levine, *Leviticus*, 89).

14. Obviously, the prohibition cannot include a man with a common discharge, since seminal emission is the definition of sexual relations.

15. I argue against Judith Romney Wegner's erroneous claim that in rabbinic literature the observance of menstrual separation, among the other commandments delegated to women, is primarily incumbent upon men, and that a wife's neglect of this religious duty makes her husband a transgressor. Her point is that "she must fulfill these commandments not on her own account, but as her husband's agent; and the sole motivation is to prevent her husband from falling into transgression" (*Chattel or Person?*, 155). Wegner's reading has been uncritically adapted by Kraemer (*Her Share of the Blessing*, 102). However, already the biblical precept in Lev. 20:19 does imply the woman as a subject of the prohibition. This underlines Boyarin's point that "the violation of the laws of menstrual sexual separation is just as much a violation for the female as for the male partner" (*Carnal Israel*, 92, note 25).

16. See also Martin Noth who translates: "When any man has a discharge *from his body*, he [his discharge] is unclean" and "When a woman has a discharge of blood which is her regular discharge *from her body*, she shall be in her impurity for seven days" (*Leviticus*, 111–12). Karl Elliger in the commentary series *Handbuch zum Alten Testament* translates: "Wenn jemand einen Ausfluss *an seinem Gliede* bekommt, so ist sein Ausfluss unrein" and "Wenn ein Weib einen Ausfluss bekommt—Blut is der Ausfluss *an ihrem Gliede*—so ist sie sieben Tage in ihrer Unreinigkeit" (*Leviticus*, 191–92).

17. Levine refers to the biblical sense of בשר as penis in Ez. 16:26, 23:20. Many medieval commentators, such as Sa'adiah Gaon and ibn Ezra explain בשר to mean the male member. See Milgrom (*Leviticus 1–16*, 907) for further references. See also D. Boyarin's discussion of the use of this metaphor in the epistles of Paul, whose use of the Greek term σάρξ is derived from the Hebrew term בשר (*A Radical Jew*, 57–85). Boyarin notes: "Σάρξ, בשר, flesh has two well attested metaphorical usages in Jewish parlance. It refers on the one hand to the penis and on the other hand to the physical connection of genealogy of filiation and of family relationship" (*A Radical Jew*, 77).

18. Similarly Hoffmann (*Das Buch Levitikus*, 427): "בבשרה ist Euphemismus für בבשר ערותה."

19. Curiously enough, this interpretation is not reflected in Milgrom's translation.

20. Milgrom, however, claims—based on the *Hizquni*, a thirteenth century midrashic commentary—that "the preposition *b* is equivalent to *min* 'from'" (*Leviticus 1–16*, 934). There is a philological legitimacy to the Hizquni's comment. See, for example, Muraoka's recent *Grammar of Biblical Hebrew*. He cites the school according to which –בּ has a double meaing as "in" and "from" (487). But the literary hermeneutical question remains, for even if we subscribe to this school and hold that both prepositions can essentially meant the same thing, the fact remains that the biblical text chose different prepositions in each case.

21. Depending on whether one reads the participle as a *hitpa'el* or a *piel*. But here both readings amount to the same effect.

22. The word is used in biblical literature as a metaphor for the interior of the body. However, biblically the corporeal use of the metaphor is not gendered, since the חדרי בטן of the proverb in Prov. 18:8 and 26:22 refer to the interior of the generic body: "The words of a slanderer are like things swallowed greedily; they go down into the chambers of the belly."

23. The term *prozdor* is a loan word and derives from the Greek προτυρα. Krauss translates *Vorhalle* (vestibule). Preuss muses that the Hebrew equivalent is חצר, "an inner court or waiting room of a house" (*Biblical and Talmudic Medicine*, 116). He states that the Hebrew term "too is used to portray the external genitalia, as opposed to *triclinium* which is used for the inner parts," but this is a misreading of his reference text in tNid 8:4 (see Lieberman, *Tosefet Rishonim*, 283), where the Tosefta does not employ a metaphor but refers to an actual inner court. I will discuss this text in the next chapter.

24. The question is whether the "chamber" is the metaphoric equivalent of the biblical "source." Most classical commentators, such as Rashi, Tosafot, Tosfei Rosh, the Meiri and Maimonides, agree that the two are equivalent. However, one medieval commentator considers "the source" to be different from the "chamber" (see Preuss, *Biblical and Talmudic Medicine*, 119), which is not completely unlikely, since the Mishnah elsewhere refers to the "blood of the source." For a recent survey of the later sources, see Tirzah Meacham's dissertation (Hebrew University, 1989) discussed in the following pages.

25. Here the mishnaic text does not seem to assume that the blood derives from the vestibule. In the case of the chamber it employs a genitivus partitivus, implying that the blood has its origin here. In the case of the vestibule it formulates: נמצא בפרוזדור—"if the blood is located in the vestibule."

26. The *terumah* is the portion of the produce to be given to the priest, which needs to be handled in a status of purity.

27. Citation according to Ms Leiden and Editio princeps. See also Tosafot, lemma ודם העליה, bNid 17b: "[We learn from this that] the blood of the upper chamber is in

the status of purity, even if it has the appearance of impure kinds of blood, since the four kinds of impure blood cannot be in the upper chamber."

28. All of these are Babylonian rabbis at the house of study in Sura, where Rav Huna was one of the most important teachers of the second generation of Babylonian amoraim, that is, in the second half of the third century.

29. The term לול is biblical, where it refers to a staircase from the ground to the middle story in Solomon's temple (1 Kings 6:8). Elsewhere in the Talmud it is described as a small room with a staircase leading up to the upper rooms of a house; compare bMen 34a לול פתוח מן הבית לעליה.

30. These are chronologically both rabbis of the fourth generation of amoraim, that is, active during the first half of the fourth century. Rav Huna is an authority in Tiberias, but lived for a while in Babylon, whereas Rav Nachman is a Babylonian authority.

31. The Meiri writes: החדר הוא חלל הרחם שהולד נוצר בו ודם נדה וזיבה יוצא ממנו והוא המקור ונקרא חדר מפני שהוא פנימי מכולן והפרוזדור הוא צואר הרחם והוא מקום ארוך שראשו מתכווץ בשעת העבור שלא יפול הולד ובשעת הלידה הוא נפתח הרבה . . . וסמוך לו וביניהם מקום הנקרא עליה ששם שני ביציה של אשה ושכבת זרע מתבשל לשם בשבילין שבה (1970, 30)—"The chamber is the space of the womb where the embryo is formed, and the blood of niddah or of zivah come out from there, and it is its origin. It is called the chamber because it is the innermost of all of these, and the vestibule is the neck of the womb which is an elongated place. Its top shrinks at the time of pregnancy so that the embryo does not fall out, and at the hour of birth it opens widely. . . . And close to it, between the two, is a place called upper chamber where the two eggs of the women are. The ejaculated semen is cooked there, in the two channels in it" (my translation).

32. He relies on Preuss. Preuss, in spite of his assertiveness about the referents of the mishnaic metaphors, despairs with respect to the talmudic interpretations and retreats by saying "this incomprehensibility of terms is shared by *all* assertions of antiquity concerning the anatomy of female genitalia" (*Biblical and Talmudic Medicine*, 116, his emphasis).

33. But she also admits that "the (talmudic) description does not fit in every detail with any of the organs" ("Mishnah Tractate Niddah," 226).

34. On the history of Western medical discourse and the changes of representations of sexual organs see Thomas Laqueur's *Making Sex*.

35. It is unlikely that the rabbis or somebody at their command dissected human bodies (Preuss, *Biblical and Talmudic Medicine*, 41–44). Evidence for exceptions might be a reference to what is considered to be the equivalent of Caesarean sections, which is extensively discussed in the fifth chapter of Mishnah Niddah. But how far this operation grants a "view" of the interior, is questionable. The purpose of this experiment was to ascertain the number of bones in a human body. On the other

hand, the rabbis were rather well-versed in the anatomy of animals of all kinds, due to the regulations of slaughtering an animal and the inspection of the firstborn animals with respect to their physical integrity. But nowhere does rabbinic literature make an explicit inference from the anatomy of the animal to that of the human, which does not exclude the possibility that their knowledge of the interior of animals served as an aid to their imagination. Nonetheless, the interior of the woman's body is primarily a product of the rabbinic imagination. Greco-Roman medical science also seems not to have engaged in dissection of human bodies. See Dean-Jones (*Women's Bodies*, 8) on the absence of dissection of human bodies amongst the Hippocratic doctors and their refusal to extrapolate from the anatomy of animals. Aristotle, on the other hand, seems to have been an avid dissector of animals, though he never dissected a human cadaver (16–17). He was willing to infer his knowledge about the interior of the human body from animals which to him seemed closer to the human on the scale of nature. From the late fourth century B.C.E. in Alexandria, Greek medical scholars engaged in dissection of human corpses. But by the time of Galen at the end of the second century C.E. human dissection was no longer possible (Temkin, *Soranus' Gynecology*, xxxix). As far as Soranus, immediately preceding Galen, is concerned, Temkin claims that it is unclear whether he himself dissected (ibid.). According to Temkin, Soranus already relied on the anatomical knowledge of his Alexandrian predecessors, enabling his elaborate description of the uterus and the vagina (8–16). For Galen, Aline Rousselle asserts that "dissection of the human body was not practised. Galen derived his (mistaken) ideas on the structure of the human womb from dissecting monkeys. . . . Physiology, the study of the internal functions of the body, was based on logic or even analogy rather than observation" (*Porneia*, 5).

36. In her presentation at the 1994 national meeting of the SBL, based on a chapter of her dissertation, Cynthia M. Baker (see notes 6 and 49) raises similar questions and briefly comments on mNid 2:1 and mNid 2:5. She argues that "whether 'the house' is a euphemism of the rabbis' invention or a slang term used by women themselves, it ultimately bespeaks an internalization, literally, of 'the house'; of that walled, enclosed, 'anoptic'—albeit inherently social—place. Women, according to these rabbis, are to internalize the practice of sexual 'domesticity.'"

37. In his commentary Albeck identifies blood as the elided object of the sentence (*Shishah Sidrei Mishnah* 6, 389). However, the context of this mishnah is the discussion of the question whether a Caesarean section is considered a normal birth, on account of which the woman would be in the status of impurity of birth. The Tosefta (tNid 4:13) understands this mishnah to refer to the placenta: Rabbi Meir on the one hand and Rabbi Yehuda, Rabbi Yossi, and Rabbi Shim'on on the other disagree on whether the placenta causes a status of impurity while it is still "in the house." Both opinions agree that the placenta in the "outer house" leaves the woman in a status of purity, but Rabbi Meir holds—against the others—that she is in the status of impurity

when it is in the בית פנימי, the "inner house." From the formulation of our mishnah at the end of the sentence, that is, the specified men "are not rendered impure until *their impurity* comes to the outside," it seems that the object in the women's case would also be their generic "impurities," such as blood, partial birth, etc., as also in the midrash from Sifra.

38. Preuss (*Biblical and Talmudic Medicine*, 120) and Meacham ("Mishnah Tractate Niddah," 237) identify the "outer house" as the vagina, which would in Preuss's system correspond to the עליה—the "upper chamber" in mNid 2:5.

39. Though this term appears in the Babylonian Talmud only (bHul 70a, bNid 3a), and always in the phrase כותלי בית הרחם, "the walls of the house of the womb," which is concerned with internal physiological processes. The use of the term רחם or "womb" by itself is the more common one. Rashi juxtaposes the החצון to the מקור—the source (bNid 2b, lemma הגס הגס).

40. I borrow this term from Margie Profet's discussion of the vagina as just that, an interface between the exterior of the woman's body and the internal organs ("Menstruation as a Defense," 348).

41. So how would the girl sit, in order to expose the "outer house"? Meacham ("Mishnah Tractate Niddah," 237) assumes that she kneels down on her knees, and sits down, which would cause her labia to open up a little bit, in accordance with Rashi (bNid41b, ד״ה כשהתינוקת יושבת). The Palestinian Talmud provides a parallel version of this discussion but specifies that she squats down to urinate (pYev 6:1, 7b).

42. *Sheretz* means literally "dead creeping thing." It is one of the eight impure kinds of vermin listed in Lev. 11. In the rabbinic context it serves as a metonym for a complex of rules concerning the transfer of a status of impurity by touch, derived from the biblical case (Lev. 11:29–47). The touch of a "dead creeping thing" in the specific place the mishnah designates as "outer house" would transfer a status of impurity to the woman. By rabbinic principles this latter impurity cannot be transferred in a hidden or interior space.

43. The Hebrew term שיניים can be derived from two words, that is either from שן for tooth, or שין for urine. Rashi comments that "inside the womb there are some warts of flesh," meaning that he probably reads the term as teeth. Preuss (*Biblical and Talmudic Medicine*, 120) identifies the labia as the referent of this metaphor, since he reads "the outer house" as the vagina. A parallel version of the Palestinian Talmud (pYev 6:1, 7b) has בית שיניים instead of בין השיניים, both of which, as synonyms, describe the spatial relationship.

44. See Rashi bNid 41b, ד״ה אותו מקום: "Is the Scriptual בבשרה entirely external, even to the touch of a *sheretz*?!" Obviously not!

45. Meacham points out that the identification of the "teeth" depends on the perspective from which exteriority is viewed. That is, the question is whether Rabbi Yohanan is imagining from the outside in or from the inside out. In the latter case his "teeth house" is interior, with the labia as its exterior border. Rabbi Yohanan's

objection to Resh Laqish is that she is in the status of impurity already when the blood has not yet reached the space between the "teeth," that is, between the labia.

46. On the equation of the two orifices, see further below, in the section on "The Metaphoric Body in Greco-Roman Gynecological Literature." On the association of the face and the genitalia in biblical visions of the divine, see Eilberg-Schwartz (*God's Phallus*, 66–80).

47. A biblical background may be found in Prov. 30:20, a denunciation of the adulterous woman: כן דרך אשה מנאפת אכלה ומחתה פיה ואמרה לא פעלתי און—"Thus is the way of adulterous woman: she eats, and wipes her mouth, and says: 'I have not done any wrong.'" This verse is cited in bYoma 75a, bKet 13a and 65b as a biblical precedent and example of לשנא מעליא or euphemism for sex.

48. For example with reference to the rectum (bHul 16b). This leads me to believe that we cannot really trace an allusion to the myth of the *vagina dentata* which famously bespeaks male anxiety about being devoured. The use of the metaphor in Rabbi Yohanan's statement is too rarefied, and too specific as to its referent in order to warrant a reading here of either a replication or even mockery of the myth.

49. For a discussion of פנים or face as a metaphoric euphemism for women's genitalia see Cynthia M. Baker's "Bodies, Boundaries, and Domestic Politics in a Late Ancient Marketplace." She analyzes the rabbinic conflicted trope of the "woman in the *shuq* [marketplace or public street]." She argues that the woman in the *shuq*, frequently a sexualized image, "likely represents on some level the threat posed to society by 'dis-placed' sexuality" (409). Baker suggests, quite convincingly, that "the rabbis' increasingly sexualized and anxiety-laden woman in the shuq embodies their growing anxieties regarding the entire 'domestic economy' of the Galilee and its large Jewish population. Just as the woman in the shuq signals the danger of the 'un-domesticated' female—specifically, the threat of sexual compromise—she at the same time encompasses the threat posed to the domestic culture of the Galilee by the larger imperial culture—that is, the threat that not only economic, but ethnic, religious, and other cultural categories, too will be compromised" (408). Baker's analysis, of course, strengthens the analysis of the metaphoric consignment of the woman to the space of the interior in this chapter.

50. The citation of this midrash in the Babylonian Talmud uses the term בנין אוצר (bBer 61a), in this case a synonym for מגורות in the Midrash, which has the connotation of silo, or reservoir. In a detailed description of the "Palestinian house" and its attachments, Krauss suggests that the בית האוצרות in rabbinic usage was understood to be a storage chamber particularly for fruit or olives (*Talmudische Archäologie*, 46). See also his suggestions that מגורות has more the connotation of dwelling than storage (44).

51. This number is widespread throughout rabbinic literature, and is accompanied by 365 as the number for sinews and ligaments. This pair of numbers is midrashically equated with the 248 days of the lunar year and the 365 days of the solar

year (bMakk 23b). Midrashic play with the numbers continues to point out that they add up to 613, the conventional number of commandments counted by the rabbis in the Bible. In his discussion of the classic rabbinic passage, Urbach points out that "it is the idea that there is a precept for every day of the year and every part of man's [sic] body ... that led to the fixing of the exact number six hundred and thirteen" (*The Sages*, 342). For an extended discussion of these numbers, and equivalent discussions in Greco-Roman gynecological literature, see Preuss (*Biblical and Talmudic Medicine*, 66–74).

52. The שיטה מקובצת, a collection of talmudic commentaries of the sixteenth century, adds for clarification of the narrative: "They [the students] came and asked Rabbi Yishma'el: How many limbs are there in a person? He said to them: Two hundred forty-eight. They said to him: Did we not conduct an examination and find two hundred fifty-two?" (see bBekh 45b, ש"ם, note 10).

53. For a graphic description of this form of execution see mSanh 7:2. mSanh 9:1 records the kinds of transgressions for which the convicted perpetrator is executed by burning. mSanh 7:2 famously also records the case of a promiscuous priestly woman who was executed by burning, to which account is appended the remark that this could only have happened because the court which imposed the sentence was not an expert court. This latter remark has often been read to indicate rabbinic reluctance as to the concept of actual execution of capital punishment. Hence, I use the term "halakhic theory" here.

54. Since this is the only story that reports experimentation with a corpse, Preuss discusses other etymological possibilities for שלק than "boiling," such as cutting open. However, in the end he insists on "boiling" as the meaning of the term and leaves his analysis of the story unresolved (*Biblical and Talmudic Medicine*, 48).

55. We will be able to observe a similar mechanism in a later chapter, dealing with the question of the examination of blood. For a more extensive discussion of the cultural mechanisms contributing to keeping women out of the study house, see Boyarin, *Unheroic Conduct*. He writes: "The study of Torah is the quintessential performance of rabbinic Jewish maleness. In other words, precisely the stylized repetitions that produced gender differentiation [ ... ] within classical Jewish praxis were the repetitive performances of the House of Study, including the homosocial bonding. At the structural(ist) level the specific performances themselves are irrelevant; what is culturally significant is the very inscription of sex through any gender-differentiating practice. The House of Study was thus the rabbinic Jewish equivalent of the locker room, barracks, or warship" (143).

56. Rashi reads צירים as "hinges," not as "birth-pangs," as the word is used in biblical Hebrew (bBekh 45a, ד"ה צירין). In a classic work, S. Krauss points out that "der ציר ein wichtiger Bestandteil des Hauses ist" (*Talmudische Archäologie*, 338). "Die Tueren hingen nicht, wie bei uns, in den Angeln, was auch in Griechenland und Rom nicht der Fall war, sondern an der beweglichen Tuere selbst befanden sich zwei

kegelfoermige Zapfen (צירים) welche in je eine Hoehlung oder Pfanne (צינור, פותה) der oberen und der unteren Schwelle (ציר עליון und ציר תחתון) eingelassen waren und sich darin drehten [Doors did not hang, as with us, in their hinges, which was not the case in Greece and Rome either. Rather, two cone-shape pins were attached to the movable door itself, each of which were fitted into a socket at the upper and lower lintel and turned in those]" (38).

57. Compare the parallel in Lev. R., Parsha 14.

58. The parallel text, with some differences as to the attribution of the individual parts of this midrash, can be found in *Leviticus Rabbah* 14:4 (Margulies, *Midrash Wayyikra Rabbah*, 306) in a homiletic midrash on Lev. 12:1. The scholarly consensus is that this midrash was edited at some time in the fifth century (Stemberger, *Einleitung*, 316).

59. For a discussion of what he calls the one-sex model of Aristotle, see Thomas Laqueur (*Making Sex*, 25–63). Laqueur traces Aristotle's representation of the female sexual organs as interior inversion of the male organs and concludes: "Claims that the vagina was an internal penis or that the womb was a female scrotum should therefore be understood as images in the flesh of truths far better secured elsewhere. They are another way of saying, with Aristotle, that woman is to man as a wooden triangle is to a brazen one or that woman is to man as the imperfect eyes of the mole are to the more perfect eyes of other creatures" (35). In *De generatione animalium* Aristotle famously expounds on his view that "it is through a certain incapacity that the female is female" (I, 20l 728 a 17f). He is committed to the idea that the female is a version of the male, but inferior and imperfect.

60. Or maybe six, if we count the two versions of the second case as different stories (Valler, *Woman and Womanhood*, 45).

61. Shulamit Valler has analyzed this collection of stories more extensively in the third chapter of her *Women and Womanhood in the Stories of the Babylonian Talmud*. She argues that "in these stories, and mainly in their [editorial] arrangement as a collection, there exists the attempt to delineate a way that would completely prevent the application of the unjust assertion that the husband is believed in his claim of absence of virginity" (42).

62. The town of Mavrakhta is mentioned elsewhere in the Talmud (bEruv 47b; 61b). According to A. Oppenheimer the town's location is west of the Tigris in the vicinity of Mahoza (*Babylonia Judaica*, 239). He points out that "the word מברכתא means 'caravan' (perhaps of camels) and was probably applied to the place because it was a way station for camels and merchants" (240), but rejects the interpretation of some scholars who interpret the word to mean merely "caravan," and not as a place name.

63. The Tosafot (ד״ה מברכתא) explain with a slightly different nuance: "They lash him because he has discredited a Jewish woman, but is certainly a liar. And since

prostitutes were lying prostrate before him, so that he became an expert, he is not believed (with his claim)."

64. The phrase באישון לילה ואפילה has it origins in Prov. 7:9. This chapter of Proverbs is an intertext for the case story here, indicating the literariness of the case, rather than presenting us with the report of an actual historical event, in which a man "really" came before Rabban Gamliel. Prov. 7 indulges in the embellishment of a scene which shows the power of female seductiveness. Wisdom describes watching the scene in which a young man wanders around in the streets in the middle of the night and is seduced by a woman who is decked out like a prostitute. This is not to say that the bride is the prostitute in the case at hand; it merely shows the rabbis' association of the phrase פתח פתוח with illicit sex.

65. This needs some supplementation. Against Jastrow, who translates the verb as "to perform coition without violently tearing the hymen," Rashi's interpretation makes more sense: "when he reaches the closed door of his house and there is something that hinders him from opening, and when he moves it aside, it [the house] is opened." In other words, Rabban Gamliel suggests that he moved his penis in a way, that he himself opened up "the house."

66. This is the point that the second version of the story makes, as Rashi emphasizes: "without intention it is impossible to move (it) aside," whereby במזיד is not merely intentionally, but also with force: במזיד—במתכוין ובכח (Rashi, bKet 10a).

67. Thus Rufus, Soranus, and Galen are all active during the end of the first century C.E. and into the second, the era when the Mishnah is collated.

68. Martin Jaffee reminds me that talmudic literature also likens the female body to a jug, for instance, in the polemic remark in bShab 152a cited above (Chapter 1, n. 48). But in the current more systematic representation of the female body and its physiology in Tractate Niddah this metaphor is not mobilized.

69. For an extensive analysis see Ann Carson, "Putting Her in Her Place," 138–39. Dean-Jones, however, differs from Carson in that according to her Aristotle does not rely on a distinction of male flesh as firm, compact, and therefore good, versus female flesh as loose, spongy, and therefore bad. She analyzes carefully the production of sexual difference through physiological explanations in the Hippocratic corpus as against Aristotle's work. According to Dean-Jones, Aristotle considers women to be less "Other" and more like men than the Hippocratics. Hence, Aristotle ties all differences to a man's naturally greater heat, whereas otherwise female anatomy corresponds to male anatomy. The difference is, therefore, one of degrees. The Hippocratics, on the other hand, "because they thought woman was a completely different creature and not simply a substandard man, . . . did not have to look for a correspondence between all male and female body parts" (*Women's Bodies*, 85). Thomas Laqueur's analysis presents a combination of these two positions, that is, he notes the paradox in Aristotle, who as a philosopher is deeply committed to the

existence of two radically different and distinct sexes, but as a biologist has a one-sex model which is later adopted by Galen and in which "the sexes were more and less perfect versions of each other" (*Making Sex*, 29; see above, note 5). Laqueur explains this paradox by the fact that for Aristotle the biological is not the foundation for the metaphysical with its implied social arrangements: "What we would take to be ideologically charged social constructions of gender—that males are active and females passive, males contribute the form and females the matter to generation—were for Aristotle indubitable fact, 'natural' truths. What we would take to be the basic facts of sexual difference, on the other hand—that males have a penis and females a vagina, males have testicles and females ovaries, females have a womb and males do not, males produce one kind of germinal product, females another, that women menstruate and men do not—were for Aristotle contingent and philosophically not very interesting observations about particular species under certain conditions" (28).

70. Translation of *hysteron*.

71. Temkin comments that here Soranus (as Aristotle in his *Historia Animalium* III, 1; 510b:13) "tries to connect the name for the uterus with the Greek name for brothers (*adelphoi*) or sisters (*adelphai*)" (*Soranus' Gynecology*, 8, note 11).

72. For example, Froma Zeitlin refers to Vernant's reading of the Pandora myth while disagreeing with it: "For Vernant, the image of the jar represents the house of *oikos* [the house], and woman is the ambiguous figure of Elpis [Hope, remaining in the jar after Pandora opens it], who resides within. In this reading, the jar replicates the domestic space of the household to which woman is consigned" ("Signifying Difference," 64).

73. A.o. bBer 44b, 44b, 56a; bTaan 23b, 24b; bHul 110a; bNid 37a; bNed 23a, 51a; bKid 45b.

74. As far as the ox is concerned, Rashi explains this by a reading of Proverbs 14:4, that "abundant crops come by the strength of the ox" (ad bShab 118b).

75. Similarly, the Rosh explains: לקנח את כל הזרע—to wipe all the semen.

76. Here I do not intend to critique Levinas's concept of the "feminine" in his work at large, which is often opaque and oscillates between essentializing not only his concept of the feminine but also women as the incarnation of the feminine, and understanding the concept of the feminine as independent from women. In this context I only concentrate on his statements in the cited essay and his lectures on the creation of woman in the "Nine Talmudic Readings," since here he makes his extraordinary claim on biblical and talmudic "primordial truth."

77. This juxtaposition raises, of course, the specter of essentializing the male as well as the female mode of relating to the world, since Irigaray explicitly does not think of the male mode as a cultural-historical one, but as a psychological-ontological one, in that man is "forever" building. However, I follow Naomi Schor's analysis of Irigaray's strategic essentializing, which enables her to think women's difference within the difference as it has always been defined by androcentrism

("This Essentialism Which Is Not One," 57–78). The point here is that Irigaray's analysis of the "male" mode of relating to the world beautifully summarizes my discussion of the woman as house in talmudic literature.

**CHAPTER 3**

1. See, for instance, bYev 77a, bGit 12a and bShev 30a. bYev 77a also alludes to the midrashic interpretation of Gen. 18:9 as a parallel tradition. The verse has Avraham's visitors in Mamre ask him where Sarah is, upon which he answers that she is in the tent. All the medieval commentators interpret this to mean that Sarah "is a modest woman" (Rashi) and "she is in the tent as is the way of modest women" (Radaq). For a more extensive discussion of the verse and its history in midrashic hermeneutics see A. Cohen, *Rereading Talmud*, 205–206.

2. Even though it shapes the Palestinian Talmud also. See Stemberger, *Einleitung*, 221; and Goldberg, "The Babylonian Talmud," 337. Both provide excellent introductions to the sugyah in their introductions to rabbinic literature. Stemberger points out that "*sugyot* as basic elements of the Babyloninan Talmud cannot be globally evaluated. Some are short and simply constructed, others are complex and hence longer; sometimes they even make use of other sugyot and hence parts of them. Although they are self-contained, sugyot may nevertheless presuppose knowledge of other sugyot and their terminology" (221). Goldberg describes the sugyah in similar terms: "The *sugyah* is an extended discussion of a particular topic which incorporates many of the *Tannaic* [sic] and other sources connected with it. The construction and form of the sugyah as well as the inner development of its dialectics, are determined by specific aims and principles. Once we gain insight into these principles we can begin to understand the reasons behind the impression of artificiality and strained logic, which at times is inescapable, as well as the forced interpretation of Tannaic sources" (337). The literature on the analysis of the sugyah as the basic literary unit of the Babylonian Talmud is, of course, extensive, and Stemberger provides a useful bibliography. Sh. Friedman's work is especially important in this respect. Aryeh Cohen coined the term *sugyaetics* as a term to describe the yet undeveloped analysis of sugyot from a literary perspective (*Rereading Talmud*).

3. On the emphasis on the process of the argument rather than on its result as the characteristic of the Babylonian Talmud, see David Kraemer's *The Mind of the Talmud*.

4. Between Rabbi Aqiva and Rabbi Ishma'el or between Abbaye and Rava.

5. For a similar approach in the case of biblical literature, see Ilana Pardes's *Countertraditions in the Bible*.

6. Whether or not this reading is really Shmu'el's, in the literary and imaginary universe of the Babylonian Talmud his name is a force to contend with.

7. If the blood is most likely genital blood, she is considered to be in a status of

impurity in this mishnah, otherwise to remain in a status of purity: "Concerning the one who sees a bloodstain on her body—if it is close to her genitals, she is in the status of impurity, if not close to her genitals, she is in the status of purity. If it is on her heel or on top of her big toe, she is in the status of impurity . . ." (mNid 8:1, bNid 57b).

8. This point will become clearer further below in the close reading of the sugyah. Classic talmudic commentaries, such as the תוספות and the תוספי הרא״ש, found in the margins of classical text editions, realize this point, as will be discussed further below.

9. I deliberately leave both formulations because they indicate exactly what I think the introduction of sensation does to the discourse. From the perspective of women's discursive objectification, the difference between the passive and reflexive formulation makes, of course, all the difference in the world.

10. This is obviously a somewhat hyperbolic claim, for technically the mishnaic tractate exists, of course, prior to the introduction of Shmu'el's midrash in the talmudic discussion. The mishnaic tractate thus sets the predominantly androcentric parameters discussed above. Nonetheless, Shmu'el's midrash presents its challenge on the level of the logic behind the discourse of menstrual impurity, and thus turns the Mishnah on its head. In his study on *Samuel's Commentary on the Mishnah*, Baruch Bokser has collated the diverse interpretations of the Mishnah attributed to Shmu'el, without, however, ever mentioning our text. Bokser concluded that "Samuel's exposition of M. [the Mishnah] enabled his disciples and later generations first to understand and then to apply M. and its laws" (237). However, it seems to me that our text shows how Shmu'el actually subverts the predominant paradigm of the mishnaic conception of the woman's body. I thank Martin Jaffee for directing my attention to Bokser's study in this context.

11. Formulated in this way, it should be clear that I do not claim Shmu'el as a proto-feminist, as if he *intended* to allow for women's subjectivity to break into the text. I focus on analyzing the discursive effects of his reading, which makes the intention of the author of the midrash irrelevant to my discussion. For a similar skepticism as to detecting the voice of an individual rabbi as proto-feminist, see the discussion of a mishnaic text by Miriam Peskowitz (*Spinning Fantasies*, 42–44).

12. In halakhic midrash, most commonly a verse or a term can only be "used" once to establish a halakhic ruling, as opposed to *aggadic* midrash, where a verse can be interpreted in multiple ways. The objection here would be that Shmu'el employs a reading of a verse that has already been "used up" in a different halakhic context. The deployment of this principle is, however, not always entirely consistent. In our sugyah the Talmud mentions only two other contexts (mNid 5:1; bNid 21b) in which the verse has been "used" for halakhic reasoning, whereas there are at least two additional contexts (bNid 40a and bNid 41b). For an excellent introduction to midrashic hermeneutics, see Stemberger (*Einleitung*, 17–35).

13. We have seen this halakhic interpretation of the verse in Sifra in the previous chapter. The Babylonian Talmud itself discusses this interpretation (bNid 21b).

14. At this point the Talmud briefly raises the point that elsewhere yet another principle has been derived from this verse, namely that the verse indicates that [she is in a status of impurity only if the blood is actually] 'in her body'—not when it is in a foetal sac [which she aborts] or in a piece [of the foetus]." This is answered with the bland "learn both principles [from this verse]."

15. For the reader who is not familiar with talmudic argumentation, it needs to be emphasized again that from a logical point of view this strategy is a classic one. It is important to keep in mind that it is in the nature of talmudic argumentation to not simply state that a position is wrong, however difficult it may appear to be, especially when it is a position held by earlier generations of scholars. On the contrary, the argumentation is often geared toward strengthening an opinion that in the end it may not necessarily agree with.

16. The distinction between sitting and standing is, of course, somewhat unclear and debated in the gemara at the beginning of the next chapter (bNid 59b) and in the medieval commentaries. The question is whether the blood could be blood from the uterus. Thus Rashi comments, based on the gemara further down, that when she is standing the urine might flow back into the uterus [מקור] and bring the menstrual blood out with it since while standing the urinal channel is squeezed. In the Mishnah itself [mNid 9:1], Rabbi Yossi disagrees with Rabbi Meir and holds her to be in a status of purity either way. In the version of this disagreement in tNid 7:7, Rabbi Meir is presented to hold that the woman who urinates in a sitting position and has a blood-flow is in a status of doubtful impurity only.

17. The citation of this case here neglects to mention that in the Mishnah this is the ruling of Rabbi El'azar, the son of Rabbi Zaddoq. The Tosefta's version of the case (tNid 7:6) adds the short comment that in the case of the round stain it can be assumed to be the blood of a louse, where in the case of the elongated stain it can be assumed to derive from her wiping.

18. I have not located this baraita in any of the tannaitic texts available to us.

19. Both touch [מגעות] and shaking (בהיסטות) are among the specified ways of contact in which the status of impurity can be transferred, not just by a woman in her impurity, but by anyone who is in the status of impurity, such as the man with an abnormal discharge, to any object by shaking it so as to move it from its place.

20. This is difficult to understand, and there is a disagreement in the medieval commentaries as to what has to be imagined as the scenario of this doubtful situation, though all agree that "the majority" has the referent "the majority of her days." Thus Rashi [ד"ה ובמגעות ובהיסטות] explains: "In the case of a woman who does not actually find a stain but only has an assumption to be in the doubtful status of menstruation, as for example where she does not have a regular period [וסת] but usually bleeds frequently, and she [establishes contact by] touching or by shaking, go after the majority of her days. If for the majority of her days [of her cycle] she usually has a blood-flow, and she touches and shakes, her act of touching or shaking trans-

fers the status of impurity—[implying that, against Shmu'el's midrash, she is in the status of impurity in this doubtful situation] even though she did not have a sensation of a blood-flow." However, the Tosafists [ד"ה ובמגעות] reject Rashi's interpretation as being too restrictive, and suggest instead that "it seems that [this case] refers back to the preceding case of the shirt, and it implies that if *after* the finding of the stains the majority of her days are impure, she is in the status of impurity [on that doubtful day also], even though [regularly in the case of the shirt we allow her to attribute the stains to an external cause, for instance when] she passed through the butcher market." According to the Tosafists, the point of this doubtful case is that the legal principle of "the majority of her days," as evidence posterior to the doubtful situation, overrides the principle of attributing the stain to whatever she can attribute it to. Whatever the case scenario to be imagined is, the point here is that the principle of the "majority of her days" is a circumstantial principle of statistics, so to speak, which seem to run counter Shmu'el's midrash.

21. Though Case IV is of course really three different case-scenarios. But the first two cases are really only subclauses in the literary structure of the sugyah. The third case, C, is the one that the gemara uses initially to think against Shmu'el's midrash.

22. Rejecting the possibility of arbitrariness out of talmudic principle, both medieval commentaries are, of course, primarily interested in the coherence of halakhic reasoning, and the consistency of talmudic literature in all of its aspects. They try to find the unifying halakhic principle that makes sense of the selection of precisely these tannaitic cases which the gemara introduces into the discussion. Hence, what in their view characterizes our cases is that they involve bloodstains on her body, which the Tosafists understand to indicate that since "it is not common for a stain to remain on the body undetected, before it dries up and 'falls off'" [bNid 57a, ד"ה הרואה]. Thus, the woman would find them quickly precisely because she had some sensation which, as we will see in the gemara, is classified as a mistaken sensation. The argument of the Tosafot can often only be followed after one has studied the entire sugyah in the gemara. It should also be remembered, however, as in so many other cases, the problem of the Tosafot as medieval commentators is not necessarily the Talmud's own problem.

23. And the argument continues: "[whereas this argument of mistaken sensation would be irrelevant in] the case of her standing [while urinating with the evidence of blood spotting] since [here we hold that] her urine might return to 'the source' [of menstrual blood, המקור] and flush it [the blood] out [with the urine]," wherefore she is now in the status of impurity no matter whether she had a sensation or not.

24. And the argument continues: "[whereas this argument of mistaken sensation would be irrelevant to] the case of the elongated [stain] where [the blood] certainly came from her body," wherefore she is in the status of impurity no matter whether she had a sensation or not.

25. The euphemistic metaphor for the penis here is "the servant." Interestingly,

the gemara in this case does not complete the argument. That is, it does not continue to argue that the argument of the mistaken sensation is irrelevant in the case of the women's examination immediately after marital intercourse. It does not offer a circumstantial reason that could apply to the case of "immediately afterwards," parallel to the backing up of the urine into her uterus in the first objection and the stretched-out stain from the second stain. Presumably we are to conclude that in this situation the blood is certainly menstrual blood.

26. A woman is sitting while urinating; a bloodstain on an examination cloth is round; a woman examined herself a while after sexual intercourse with her husband.

27. A woman is standing and urinating; a bloodstain on an examination cloth is drawn out; blood is found either on the husband's examination cloth after sexual intercourse, or on hers when she examines herself immediately afterwards.

28. This methodology is, of course, what some Jewish feminists from various perspectives employ for reading talmudic literature. See, for instance, Judith Hauptman's *Rereading the Rabbis* and Blu Greenberg's *Women and Judaism*.

29. The Tosafot seem to read this phrase not quite as oxymoronic. In their reading this argument applies only to situations when some time has passed between the discovery of a bloodstain and the woman's supposed genital bleeding. Thus, they understand the phrase to mean that she had a sensation but she forgot about it and, due to the time passed, can no longer recall it (ד"ה הרואה כתם and ד"ה קתני מיהא).

30. And not just these specific cases, but the mishnaic discourse on the status of im/purity of a woman's menstruation in its totality.

31. The first, attributed to Rav Yirmeyah from Difti, a Babylonian rabbi of the fifth generation, that is, approximately the latter half of the fourth century, is even more complicated than the following and engenders disagreeing readings in the medieval commentaries. This would lead my discussion too far afield into the labyrinth of halakhic reasoning. In brief, his solution to the problem is to introduce a classic theoretical talmudic distinction between types or levels of halakhic reasoning between biblical [מדאורייתא] and rabbinic law [מדרבנן]. Both levels usually have equal practical force (Roth, "The Concepts"). In our context Rav Yirmeyah solves the problem by claiming that "Shmu'el would agree that 'she' is in the status of impurity rabbinically [מדרבנן]" (bNid 57b, bottom). Rashi and the Tosafot have different readings of this statement.

32. That places him chronologically at the beginning of the fifth century. Again, the problem of historical attribution is not central for my discussion. For an introduction to Rav Ashi's supposed role in the organization of the talmudic material, see Stemberger, *Einleitung*, 211–13.

33. The Meiri suggests the following explanation of the case of the anonymous majority opinion: "This is a small bench, and they sit on it one after the other" (*Beit ha-Behirah*, 249). That is, in such a case we could not ascertain from whom the blood stems. "And even if all of them sat together at the same time, only she under whom

the blood is found is in the status of impurity, because it would be evident to her that she has not sat in her friend's place; but if the blood is found between them, they are all in the status of impurity" (ibid.). Hence Rabbi Nehemiah's reasoning could be that if the women sat on the bench one after the other, the material of the bench would play a role, in accordance with Lev. 15:20–22: "and everything that she sits upon shall be impure . . . and whoever touches anything that she sat upon shall wash his clothes, and bathe himself in water, and be impure until evening." If the first woman had the blood-flow, her blood on the bench would have rendered the bench impure, and then transferred the status of impurity to the following two women (who did not examine the bench before they sat down). In the case of the stone bench, this point would be rendered moot. Nonetheless, the mishnaic case is evidently one that decrees a status of impurity on the women because we don't know from which of the women the blood derives. The logic of Rabbi Nehemiah's principle rubs against this by thinking in terms of a physical transfer of the status of impurity. In Shmu'el's case this would certainly not make sense, since it deals with one woman.

34. Daniel Boyarin suggests to me a possible reciprocal relationship. Not only does Shmu'el agree with Rabbi Nehemiah, but vice versa, conceptually, that is, since Rabbi Nehemiah precedes Shmu'el by about two generations. Rabbi Nehemiah would agree with Shmu'el as well that women enter a status of impurity only if they have a sensation of their menstrual bleeding. This would explain why Rabbi Nehemiah rules all three women to remain in a status of purity, including the one from whom the blood on the stone bench must have originated. Why that woman also? Because Rabbi Nehemiah holds like Shmu'el, for in a case in which the bench is made from a material that transfers impurity, Rabbi Nehemiah would agree that all three women are rendered impure, regardless from whom the blood originated, since the blood on the bench would have transferred the impurity of the bloodstain to all three sitting on the bench! If we read Rav Ashi's comment in this way he would not dismiss Shmu'el's midrash but instead lend it tannaitic authority, a very powerful way to strengthen the opinion of an amora!

35. This is how Rashi reads Rav Ashi's comment: "Shmu'el's reason . . . was not [dependent on] her sensation. Rather he ruled in accordance with Rabbi Nehemiah. . . . Therefore, all these objections [raised previously with the four cases] do not present a difficulty, since Shmu'el did not deal with [the question of her] sensation at all" (bNid 58a, ד"ה רב אשי אמר). Textually it is possible to read the two units, Shmu'el's case and the midrashic reading of Lev. 15:19, as separate units, though the latter cannot stand by itself. I should point out also that we have seen a similar splitting between the halakhic and the discursive effects of the argumentation with respect to gender. Halakhically, as mentioned in the preceding note, Rav Ashi can be read to actually lend Shmuel's midrash more authority. Discursively, however, he circumvents the question of a woman's sensation altogether and shifts the discussion to circumstantial, "objective" reasoning.

36. The sugyah has a short Coda, in which it weighs Rav Ashi's and Rav Yirmeyah's opinions against each other. Here, Rav Ashi is the favored, or at least unchallenged opinion, who has the last voice.

37. In his effort to distinguish the ideological precepts of midrashic interpretation and poststructuralist literary theory, David Stern attempts to explain the function of the multiple interpretations of a biblical verse in midrash. His explanation is applicable to my reading of Shmu'el's halakhic midrash: "The object of midrash was not so much to find the meaning of Scripture as it was literally to engage its text. Midrash became a kind of conversation the Rabbis invented in order to enable God to speak to them from between the lines of Scripture, in the textual fissures and discontinuities that exegesis discovers. The multiplication of interpretations in midrash was one way, as it were, to prolong that conversation" ("Midrash and Indeterminacy," 153).

38. The discussion of the first mishnah of the tractate extends from bNid 2a to 7a.

39. Already Sherira, the Gaon of Pumbeditha (906–1006), in his famous *Epistle* (אגרת) of 987, pointed out that the opening sugyah of Tractate Kiddushin (2a–3b) is entirely a product of the last, anonymous group of redactors of the Babylonian Talmud, called the *saboraim*, the "examiners" or "reflectors." Little or nothing is known about their history and their work. Modern scholarship on the saboraim and their role in shaping the Talmud is, of course, extensive, with differing opinions as to the extent of their role. Again, Stemberger's as well as Goldberg's introductions provide accessible entries to these discussions. As to the opening sugyot of tractates Goldberg writes: "Rav Sherira Gaon mentions the fact that the opening sugyah in Tractate Kiddushin (2a–3b) is a completely *Savoraic* creation. This has been extended by [I. H.] Weiss (1954) who showed that in almost all tractates the opening sugyot are *Savoraic*. These serve as a kind of 'introductory lecture' to the tractate in which a plethora of sources are introduced" ("The Babylonian Talmud," 339).

40. I am borrowing this formulation from Mieke Bal (*Lethal Love*, 83), from whose work on reading differences in biblical literature I have learned a lot.

41. The attribution of this dispute to Hillel and Shammai serves as one of the key passages for Neusner's theory that "at the time of Herod, the Pharisaic group, formerly a political party in Hasmonean politics, begins to reshape itself into something quite different, a sect devoted to, and defined by table-fellowship" (*A History of the Mishnaic Law of Purities*, 209). This table-fellowship is defined by its requirement to keep the im/purity rules outside of the Temple, then still in existence. Neusner continues to argue that "if, as seems clear, the laws of Niddah go back to the times of Shammai and Hillel, then Niddah should represent one of the earliest topics to which the Pharisees of that period devoted attention" (ibid.). This contention leads him to the somewhat hyperbolic contention that "Pharisaism begins in menstrual blood" (11).

42. Chronologically Hillel and Shammai would be located at the beginning of the

first century C.E. But already Neusner points out that "the only firm conclusion is that Hillel was likely to have lived sometime before the destruction of the Temple and to have played an important part in the politics of the Pharisaic party. We may further hypothesize that traditions about his teachings on the festivals, on purity laws, and on legal theory may go back to him. But the materials before us are so highly developed and sophisticated that we cannot recover anything like his own words" ("From Scripture to Mishnah," 43). There are only four differences of opinion attributed to Hillel and Shammai themselves in all of rabbinic literature, one of which is this one (mEd 1: 1–3, bShab 15a; see Urbach, *The Sages*, 588). If we accept the attribution of this disagreement to the historical personalities, it would function as a dispute on practical halakhah, since at the time of Hillel and Shammai the Temple was still standing. But again, this historicizing argument is unimportant to my current analysis, since I take Shammai's and Hillel's disagreement as a conceptual framework for talmudic thinking on menstrual impurity, and beyond that on female corporeality. As the opening mishnah of the whole tractate the disagreement has no longer merely a value as an individualized dispute that supposedly took place at the beginning of the first century, but has to be read in the context of and with respect to its function within the tractate as a whole. The talmudic discussion itself is not interested in such a historicizing reading but deals with the Mishnah as an integrated whole.

43. This mishnah is also cited as the opening mishnah in Mishnah Tractate Eduyot, a tractate differing from the rest of the Mishnah, since it orders its literary material by names of rabbis and not by contents. According to Albeck, Tractate Eduyot cites the mishnah from Tractate Niddah (*Shishah Sidrei Mishnah*, השלמות על עדויות).

44. Rashi similarly comments that the reference point for this mishnah is the Temple: "[Shammai holds that] if she has a blood-flow, it is sufficient for us to consider her to transfer a status of impurity to the heave-offering [or terumah] and to other Temple-related objects which she touches only from the time of her flow onward" (Rashi bNid 2a, ד"ה שמאי).

45. The Babylonian Talmud (bNid 4b) cites a baraita, which comments on the compromising ruling of this mishnah: "The sages say: Neither according to the words of him nor according to the words of him, [meaning] neither according to the words of Shammai who did not make a fence for his words, and neither according to the words of Hillel, who went beyond his measures." That is, Shammai's opinion is rejected by the majority ruling because he does not provide precautionary measures, one of the classic rabbinic principles vis-à-vis biblical rulings, whereas Hillel's opinion is rejected because his use of the principle of retroactivity is far too restrictive. This baraita does not exist in the Tosefta. However, the Palestinian Talmud (pNid 1:1, 48d) gives the same explanation, almost word for word, with the one difference that Hillel "disagreed with his own principles" [הפליג על מדותיו] instead of "went beyond

his principles" [הפריז על מדותיו] in the Babylonian Talmud, which is only a stylistic difference. The Palestinian Talmud does not cite this as a baraita, however. This is not a singularly occurring phenomenon (for instance, bBM 59b and pMQ 3:1, 81c) and has triggered an extensive debate among scholars, both in terms of the implications for the redaction of the Babylonian Talmud, and of the literary relationship between the Babylonian and Palestinian Talmud. As to the former, Judith Hauptman has most recently argued that such baraitot as the current one, which are more or less commentaries on the Mishnah, belong to the earliest redactionary layer of a sugyah in the Babylonian Talmud (*Development of the Talmudic Sugyah*). She argues against earlier contentions that indeed such baraitot are later Babylonian inventions. As to the latter, I would suggest that the current textual examples do not present a conclusive source for defining the relationship between the Palestinian and the Babylonian Talmud, since the hermeneutic options for the explanation of a compromise solution in mNid 1:1 are limited in the first place. Any commentary would have to come to such a conclusion as suggested in the baraita in the Bavli or in the commentary in the Palestinian Talmud. Before we could ascertain that Jaffee's conclusion applies to our tractate, namely, that "the Yerushalmi, in more or less its extant form, shapes the Babylonians' conception of their own task and, moreover, supplies the dominant exegetical themes appropriated by them for amplification or revision" ("Babylonian Appropriation," 7), we would have to compare the chapter as a whole. For a nuanced discussion of the various factors producing specifically halakhic differences between the Babylonian and Palestinian gemaras on Mishnah Tractate Avodah Zarah, see C. Hayes, *Between the Babylonian and Palestinian Talmuds*.

46. Therefore, the rabbinic consideration of the retroactivity of the impurity of menstruation cannot be pathologized as if the assumption of retroactive impurity were characteristic to the discussions of menstruation only. It is an integral part of the complex rabbinic system of impurity as a whole and even beyond the issue of impurity.

47. In talmudic terminology the term חזקה—"presumptive status"—is used, which is operative not just in the context of impurity. The current proven status of a thing or person is designated as its presumptive status, which extends backward to the last previous point of a proven different status. For an extensive treatment of the halakhic principle, see *Encyclopedia Talmudica*, vol. 13, pp. 453–753 and vol. 14, pp. 1–423. See also Louis Jacobs (*The Talmudic Argument*, 110–14) for a discussion of an exemplary sugyah (bHul 10b) dealing with this principle. Jacobs formulates: "*Hazakah* determines the law in all cases of doubt so that the matter is no longer treated as doubtful . . . [it] is a matter of procedure. Where the case is in doubt, the *hazakah* principle informs us, the correct procedure to be adopted is to leave it in the state which previously obtained" (110).

48. The case is cited in bGit 31b, in the discussion of another mishnah that is concerned with the principle of twenty-four-hour retroactivity. In this context the

Talmud uses mMikv 2:2 to emphasize that in the case of the miqveh the assumption is that we are dealing with undefined, that is, unlimited retroactivity. Further it is cited in bKid 79a, here in conjunction with the following case of the wine jugs. In bKid 79a the introduction of the tannaitic texts is attributed to Shmu'el, a first-generation Babylonian amora, in a dispute with Rav. In our context, however, the discussion is anonymous. It seems to me that the original use of the tannaitic cases by the Talmud is the context of bKid 79a, from where the redactors of our sugyah adopted the two cases as illustrations for the discussion of menstrual impurity. Interestingly the debate in bKid 79a also centers around the woman's body, here, however, in its exteriority.

49. Usually in the public domain more leniency is applied than in the private domain in matters of doubt concerning im/purity. The distinctive point of this case would be that the location of the miqveh does not matter. This becomes evident in the version of this case in tMiqv 1:16, which records a disagreement of Rabbi Shime'on. According to the latter, the items are in the status of impurity only if the miqveh is located in the private domain, but where it is located in the public domain they should be considered to be in the status of purity. The sugyah cites this baraita further down (bNid 2b), and in a parallel sugyah in bKid 79a. The baraita differs slightly from the version in the Tosefta. In the baraita Rabbi Shime'on is said to hold that where the miqveh is located in the private domain the status of the items would be held in a suspended status, instead of in a status of purity. The practical difference of this would be that Temple food in such cases would be neither burned nor eaten.

50. The sugyah here introduces the case as a mishnaic case with דתנן, as witnessed also by the manuscripts. However, both in bKid 79a and bB.B. 96a the case is "properly" introduced as a baraita with דתניא. Nonetheless, we do not find the case in this form in either Mishnah or Tosefta. The closest case is mTer 3:1, which has an almost identical parallel in tTer 4:7: "[Concerning the case of] one who separates [from his stock of wine] a barrel of wine for the obligatory contribution to the priests and it is found to be a barrel of vinegar: if it is known that it was vinegar before he made the separation, it is not considered as a valid offering; if the wine turned sour after he made the separation, it is considered a valid offering. If there is a doubt, it is considered a valid offering, but he has to make another separation [for the obligatory contribution to the priests]." The Tosefta adds that the latter is the opinion of Rabbi (Yehuda ha-Nassi), and not an anonymous opinion because "Rabbi holds the opinion that wine and vinegar are two different species," implying that one cannot make a separation for the *terumah* from one kind for the other, but that both would have to be tithed separately, whereas in an opposing opinion, "the sages say that they are one species."

51. All the manuscripts consulted (Vat Ebr 111, 113, 127, Munich) have the grammatically correct נמצאת.

52. None of the manuscripts consulted, nor the parallel citations of this baraita in bB.B. 96a and bKid 79a, has this insertion of the curly brackets in the printed edition.

This seems to be an attempt on behalf of the editors of the printed edition to clarify the referent of the "three days," possibly with the discussion of this case in bB.B. 96a in mind, where this is an interpretation of the baraita by Rabbi Yochanan. Vat Ebr 113 has כל שלושה ימים מכאן ואילך ספק and a marginal note fills in ודאי after the three days.

53. The case is discussed extensively elsewhere in the Talmud (bB.B. 96a). There is a disagreement between Rabbi Yochanan and Rabbi Yehoshua ben Levi, two Palestinian amoraim of the second and first generation, at the beginning of the third century, as to those three days. According to the former, the three days of the baraita refer to the first three days after the last examination when we assume the liquid to be certainly wine, "since it takes wine three days to turn sour" (Rashi, ad. loc.), whereas the latter holds that they refer to the last three days before the current examination, during which the liquid would be considered to be vinegar with certainty.

54. The case of the alleyway is discussed more extensively in bNid 56a. Further, this is the only one of all of these test cases adduced by the Babylonian Talmud that the Palestinian Talmud takes up as a test case (pNid 1:1, 48d).

55. Compare Albeck, *Shishah Sidrei Mishnah*, on mToh 3:6.

56. Miriam Peskowitz's approach to tannaitic texts raises similar questions. She claims: "Gender can be as powerful in its apparent absence as in its presence" (*Spinning Fantasies*, 41). It is exactly this apparent absence of gender that creates the effect of what she calls "patriarchy's ordinariness," the title of her first chapter. In the terms of contemporary literary and cultural studies, it is this analysis of the hidden structures of a text or its implied rhetorical choices that creates an effect of naturalizing certain ways of thinking gender difference. The concept of naturalizing certain ways of seeing and thinking is born from Walter Benjamin's work, as Peskowitz herself explicates: "The idea of gender was embedded in things used daily, in things that were background and commonplace, in acts that were so boring that, in Benjamin's terms, the retelling of their meanings is not conscious, but comes 'all by itself'" (81).

57. The case of the dead vermin in the alleyway does not involve fluids. However, interestingly enough the Palestinian Talmud (pNid 1:1, 48 d) introduces fluids even in this case. Two Palestininan rabbis of the third generation, Rabbi Ammi and Rabbi Yossi, discuss this case. According to Rabbi Ammi the mishnaic case is (obviously) contradicting Shammai's opinion, whereas according to Rabbi Yossi this case also contradicts Hillel: ולא מודה הלל במבוי שהוא מתכבד ושטף של גשמים עובר בו שהוא טהור שמאי אומר הדא אשה על ידי שהיא רגילה במי רגלים עשו אותה כמבוי שהוא טהור—מתכבד ושטף של גשמים עובר בו והוא טהור "Does not Hillel agree in the case of an alleyway which is swept and through which a rain-flood passes, that it is in a status of purity [when the vermin is found]? Shammai says: Since the woman (in mNid 1:1) regularly urinates, they equate her with a gateway which is swept and through which a rain-flood passes, so that it is in the status of purity." Thus even the case of the gateway turns into an illustration of how the woman's physiology might be imagined.

58. Exactly the same structure of discussion is repeated for the case of the wine jug, so that the two sections of the sugyah could be superimposed on each other, with the one obvious difference that instead of the lacking quality of water we fill in the souring of the wine, so that one could argue that the wine sours only gradually, but would that be applicable to the woman?

59. This is reiterated in a somewhat different formulation further down in the sugyah (bNid 3a bottom), where the Talmud suggests as a possible alternative explanation for Shammai's position that his reason was דאם איתא דהוה דם מעיקרא הוה אתי—"for if there had been blood [before it appeared outside], it would have flowed out immediately." Hillel's counter-position in these terms would be that כותלי בית הרחם העמידוהו—"the walls of the house of the womb held back the blood (and it did not flow out right away)." Though this is presented as an alternative explanation of the disagreement of opinions of the fathers, that is, as being based on different understandings of anatomy rather than halakhic principles, at the same time it is the presumption of our current discussion.

60. Rashi comments on the argument that "she observed the blood-flow only when it came in large quantities" (bNid 2b): "when the blood has proliferated in the source, that which the source [מקור] cannot contain anymore begins to exit from there very slowly, in the quantity of a mustard seed, and slowly exits to the 'outer house' [בית החיצון] and this process can last several days, but she will be in the status of impurity on account of a drop of blood of the size of a mustard seed, as we learn further down (in the tractate, on bNid 40a)." Rashi here anticipates what we learn later in the tractate. On the mishnaic terminology of "outer house" (mNid 5:1), see the previous chapter. However, this explanation seems somewhat difficult to me and to be the product of an attempt to homogenize various mishnaic ideas, because the point of the discussion is the visibility of the blood and the interpretation of this visibility. Given the ambiguity of the term "outer house," the distinctions within the woman's "interior" are not necessarily the issue here.

61. See also Rashi's explanation in the previous note.

62. In her *Volatile Bodies* Grosz devotes a chapter to the analysis of Merleau-Ponty's "Corporeal Phenomenology." In his unfinished *The Visible and the Invisible* (1968), Merleau-Ponty attempts to reverse this traditional understanding of vision, by claiming the reversibility of seer and seen, similar to that of the toucher and the touched, since for him "the seer's visibility conditions vision itself, is the ground the seer shares with the visible, the condition of any relation between them" (*Volatile Bodies*, 101), although he has to admit the asymmetry of this reversibility. However, for the current discussion Irigaray's critique of Merleau-Ponty is extremely relevant. She points out that Merleau-Ponty's privileging of vision, in having it act as a model for all other perceptual relations, "submits them to a phallic economy in which the feminine figures as a lack or a blind spot" (104) and "can be understood [as] a desire for mastery" (Irigaray, *An Ethics of Sexual Difference*, 163). It seems to me that the

discursive effect of the rabbinic inscription of the blood-flow itself with visibility is another of those discursive mechanisms to enable the displacement of the women from the discussion.

63. This argument is not central to my discussion. The basic claim is that in the case of menstrual bleeding only one factor of doubt, called the "unfavorable factor" [ריעותא] in the sugyah, is involved, versus two factors of doubt in the three other cases. In the case of menstrual impurity, the only factor that indicates her change from a status of purity to a status of impurity is the visual evidence of blood, whereas in the three test cases two such factors exist: in the case of the miqveh it is the lacking quantity of water *and* the uncertain status of the person or the things that were immersed; in the case of the wine barrel it is the wine that turned sour, *and* the uncertain status of the other wine barrels as improperly tithed food; in the case of the dead vermin in the alleyway (bNid 3a) the construction is somewhat forced. Here the sugyah suggests that "there is vermin that has its origin inside the alleyway and vermin that comes in from the outside, the case resembles one in which there are two negative factors," that is, the two previous ones.

64. This second approach is introduced by the formula אי בעית אימא—"if you want I could argue," which signals an alternative hermeneutic angle to the one presented previously. Thus, it signals simultaneously the end of the part of the sugyah discussed so far. In and by itself, this alternative approach is not necessarily better or worse.

65. Rashi comments: "She knows herself when blood exits from her, and since she did not sense it yesterday it certainly came out only now with the current examination (when she found the blood)."

66. Names of rabbis are signifiers more of certain positions and arguments than of individual, historical persons.

67. None of the classic commentaries explicitly cross-references the two texts. However, the Tosafot curiously seem to allude to the latter text, without citing it. The Tosafot (ד"ה מרגשת, 3a) argue against Rashi's interpretation that "Shammai holds the opinion that a woman always has a sensation [of her blood-flow] and is not worried about [misidentifying it as] a sensation of the testing-rag or of his penis, just like she is not anxious about [misidentifying it as] as sensation of urine." The commentary clearly must have the sugyah related to Shmu'el's case in the back of their mind.

68. The phrase in bNid 57b is עד שתרגיש בבשרה—"[she is not in a status of impurity] unless she has a sensation in her body." Body and self here are virtually synonymous.

69. On the question of a "Hillelite" edition of the Mishnah, and reading Shammai halakhically as a minority opinion, see Stemberger, *Einleitung*, 34.

70. This is Rashi's reading of Rabbah's argument, because he adds "[since they held that she had a sensation] they fixed the retroactivity at only twenty-four hours [rather than postulating a potentially longer period as in Hillel]." However, this does

not make sense as Abaye's answer indicates, unless we assume that it was so impossible to agree with Shammai against Hillel that the rabbis had to find a rather unsatisfactory middle ground. Rabbah's answer could also be read as an objection, if it were read as an exclamation rather than as an explanatory statement. He would argue: how could they declare a retroactive status of impurity for the woman at all, seeing that she has a sensation of her blood-flow and, therefore, would have felt the blood-flow if it had started earlier? In this case, we would have yet another voice added to the counter-discourse. But then Abaye's answer would have to be read as an agreement with Rabbah, which does not work either, since the Talmud clearly understands it to be an objection to Rabbah.

71. This is a topos that occurs in many places in the Babylonian Talmud in debates between Rabbah and Abaye, for instance, bHul 43b, bBer 33b, bNid 45a, bZev 13a, bNaz 59bb, bEruv 13b.

72. Here I am thinking along the lines of Judith Butler's strategy of reading Freud in *Bodies That Matter*. She suggests that "the point is to read Freud not for the moments in which illness and sexuality are conflated, but rather, for the moments in which that conflation fails to sustain itself, and where he fails to read himself in precisely the ways he teaches us to read" (65). This is a cogent formulation of what it means to "read against the grain."

73. The truncated Palestinian gemara on Niddah never raised the issue of women's sensation of their bleeding.

**CHAPTER 4**

1. For the biblical texts I am using Jacob Milgrom's translation (*Leviticus 1–16*, 903).

2. This would seem to assume that a woman establishes something like a fixed cycle. Certain seven-day periods are assigned to menstrual impurity, and any bleeding that occurs outside of those periods makes her a zavah.

3. This term is difficult to translate. Gonorrhea is an inappropriate term, though even Jacob Milgrom chooses this term. In terms of biblical law the most appropriate way to render this term into English seems to me to be "a woman who has a discharge not during her regular cycle" (Cohen, "Menstruants and the Sacred," 277). Thus, Preuss explicitly does not deal with the zavah under his rubric of gonorrhea. He only goes as far as calling her bleeding what it is, that is, either "protracted" or "atypical" (*Biblical and Talmudic Medicine*, 375).

4. I have dealt with the parallel between male and female impurity in Lev. 15 in Chapter 2, as a feature of the priestly text. However, the repetition of this point is important. In her recent book Judith Hauptman reminds us that "since many people do not read the verses or mishnahs about the *niddah* and *zavah* in conjunction with those about the *zav* and ejaculant, they assume that only women can become a source

of impurity, and not men. Thus they conclude that these rules treat only women as object. But this is incorrect.... In fact, the purification ritual for the *zavah* is similar enough to that of the *zav* to say that the Torah draws little distinction between men and women as sources of impurity" (*Rereading the Rabbis*, 54).

5. Judith Hauptman emphasizes this effect in her recent work. Reading the rabbis diachronically and comparing them to the biblical text, she emphasizes that we have to take note of the positive trajectory: "A remarkable feature of tractate Niddah is the attempt to minimize the number of cases in which the dry blood stain a woman sees—not at the time of her regular menstrual period—renders her impure" (*Rereading the Rabbis*, 158). Reading this way, rabbinic texts appear to limit the patriarchal circumscription of women's life in biblical law.

6. This double effect is adumbrated in Boyarin's discussion of the case of wife-beating. Concerning the almost universal condemnation of all husbands toward their wives at least in Ashkenazi tradition, Boyarin argues against an apologetic reading of rabbinic culture as "good for women." Instead, he writes, "the very terms within which the condemnations of violence against wives occur in rabbinic literature demonstrate how that condemnation served as a technology for the control of women by men" (*Unheroic Conduct*, 167).

7. See also mEduyot 5:6 and Sifra Metzora, 4:4, 78a. The characters mentioned in this mishnah, the school of Shammai, the school of Hillel and Aqavia, are all of the same first generation of mishnaic teachers, that is, attributed to the first century C.E.

8. See, for instance, the popular handbook on the *Halachos of Niddah* by Rabbi Shimon D. Eider, who notes with reference to our mishnah and subsequent halakhic sources: "What color discharges and stains render a woman a *Niddah*? If a woman discovers a red or black discharge or stain, regardless of how light or dark a hue or shade [unless attributed to other causes] she is considered a *Niddah*. If a woman discovers white, blue, green, or pale yellow discharges or stains she is not considered a *Niddah*" (8–9).

9. Introduction to Foucault, *The Order of Things*, xv.

10. Judith Wegner, for instance, writes that "the ancients saw this phenomenon as embodying the dangerous power of contamination that lurks within women" ("The Image and Status of Women," 77).

11. See, however, the Samaritan halakha, which is also based on a reading of the biblical text. According to Boid in the Samaritan halakha "blood itself, as opposed to a discoloration of the vaginal fluid, is recognised as being pure red, blacky-red, or yellowy" (*Principles of Samaritan Halakhah*, 299f). The Samaritan texts Boid discusses stem from the tenth to the nineteenth century. The colors of genital blood in these texts are apparently the same as the ones recognized by the Karaites. A point of discussion, however, would be in how far the Samaritan and Karaite discourse can really be considered as separate from rabbinic discourse, or whether not, in fact, their texts could be considered a part of the same discourse of biblical hermeneutics. Thus

Boid claims that "the Samaritan, Karaite and Rabbanite systems have more points of agreement than disagreement, and are three variations of one system" (17).

12. In this discussion I disagree with Jacob Neusner. In his extensive work on what he calls the "idea" (1973) of purity Jacob Neusner has claimed that the mishnaic order of purities relies more heavily on biblical law than other sections of the Mishnah (*The Idea of Purity*). Particularly Tractate Niddah, according to Neusner, does not present any innovations (1978, 135–48). However, I would argue that the point is not to realize that "the Written Torah's system of uncleanness and cleanness is augmented and enriched by the Oral Torah, not revised or overturned" and that "nothing declared by the Written Torah to be a source of uncleanness is held to be clean in the Oral Torah" (148), though these observations are undoubtedly true. This insight does not particularly further our understanding why the rabbis read the biblical text the way they did and how the ways they read provided for new constructions of sexual difference and consequently, for new structures of gendered authority.

13. bNid 19a; compare yNid 2:6, 50a.

14. What the biblical text discusses as *zara'at* is not necessarily leprosy, as it is often translated, but some kind of skin disease that becomes a source for impurity. Rabbinic rules pertaining to this kind of impurity are discussed in the mishnaic tractate Nega'im, which does not have a gemara.

15. I am grateful to Martin Jaffee for directing my attention to the discussion of colors in Mishnah Nega'im.

16. By not explicating the move to force the discussion of menstrual impurity into the avenues of the impurity of skin lesions, the Mishnah also does not allow this move to be debated.

17. אומנא literally means skillful person or artisan, but is often used to designate the bloodletter, and sometimes the circumciser. On the role of the bloodletter in rabbinic culture see Preuss (*Biblical and Talmudic Medicine*, 33ff).

18. The Palestinian Talmud reports a similar incidence in which Rabbi Abbahu brought to the study session of Rabbi Eleazar various sorts of animal blood contained in bloodletter's vessels, which Rabbi Eleazar, however, invalidates, since כבר דהוא מראיו—"the color has already dimmed"(yNid 2:7, 50b).

19. Usually attributed to the turn of the fourth to the fifth century c.e.

20. For instance, according to Rachel Biale "the Talmud reflects the gradual disappearance of this expertise (Niddah 20a–b). The custom of relying on expert examination was gradually abandoned" (*Women and Jewish Law*, 153).

21. The one exception in the Bible is Jer. 2:22 כי אם תכבסי בנתר ותרבי לך בורית נכתם עונך לפני נאום אדני יהוה—"for though you wash yourself with lye, and increase your use of soap, the stain of your iniquity remains before me, says the Lord God." Here the prophet uses the term in verbal form in its figurative sense. It is interesting that the two kinds of lye in this verse, rare terms in biblical Hebrew, are later

prescribed in the Mishnah to wash out and distinguish a bloodstain from mere color (mNid 9:6, tNid 8:10).

22. For a discussion of the concept of retroactive impurity see the previous chapter.

23. This is also parallel to the issue of the colors. The Mishnah is primarily interested in the aspect of impurity. But conceptually it often extends into the issue of prohibited sex. As such it remains a practical legal discourse, relevant to current halakhic handbooks on laws of menstruation. I cite once more the popular handbook by Rabbi Eider: "If [a woman] did not feel any menstrual flow . . . but discovered a stain on her garments, nightclothes, or linen she would be considered a Niddah only if" certain conditions as to the location and shape of the size are fulfilled (20–21). If the stain fulfills those conditions, the woman has to abstain from marital intimacy.

24. For a discussion of the distinction between concepts originating דאורייתא and דרבנן, and the leniency connected with the latter, see most recently Joel Roth, "The Concepts of De-Oraita and De-Rabanan" (13–49).

25. Again one may argue that this is not so surprising since it is in the nature of rabbinic literature that rabbis are represented as the experts in all the areas discussed in that literature. Since there is virtually no woman sage among the rabbis, it is only logical that women are represented as advisees only even in cases of menstrual impurity. However, it is important to consider that in the case of women's bodies this process of rabbinic self-fashioning is even more drastic.

26. See for instance tNid 4:3, 4:4 and 4:6. Or the case is structured as a) describing the case, b) the case בא לפני חכמים—before the (collective) sages, and c) the way they rule (compare tNid 4:6).

27. See Judith Hauptman's reading of this story in her recent book. In her reading she focuses on Rabbi Aqiva's leniency and makes a case for his intentionally ruling with leniency. She writes: "This set of *mishnahs* is amazingly self-critical. The rabbis are fully aware of their knowing and intentional avoidance of declaring a woman to be ritually impure. R. Akiva goes so far to place words in a woman's mouth about the origin of a spot in order to dodge the most likely explanation that the blood came from the uterus. . . . For R. Akiva, this meant that any stain that could possibly be explained as anything other than uterine blood should be explained in that way" (*Rereading the Rabbis*, 154). Her reading is convincing, especially since she provides a parallel from a discussion in the mishnaic tractate on the ritual impurity of male seminal discharges, Tractate Zavim 2:2. I take a somewhat different approach by focusing on the position of the woman.

28. To make the point, we can exaggerate the rhetorical force of Rabbi Aqiva's position as saying: "My daughter, I appreciate your zealousness with respect to observing menstrual impurity laws. But you should not exaggerate, since you make marital life impossible."

29. Again, if we exaggerate in order to clarify the rhetorical force of the woman's

reluctance in this perspective, what she really is saying is this: "Yes, rabbi. There, indeed, was a wound, but, please, don't allow for such an unlikely excuse. Please, declare me to be in a status of impurity so that I do not have to engage in sexual relations with my husband." I admit that this second possibility of reading is not as strong as the first, but it shows that whatever way we read the story the woman is really at the mercy of somebody else's interpretation of her body.

30. This point will be discussed in the next chapter.

31. This phenomenon is structurally paralleled in the development of Greco-Roman gynecological literature, as will be discussed in the following chapter.

32. In the preceding sentence Jerome writes about the multitude of the "traditions of the Pharisees," too many to be accounted for in his epistle, which now are called *deuteroseis*, a term which in Jerome's language refers to the Mishnah. On the term and its polemical use in Christian literature see Chapter 6. The "Pharisaic traditions" are the implied subject of our sentence.

33. According to Rebenich (*Hieronymus*, 276), Jerome composed this epistle in the year 406, at a time when he resided in Bethlehem. This would place this remark at one or two generations later than Yalta and Rabbah bar bar Hana, who would have lived at the beginning of the fourth century according to traditional rabbinic chronology.

34. For a discussion of the possible motivation Jerome might have had with this polemical distortion, see my dissertation "Women's Bodies, Women's Blood: On the Politics of Gender in Early Rabbinic Culture." Michael Williams carefully discusses Epiphanius's charge against some "gnostic" sects that they consumed menstrual blood and semen, supposedly as a eucharistic meal. He argues that "we are dealing with instances in the life history of a rumor, much like other widely circulated and richly embroidered rumors about obscene practices among Christians and others in antiquity" (*Rethinking "Gnosticism,"* 184). Jerome's charge against the Pharisees is, then, part of the life history of this rumor.

35. Gafni discusses the difficulty of identifying Ifra Hormiz as a historical pesonality (*The Jews of Babylonia*, 44–45, 253–54). Neusner notes that "no other sources report Shapur's mother's name as Ifra Hormiz. His father's name of course was Hormizd" (*History* IV, 36). According to a tradition cited in the Nestorian Chronicle, Shapur's mother's father was a Jew, whereas Shapur's mother was converted to Christianity, which subsequently led to the persecution of Christians. That tradition would not accord well with the rabbinic tradition, in which she appears as a sympathizer of the Jews (bB.B. 8a–b; 10b–11a; bZev 116b; bTaanit 24b). Neusner speculates that "either the rabbinical academies had no very good traditions on the subject, or that some other Ifra Hormiz, later on called 'mother of Shapur the King,' was involved. But I do not think the king's mother figured in whatever actual events underlay these stories" (*History* IV, 38–39). This only seems to corroborate the impossibility of reading the story historically.

36. It is curious that this presumably non-Jewish woman, who obviously does

not have to observe the commandments of Niddah, should be portrayed as sending in her blood sample to a rabbinic expert. Already Rashi recognized the curiosity of the narrative and comments that נכרית היתה ואעפ"כ היתה משמרת עצמה מנדות וקרובה להתגייר—"even though she was a gentile she observed the commandments of Niddah and was close to conversion" (Rashi ad loc., bNid 20b). However, the gist of the story, especially in light of its end, seems to be that she did not send the blood because she wanted to know what it was for purposes of practice, but rather in order to test Rava or the wisdom of the Jews. Neusner only writes that "the consultation about the meaning of a vaginal excretion does not appear unlikely, since the rabbis achieved a widespread reputation for their expertness in interpreting just such phenomena. But why a non-Jew should inquire I cannot say" (*History* IV, 37). Widespread reputation among whom? He does not provide support for that statement, though Jerome's statement would perhaps serve as evidence for such an assumption. Nonetheless, Neusner assumes that this story indicates that "someone at the court of Shapur II believed the Jews were good magicians and physicians. That does not prove that the Jews had a friend at court, only that the rabbis' reputation as people possessing supernatural power was taken seriously" (38). But ultimately his distinction between those stories about Ifra Hormiz that are "of little historical use" (38) and those with historical value (however limited) that "are preserved in a more narrowly historical framework" (37) is entirely arbitrary.

37. The number sixty is a narrative topos. Compare, for instance, the story in bB.M. 84a, in which sixty different kinds of women's blood are shown to Rabbi Ele'azar, all of which he declares to be pure, and though he meets disbelief by his colleagues, he is miraculously proven to be right. For a reading of this story see Boyarin (*Carnal Israel*, 204–6).

38. Aside from a short case story that introduces this story.

39. This is a *hapaxlegomenon* in rabbinic literature. The Talmud suggests elsewhere in the same tractate (bNid 66a) that a woman who had a marriage proposal might bleed מחמדא—"because she desires." In the short incident that introduces the Ifra Hormiz narrative, the anonymous woman acknowledges that וחמדתיו בעלי היה בדרך—"my husband was away and I desired him" (bNid 20b). Preuss in his *Biblical and Talmudic Medicine* merely lists, without further commentary, this type of blood under a list of "external stimuli" that can cause bleeding in a woman (124). None of the commentaries on the text seems to wonder about the concept of "blood of desire." However, Tirzah Zechurah Meacham emphasizes in her dissertation: "We have not found a remark of the existence of 'blood of desire' in medical literature. I have mentioned that from a realistic perspective excitement of an approaching wedding marriage and all the changes that it stands for is prone to cause tension and can therefore upset the cycle" ("Mishah Tractate Niddah," 182). This latter explanation is consistent with her general endeavour to support rabbinic physiology by modern medical knowledge in an attempt to prove its medical-scientific accuracy. However,

she also suggests somewhat more convincingly that here "male physiology serves as a model for female physiology" (182), according to which male ejaculation as a result of excitation would serve as the model for the "blood of desire." Finally, it should be mentioned that in Greek medical literature—for instance, in Hippocrates (cited in Preuss *Biblical and Talmudic Medicine*, 124)—it was assumed that women before their weddings bleed more heavily, which still would not render this bleeding as something distinct from menstrual blood.

40. The ability of certain rabbis to smell, however, has a literary aftermath in Jewish mysticism, that is in the famous story of Rabbi Nehunyah's deposition from heaven in the *Hekhalot* literature (Lieberman, "Knowledge of Halakhah," 243; Swartz, "Like the Ministering Angels," 162–64).

41. According to some medieval commentators, such as the Tosefei' Rosh and the Meiri (*Beit ha-Bechirah*, 71) it is impure. Both of them reason from Rava's ruling at the end of the tractate (bNid 66a) that a woman who received an offer of marriage and accepted, should wait seven clean days previous to the wedding night חשש חימוד משום—"because of the suspicion of [a bleeding because of her] desire." The Meiri, however, mentions some authorities according to whom the דם חימוד is impure not in itself, but only because of the suspicion that it might be mixed up with menstrual blood. These authorities hold accordingly that if it is known that there is only חימוד דם it is pure.

42. According to yGit 9, 50 ערוה has an odor. From the poetic vision of the messianic future in Hos. 14:7–8 the midrash expands that Israel will give forth the sweet smell of purity (LevR 30). And finally the Messiah has the capacity to distinguish between righteous and wicked (bSanh 93b), which is how according to a later midrash (Yalkut Is. 284), Bar Kokhba was detected as a false messiah, when he was found to be unable to judge by smell.

43. This story deserves a much more extensive treatment than the current context can allow. In a future study I am hoping to analyze the aspect of double-mirroring in rabbinic narratives, of how such narratives in rabbinic literature project the rabbis' reflection of themselves in the eyes of outsiders back into their own texts.

44. I would like to emphasize once again that I will not be making a historical claim about an actual woman consulting with actual rabbis. My interest here is not to read these case stories as representing the historical reality of Babylonian Jewish culture, as if here the texts in the Talmud could be read as some quasi-ethnographic reports. In his *History of the Jews in Babylonia*, Neusner reads Yalta's and the other case stories similar to hers as an indication that in fourth-century Babylon the menstrual prescriptions of the rabbis were widely followed among the Jewish populace (*History* III, 352). However, as with most other issues we have no historical means external to rabbinic literature to ascertain whether the Yalta in the narrative mirrors an actual historical woman called Yalta, though we also do not have any reason to reject outright the possibility of a historical Yalta. More importantly, and in

line with my project, even if we accepted a historical reading of the narrative as accurate, we still would have to think about why among all the possible options the Babylonian Talmud tells this story. That is, we still would have to think what the story is reflective of and what the function of the narrative is once it becomes integrated into the larger framework of the Talmud.

45. Kohut suggests that the name is derived from יעלתא, the Aramaic form of יעלה, a mountain goat. He mentions that another possible etymology is to derive it from אילתא, the Aramaic form of אילה, a doe (*Arukh ha-Shalem* 4:134).

46. According to Geonic chronology he died around 320 C.E. In her recent discussion of the Yalta corpus in the Talmud, Tal Ilan points out that the exact relationship between Rav Nachman and Yalta is never spelled out. That is, she is actually never explicitly designated as Rav Nachman's wife. Ilan suggests that she was perhaps his sister or just a friend (*Mine and Yours Are Hers*, 129). This is an interesting suggestion, but the fact remains that the earliest talmudic commentators already understand Yalta to be Rav Nachman's wife.

47. Here we find a pattern opposite to the one in Rabbi Aqiva's case story in the Mishnah above. Whereas in the mishnaic case the woman is represented as resisting being declared to be pure by Rabbi Aqiva, here Yalta is represented as resisting being declared impure.

48. But the *Tosafist* (bNid 20b, ad.loc., ד"ה אגמריה) mentions that "one could raise an objection in the case of Yalta: how could *she* have acted this way? Don't we say in the first chapter of Tractate Avodah Zarah (bA.Z. 7a) that if one consults a scholar for a decision on an issue in a ritual case and he declares it impure, one should not consult another scholar to have it declared pure"? However, the Tosafot maintain that to this objection "one has to answer that the onus does not lay upon the person who inquires, but on the scholar, whereas the inquirer can ask as much as he [sic] wants to. For because of this they [the scholars] will be thorough in the matter to be examined, since sometimes the first [opinion] errs, and thus the mistake will come to light."

49. bHullin 44b, bBer 63b. The basis for this baraita can be found in tEduyot 1:5, which is cited also in bA.Z. 7a (see preceding note), as well as in yShab 19:1, 16d. Rachel Adler has claimed that the point of the baraita is to secure a solidarity among the judges which would protect them from critique: "Yalta exposes the hidden relativity of the law and the hidden fallibility of its interpreters. The purportedly divine Torah must be translated into human authority. The baraita seeks to protect this authority and its appearance of objectivity through a policy of judicial solidarity" ("Feminist Folktale," 54). But she errs in that the principle of halakhic decision-making is not questioned here. The gemara's problem is how this principle "works" in the Yalta narrative.

50. For a theoretical discussion of the trickster figure, see James C. Scott's *Domination and the Arts of Resistance* (1990, 162–66). He writes: "Typically the trickster makes his successful way through a treacherous environment of enemies out to

defeat him—or eat him—not by his strength but by his wit and cunning. The trickster is unable, in principle, to win any direct confrontation as he is smaller and weaker than his antagonists. Only by knowing the habits of his enemies . . . does he manage to escape their clutches and win victories" (162). As we will see, Yalta is presented as knowing and making use of the habits of her narrative antagonists by engaging Rav Yitzhaq in a halakhic argument.

51. In her short essay on the "Feminist Folktale of Justice: Robert Cover as a Resource for the Renewal of Halakha," Rachel Adler has called Yalta a "legal guerilla" (52).

52. Compare Sifra Tazria 4:4, 95b, which cites this mishnah.

53. It is, then, not necessarily helpful to characterize the narrative character of Yalta as the "woman the rabbis love to hate, the Leona Helmsley of rabbinic legend" with Rachel Adler ("Feminist Folktale," 49), because such a strategy of reading reinforces the marginality of Yalta rather than subverting it. It does not sufficiently establish what it is that troubles those who integrate the story into the Talmud, and how they attempt to resolve that trouble, however unsuccessfully. Further, I do not see any evidence that the rabbis hated the character of Yalta (see also bShab 54b and bGit 67b).

54. The printed edition makes grammatically no sense, since it asks the question in the masculine plural. However, most manuscripts have either the singular feminine participle, or an abbreviation that leaves out the suffix.

55. Rashi's commentary is based on a reading of the gemara text which has "(that case is different) because the blood is not in front of us," whereas our text edition reads "not in front of him." Some manuscripts, such as Vat. Ebr. 111 and 127 read "in front of us," whereas Vat. Ebr. 113 and Munich Ms read "in front of him." It seems to me that a "we" against the woman would have a much greater exclusive force than a singular "him" over and against the woman.

56. The second chapter in Mishnah Tractate Ketubbot, for instance, discusses the credibility of witnesses and testimonies of both genders in different circumstances inscribed by desire.

57. There is no gemara on this mishnaic tractate that would discuss the reasons for this Mishnah.

58. Interestingly the Tosafot also read mNeg 2:5 as an intertext but from a rather different angle. The Tosafot draw the parallel between the subject of *Mishnah Nega'im* and the woman's husband, not, as I have suggested, between the subject of *Mishnah Nega'im* and the woman herself. With the guiding question why Yalta actually did not show her blood to her husband Rav Nahman, who has previously in the Talmud appeared as having some expertise in the new science, the commentary remarks: "But one cannot say that it is forbidden to inspect the blood of one's wife, because we learn in Tractate Nega'im 2:5: 'A person may inspect any leprous lesions, except his own. Rabbi Meir says: Not even the leprous lesions of his relatives. A

person may absolve any oath except his own. Rabbi Yehoshua says: Not even his wife's.' Whereas it does not teach: A person may inspect any kinds of blood, except his wife's." The Tosafot read mNeg 2:5 exclusively: since the text does not explicitly teach that men should not expect their wives' blood, it follows that they must be allowed to do so. However, it appears to me that the gist of the sugyah's question about women's credibility in our case-scenarios of judging women's genital blood would suggest a parallel between the subject of *Mishnah Nega'im* and the woman herself: just as a person should not judge his own leprous lesions, we might think that a woman should not judge her own menstrual bleeding when in doubt, nor should a husband evaluate that of his wife, because his own desire is at stake.

59. From a structural point of view this last statement of the sugyah is analogous to Rav Ashi's statement at the end of the sugyah on Shmu'el's midrash discussed in the previous chapter. In both cases, the sugyah follows one type of argumentation for a while, before it arrives at a certain impasse and then suggests a totally different type of argumentation.

60. Indeed, currently there is a push in more traditional circles to promote the technical training of women as experts in halakhic issues related to menstrual bleeding. Such programs may contribute to the transformation of the "face" of talmudic literature.

**CHAPTER 5**

1. With the exception mentioned above, that is, the push even in some orthodox circles to train women as experts in halakhic matters concerning menstruation.

2. A possible exception might be mNeg 2:4, which prescribes the positions men and women are supposed to take in order to be examined for skin lesions. This imagined examiner here, however, is the priestly examiner of the biblical precedent in Lev. 13. For a recent discussion of this text in a different context see M. Peskowitz (*Spinning Fantasies*, 84–92). I am excluding incidents of rabbinic fantasies about women's bodies from this, since those don't involve concrete situations of examinations of women's bodies.

3. Thus G. R. E. Lloyd points out for the period of the fifth and fourth centuries B.C.E. that "when we turn to the history of science there is no Hippocratic author, and no prominent biologist, who is a woman, just as there is no astronomer, mathematician or physicist" (*Science, Folklore, and Ideology*, 60). See also Aline Rousselle, *Porneia*. And even though Pliny (23–79 C.E.) and Galen (131–201 C.E.) cited certain female authorities even by name, mostly called μαῖαι (midwives), obstetrics, and in some cases also *medici* or ἰατρίναι, that is, female physicians, "there is no indication that any was responsible for any known extant writing" (*Science, Folklore, and Ideology*, 61, note 11).

4. Lloyd cites various examples. In some cases doctors might choose a remedy, as

the Hippocratic writers criticize, "to make the vulgar herd gape, for to such it seems marvellous to see a man suspended or shaken or treated in such ways; and they always applaud these performances, never troubling themselves about the result of the operation, whether bad or good." Lloyd comments himself that "certainly the prescription of some of the more elaborate, exotic and expensive drugs . . . seems designed partly to add to the doctor's prestige, not to mention to the cost of the treatment" (*Science, Folklore, and Ideology*, 82).

5. Lloyd observes that "the development of the scientific text book can . . . be followed broadly both in mathematics (where Euclid came to occupy the dominant position) and in medicine (where Galen, for instance, composed a series of special works designed as introductions 'for beginners')" (*Science, Folklore, and Ideology*, 116).

6. Lloyd, however, is much more cautious: "A male orientation of interest may be detected in the heavy concentration, in these works [the Hippocratics], on the woman's reproductive role—on questions relating to how to overcome sterility, on determining whether a woman could conceive or had done so, and whether the child was going to be male or female—not that these questions were not also concerns (and not just for reasons that reflect their position in society) of Greek women as well as of Greek men" (*Science, Folklore, and Ideology*). He admits, however, that a more obvious "male bias" is reflected in the explanations of sterility, since "there is, on the whole, little recognition, in the gynaecological works, that failure to conceive may be due to the male as much as to the female."

7. This *Tendenz* of the gynecological literature of later antiquity is further corroborated by the fact that by the first and second centuries C.E. Aristotelian metaphysics and concomitant gender politics had become rather authoritative and pervasive (Rousselle, *Porneia*, 24–46).

8. Ann Ellis Hanson also presumes the preservation of women's oral tradition within the Hippocratic corpus: "Elements of the oral tradition among women are no doubt preserved in the recipes of the gynecologies, for the medical writers refer to therapies for the care of women as γυναικεῖα (gynaikeia)" ("The Medical Writers' Women," 310), meaning therapies for women's diseases. She explains that the technical meaning of γυναικεια as a name for a genre of literature is much younger. However, Paola Manuli has made the exact opposite claim: that the same gynecological material is derived from "male practice and theory" (Manuli, "Fisiologia e patologia," 393–408; and compare Hanson, "Continuity and Change," 78, 101).

9. Compare also Lloyd who argues somewhat differently: that our answer to the question of how far the women healers referred to in the Hippocratic texts offered an alternative, rival service is bound to be impressionistic (Lloyd 1983, 70).

10. Dean-Jones likewise suggests that even though what she calls a medical wisewoman might be more sympathetic to women's health care than a male doctor, especially in matters concerning midwifery, it should be assumed that in matters of

pathology "a wise-woman was simply a receptacle of received wisdom which could be assimilated by a male as easily as by a female. The existence and continuity of a traditional medicine for women side by side with the scientific medicine, therefore, need not imply that the Hippocratic gynaecology was less effective or compassionate or less informed by female experience" (Dean-Jones, *Women's Bodies*, 35). This is true but it still represents a shift in authority at least potentially. The modern shift from midwives to obstetricians might illustrate this.

11. Medieval gynecological literature is, of course, embedded in a different historical, social, and cultural context. Nonetheless, the questions pertaining to the gender politics of women's health care are similar. Thus, Monica Green advances this argument in a discussion of gynecological treatises of the eleventh and twelfth century in Italy ascribed to a woman by the name of Trotula. Previously, it had been argued that these treatises were written both by and for men, and were falsely attributed to a woman only to aid toward the takeover of women's medicine by male physicians and the gradual exclusion of women themselves from medical practice. This argument is quite similar to Rousselle's analysis of the cultural function of the Hippocratic corpus. Green, however, believes "that the victimization of women both as practitioners and as patients was not so absolute" ("Women's Medical Practice," 460). Rather, she wants to keep open the possibility of women's authorship and intended readership.

12. This is, however, a monistic characterization of the Talmud and an example for what Hasan-Rokem has seen at work in most scholarship on rabbinic literature, "a projection of Western scholastic and academic models of discourse" ("Narratives in Dialogue," 128).

13. They are more limited in scope, monolithic in purpose, and more specifically aimed at creating an art—a τέχνη (Lloyd, *Science, Folklore, and Ideology*, 87)—of both literary medicine and medical literature.

14. Daniel Boyarin has aptly expressed this point: "The Talmuds are complexly authored works, and any given passage does not necessarily reflect social practice or even theory of any more than the redactors of that particular passage" (*Carnal Israel*, 179).

15. Based on her research on the tractate dealing with divorce law Hauptman does indicate that the Tosefta has "a more liberal stance" and argues that "it may be true that the document that assumed ascendancy and became the canon for later generations [the Mishnah] was more pietistic and less feminist than others that existed at roughly the same time [the Tosefta]" ("Feminist Perspectives," 55). The rhetorical choice of feminism in connection with a rabbinic text is perhaps somewhat too strong. If the semantic range of feminism is stretched to such a degree that it includes rabbinic texts of whatever propensity, the term may come to mean everything and nothing, and thus become rhetorically ineffective.

16. Most prominently, H. Albeck and J. N. Epstein have taken the two opposite positions. Albeck's claim is that the Babylonian Talmud did not know our Tosefta, a

Palestinian text (*Mehqarim ba-baraita*, 93), and that where both provide different versions of a textual tradition, the Babylonian Talmud draws on a different textual source (130). In fact, he argues that the Tosefta is a late amoraic collection (73–75). By contrast, Epstein maintains that there was an "ancient" Tosefta from which two literary branches developed. One branch is that of our Tosefta and the almost identical baraitot in the Palestinian Talmud; the other is that characterized by the Babylonian baraitot (*Introduction to Tannaitic Literature*, 246). For a more extensive discussion see A. Goldberg, "The Babylonian Talmud." Judith Hauptman analyzed a number of sugyot of the Babylonian Talmud with respect to the baraitot they use. She concludes that these baraitot, especially when they also appear in tannaitic collections such as the Tosefta and halakhic Midrashim, represent the earliest stratum of a given talmudic sugyah. Thus, she argues that "although we might not know whether or not the Tosefta of the Babylonian amoraim was identical to ours, it is rather clear that they possessed a Tosefta, or at least a collection of *baraitot*, which they studied along with the mishnah as a commentary on it" (*Development of the Talmudic Sugya*, 54, note 42). Though her analysis is restricted to baraitot which the Talmud introduces with a particular formula (תניא נמי הכי—thus it is also taught) Hauptman claims that her conclusions have implications for other baraitot as well (216).

17. Preuss in general tends to exclude the possibility that anybody other than the examined woman herself performed examinations for forensic purposes: "In the explanation of [these] Talmudic statements, one must always keep in mind that the 'examination of women,' of which the Talmud speaks, is, with rare exception, always performed by the woman herself" (*Biblical and Talmudic Medicine*, 115). The question, of course, is which of the few incidents of physical examinations dealt with in rabbinic literature should be regarded as the exception, and which as the rule. However, Preuss is subject to his own ideas about gender and about the respectability of rabbinic literature. He does not carefully read the texts as to difference between different textual version and what such differences imply for his historical "reconstruction" of talmudic medicine.

18. Zuckermandel, as well as the citation of the baraita in the Babylonian Talmud (bNid 10b) in all manuscript versions, has בחזקת טמאה, or טומאה (compare Rashi ad loc.; Meiri, *Beit ha-Behirah*, 38). But in his preliminary commentary on Tosefta Niddah, Lieberman corrects the text based on the Vienna manuscript of the Tosefta, which has הרי הן בחזקת טהרה—"they are, indeed, in the status of purity." The rhetorical structure of the baraita would indeed let us expect a contrast: that is, before girls reach puberty they are in the status of purity, but then they are in the status of impurity. Therefore, they should be examined from then on. According to Lieberman, however, "as long as she has not had as a blood-flow, a woman is considered to be in the presumptive status of purity *even though she has reached her puberty*" (1939, 269, my emphasis). He emphasizes that the difference between her

pre- and post-puberty phase lies merely and exclusively in the way of examination (1939, 269): Pre-puberty, women do not examine the girls, post-puberty they do. Lieberman's reading seems to be corroborated by Maimonides who omits any remark on a girl's change of status of im/purity and rules: חזקת בנות ישראל שלא הגיעו לפירקן בחזקת טהרה ואין הנשים בודקות אותן אבל משהגיעו לפירקן צריכות בדיקה ונשים בודקות אותן "The assumption is that Israelite women who have not reached their period are assumed to be in the status of purity and (other) women do not examine them. But from the time when they have reached their puberty, they require an examination, and (other) women do examine them" (Mishnah Torah, Hilkhot Metam'ei Mishkav u-Moshav, 4:8).

19. The more accurate translation for פרק is "period of time." According to tannaitic halakhah, the halakhic thinking represented by the rabbis of the Mishnah and the Tosefta, this period lasts from the age of eleven years and one day until twelve years and one day for girls, for the boy from twelve years and one day until thirteen years and one day. This is a kind of in-between stage, between the status of legal minority and adulthood to which certain rights and obligations apply (see for instance mNid 5:6). At the same time, the context of the baraita's citation in the Babylonian Talmud seems to suggest that here the פרק is understood to be simply potential menarche or physical maturity. The expression used in the other case-stories which the Talmud quotes in context with this baraita is תינוקת שלא הגיע זמנה לראות—a young girl whose time to have a flow of blood has not yet arrived (bNid 9 and 10b; see also tNid 1:8–9). In the following texts, I will retain the rabbinic expression "season."

20. See, however, the different manuscript traditions discussed in note 18.

21. On a philological note, the verb קלקל literally means "to spoil" or "to damage." The implication could be either that women examiners might in a general sense hurt or wound the girl and thus cause premature bleeding, or that they might damage her hymen accidentally, and thus destroy her virginity. However, it is not totally out of the realm of possibility that the moral connotation of the term plays some role here. That is, the verb often appears in the context of sexual corruption (bSanh 108b, bRH 12a a.o.). Hence the women might teach the girl about sexual pleasure.

22. The context is the determination of the status of menstrual im/purity of "other" women, dependent on the im/purity practice of the "other" communities, such as the Samaritan, the Sadducean, and the non-Jewish communities. Hence, Samaritan women are considered to be in a status of *perpetual menstruous impurity* [בנות כותים מעריסתן נדות] (tNid 5:1; compare mNid 4:1; bNid 31b ff). Women from the Sadducean community are considered to be like Samaritan women and therefore "different," as long as they follow the ways of their fathers. But as soon as they abdicate those traditions and follow "the ways of Israel," that is, the true tradition as defined rabbinically, they are considered to be one of "us," of the rabbinic commu-

nity or the *verus Israel* [בנות הצדוקים בזמן שנוהגות ללכת בדרכי אבותם הרי אלו
ככותיות פרשו לדרכי ישראל הרי אלו כישראל] (tNid 5:2; compare mNid 4:2; bNid 33b
f). The menstrual blood of non-Jewish women, however, just like the nonmenstrual
blood of a leprous woman, is considered to be like the blood from a wound, at least
according to the Shammaite school, and does, therefore, not fall under the concern
of purity regulations [דם נכרית ודם הטהרה של מצורעת בית שמאי אומרים הרי הן כדם
מגפתה] (tNid 5:5; compare mNid 5:3; bNid 34a). Incidentally, this collection of baraitot shows how im/purity practices and traditions are used to determine women's
"ethnic" difference in rabbinic literature. This passage, which I cannot fully discuss
here, deserves a separate study of rabbinic constructions of "other" women.

23. Against Lieberman's suggested emendation of the Tosefta as discussed in note
18. I follow here the version of the baraita in the Babylonian Talmud, attested by all
manuscripts, as well as by Rashi's commentary and other commentaries on the
Talmud. According to this version, the girl changes from a presumptive status of
ritual *purity* to a presumptive status of ritual *impurity*. However, this version harbors
some difficulties. For one, it remains unclear why she should be in a status of
*presumptive impurity*. This problem has moved numerous medieval talmudic commentators and is one of Lieberman's arguments to emend the text in the Tosefta (see
note 16). Since a discussion of this problem will digress too far from my question at
hand and, in any case, is the theoretical one of potential retroactive impurity, I want
to note only the very basics. The question that the early rabbinic texts raise is the
establishment of a regular cycle. A regular cycle (וסת) is established after three times
of bleeding at the same time. Once a woman has a regular cycle, she does not have to
consider a possibility of retroactive impurity with respect to Temple-related items.
However, before regularity is established the question arises again, how long blood
possibly was present in her body without her being aware of it, raising the specter of
retroactive impurity. With her menarche, a girl is subject to the possibility of retroactive impurity for the first two cycles, but no longer from the third one onwards.

24. Such a model can be recognized by now as the Aristotelian model of the
physiology of menstrual blood. As discussed in Chapter Three above, the Talmud
employs such a model to explain the position of Hillel at the opening of the tractate.

25. The translation of this last part is awkward. But it should be noted that here
the Hebrew text remains ambiguous with regard to the agency behind this expression.

26. Compare Rashi bNid 10b, ד״ה מבפנים. The text does not explain, however,
how the women would apply the oil internally without using their hands. See,
however, the next text.

27. See Kohut, *Arukh ha-Shalem*, on עות.

28. See also Bernadette Brooten's discussion of the rabbinic category of "women
who rub each other [מסללות or מסלדות]" (*Love Between Women*, 66–71), appearing
in both the Palestinian and the Babylonian Talmuds (yGit 8:10, 49c; bYev 76a). The
question the Talmuds ask with respect to women engaging in homoerotic sexual

contact is whether this disqualifies such women from priestly marriages. That is, the question is whether the rabbis imagine women's homoerotic sex as involving penetration (68–69). Brooten discusses the different opinions attributed to various rabbis and also notes their convergences with the opinions of Greek and Latin writers. On the whole, she argues, the emergent Jewish discussion of sexual relations between women can be read as part of the larger discussion within the Roman world (70). In this context we find a possible textual echo of the anxiety about older women corrupting younger girls. Brooten briefly discusses a passage in the Babylonian Talmud (bShab 65 a–b) according to which the father of Shmu'el, a Babylonian rabbi of the early third century, prohibits his daughters from sleeping together. Inquiring into the reason for this prohibition the Talmud rejects the suggestion that the father might have been worried about the possibility of their erotic intimacy: "Shall we say that this [prohibition] supports Rav Huna [a third century Babylonian rabbi] who held the opinion: 'Women who rub each other are disqualified from the priesthood'? No. [Rather,] he held the opinion that they should not become accustomed to a foreign body—כי היכי דלא לילפן גופא נוכראה." The Talmud does not provide a reason why they should not become used to another body in their bed. Brooten suggests that "the rabbinic sages probably were thinking of the laws of menstruation, according to which a married woman has to sleep separately from her husband for a good part of the month. If a young woman grew used to sleeping with another person, she might have difficulty abiding by the menstrual laws in the future" (68). Rashi, on the other hand, reads this passage as a preventative measure, typical to rabbinic thinking. He understands the Talmud's reasoning to be that once the girls get accustomed to another body in their bed their sexual desire for a man is awakened (bShab 65b). Both are possible readings, but I want to emphasize a slightly different nuance. The term נוכראה or *foreign* body suggests that the emphasis is that they should not get used to any body other than the one they are meant to be intimate with, that of a husband. Thus the practice of Shmu'el's father supports the rabbinic ethos that women's desires should be one-directional and exclusive. Women's intimacies of whatever kind could present a possible threat to that ethos.

29. Thus according to most commentators, beginning with Rashi. Compare also *Hidushei ha-Rashba* (Metzger, ed., 327). See above, note 19. The girl's twelfth year and the boy's thirteenth year constitute an in-between stage, and from the girl's age of twelve years and a day, and the boy's age of thirteen years and a day they have come of age legally. The Mishnah remains silent as to the reason of the girl's supposed earlier maturation than the boy's. Wegner suggests that this reflects reality (*Chattel or Person?* 36). For the midrashic explanation, see GenR 18:1 (Albeck and Theodor, *Midrash Bereshit Rabba*, 160), also cited in bNid 45b. The Mishnah (mNid 5:6; compare tNid 5:15–17) makes these distinctions with respect to the validity of oaths. As minors the children's oaths are invalid. When they reach adulthood, the oaths are valid even if they later claim ignorance as to the possible consequences. But in the

intermediate phase the validity of their oaths needs to be examined. That is, it needs to be ascertained that the children know in whose name they took the oath. The Mishnah (mNid 5:7) continues with differentiation of age limits with respect to the father's control over his daughter's property. Here it distinguishes between the קְטַנָּה, the minor girl, the נערה, the girl in her youth, and the בוגרת, the fully matured woman. These stages apply only to girls. Further, in the famous baraita on the three kinds of women who may use birth control, the minor (קטנה), the pregnant, and the nursing woman, the age of the girl's minority, during which she is capable of conception but is assumed to die from pregnancy, is defined as "from the age of eleven years and one day to the age of twelve years and one day" (bYev 12b, 100b; bNid 45a, bNid 45a, bKet 39a). See Feldman, *Marital Relations*, 169ff; and R. Biale, *Women and Jewish Law*, 203ff. For a fuller discussion of this complex distinction of age limits, see my "Women's Bodies, Women's Blood" (1995).

30. Hence, we perhaps can make sense of the fact that the signs of puberty are discussed almost exclusively in the context of *levirate marriage*. According to biblical law and subsequently rabbinic law a woman is obligated to marry the brother of her deceased husband, if her marriage remained childless (Deut. 25:5ff). The rabbis understand the sole purpose of the secondary marriage to be the production of offspring for the dead brother. Hence, if either of the potential candidates for such a marriage is deemed to be incapable of reproduction, the obligation cannot be fulfilled and hence is invalidated altogether. The rabbinic discussions of levirate marriage have not yet been analyzed adequately as to rabbinic constructions of gender. In every instance in which the Mishnah discusses the appearance of the two pubic hairs it cites as the prime consequence for the girl that she can or cannot contract, and can or cannot be released from the obligation of levirate marriage, depending on her physical signs of maturity, with one exception (mNid 6:11, compare tNid 6:5–6). What this means, ultimately, is that the whole question of signs of physical maturity is raised as external evidence for the capability of reproduction. Such capability, obviously, does not depend on chronological age.

31. According to the Mishnah, the growth of pubic hair may not concur with the expected chronological age of puberty and legal adulthood. Thus, a girl who is still a minor, but has grown pubic hair, is legally considered to be an adult (mNid 6:1). Further, it rules that if a man or a woman has not grown pubic hairs by the age of twenty, or according to one opinion, by the age of eighteen (mNid 5:9, tNid 6:2), they are deemed to be incapable of reproduction. As usual in its endeavor to categorize life, the Mishnah devises a terminology to name such uncommon cases. As to the man considered incapable of reproduction, he is called a סריס, a term commonly commonly translated as eunuch or castrate and derived from the verb סרס "to mutilate." A woman is called an אילונית, a word most likely derived from איל, or ram, hence the ramlike woman. Finally, the Tosefta adds that if a boy has not produced pubic hair by the age of fourteen or fifteen, he is legally considered to be a minor

(tNid 6:2). Thus the Tosefta suggests that if pubic hair appears before its expected time, it might be considered to be mere mole. This indicates that the corporeal signs of puberty are just that, that is, "signs" (סימנים), and as such always require interpretation. The hermeneutics of the body's language get even more complex when the Mishnah rules with respect to the girl and the "upper" and "lower sign." To the rabbis the expected and normal sequence, indicating legal adulthood, is the appearance of the lower sign before the upper one (mNid 6:1; compare tNid 6:4). The relationship between the two engenders long and extremely interesting discussions which I discuss in more detail in my dissertation, "Women's Bodies, Women's Blood."

32. Textually, this Rabbi Yehuda need not be the same as in the previous baraita, or consistent with him. Even if the redactors of both *baraitot* refer to the same "historical figure," they might both present different readings of him, or different traditions. There would, indeed, appear to be a contradiction between the two sources if we insisted on the coherence between both texts: the "previous" Rabbi Yehuda holds, at the very least, that before menarche other women do not examine the girls. By contrast, the current Rabbi Yehuda holds that both before and after their menarche other women do examine the girls. On the other hand, the context of the examinations needs to be considered here as well. The previous baraita and the current baraita both refer to different examinations, to which different rules apply. That is, whereas in the previous baraita Rabbi Yehuda refers exclusively to examinations with respect to menstrual impurity, here he refers to examinations with respect to establishing the girl's legal minority or majority.

33. The ceremony of taking off the shoe of a brother of her deceased husband (Deut. 25:5–9), to circumvent the obligation of levirate marriage (see mYev 12:6; Wegner, *Chattel or Person?* 109). A minor does not have the right to perform this ritual. The stricter ruling in this context would, therefore, be to classify the examinee as a minor and thus to prevent her from bypassing levirate marriage, whereas, if she were judged an adult, she could perform the ceremony and bypass the obligation.

34. See mYeb 13:1ff. According to mishnaic halakha, the woman who has been married off not by her father, but by her brothers or mother as a legal minor, has the right to protest and dissolve the marriage without having to get a divorce bill from the unwanted husband, but only before the age of twelve years. See also Wegner, *Chattel or Person?* 33.

35. It seems that the examination of boys with respect to their corporeal signs of puberty was undertaken by men, presumably by the rabbi himself, to whom a case in question was brought (see tNid 5:14).

36. See Tal Ilan's brief reference to this statement (*Jewish Women in Greco-Roman Palestine*, 194). In her survey on the question of women and Torah study she writes: "Even Rabbi Eliezer [who famously denounces the idea of fathers teaching their daughters Torah in mSot 3:4, Ch.F.] thought that some matters of halakhah were more suited to women than men, for he taught his wife about the signs of sexual

maturity in an adolescent girl so that she could perform examinations and help him in his own work (tNid 6:8; bNid 48b). R. Ishma'el is said to have done the same thing with his mother. Thus there were some areas of the law in which women not only were permitted to be involved but even gained more expertise than men" (1996, 194). Taking the statement out of the context of the baraita as a whole, Ilan reads this passage as a positive indication of the historical reality of women's learning generally.

37. On Rabbi Yishma'el's mother see pPeah 1:1, 15c. Lieberman (*Tosafet Rishonim*, 279) mentions that in *Halakhot Gedolot* the text version reads ור׳ יהושע מוסר לאמו—"and Rabbi Yehoshua transferred [physical examinations] to his mother." Rabbi Yehoshua's mother is equally known as a particularly virtuous woman, see pYevamot 1:6, 3a.

38. See also the Meiri's commentary (*Beit ha-Behirah*, 176). He uses the expression על ידי כשורות ובקיאות—"on account of proper and expert women." According to the Meiri the general statement articulates the halakhic principle. That is, against what we might expect women can indeed in this particular case serve as witnesses, so that even one examining woman could be considered a reliable witness, and even if she is a relative of the examinee. The "properness and expertise" then are merely qualifiers of the halakhic acceptability of women as witnesses in this case. The formula of the נשים נאמנות, however, has an earlier linguistic history. Jeffrey Tigay has kindly referred me to his article on the "Examination of the Accused Bride in 4Q159: Forensic Medicine at Qumran." The purpose of his article is the reconstruction of a Qumran text fragment from 4Q159 which reads [כי יוצי איש שם רע על בתולת ישראל אם ב]יום קחתו אותה יואמר ובקרוה [ ] נאמנות ואם לא כחש עליה והומתה ואם בשקר ענה בה וענש שני מנים [ולוא] ישלח כול יומיו...—"If a man defames an Israelite virgin, if he speaks out on [the day] he marries her, trustworthy [ . . . ] shall examine her, and if he has not lied about her, she shall be executed. But if he testified against her false[ly], he shall be fined two minas [ . . . ] and he may [not] divorce (her) for his entire life." Tigay shows convincingly that the original reading of the text was ובקרוה נשים נאמנות—"trustworthy women shall examine her" (131). Further, the Damascus Document from Qumran Cave 4 demands that under certain circumstances a man should not marry a girl except after examination by נשים נאמנות וידעות ברורות ממאמר המבקר—"trustworthy, knowledgeable women chosen on the instructions of the מבקר (examiner)" (134). This latter citation makes the issue of control over women examiners even more explicit.

39. The omissions spell out the halakhic consequences of the case with respect to levirate marriage. If pubic hair has grown, the girl is considered to be an adult. She cannot protest against a marriage arranged by her mother or brothers while she was still a minor, a privilege of legal minors only.

40. The Meiri makes a distinction between purposes of examinations. Consequently, he exempts from the requirement of corporeal examinations the issue of

*mi'un*, or protest of the minor daughter against the bridegroom chosen for her by her mother or her brothers in absence of a *pater familias*. In such a case, the Meiri claims, we strictly follow absolute age and the empirical evidence of pubic hair becomes irrelevant. But with respect to *chalitzah*, the ceremony of circumventing levirate marriage, the establishment of physical evidence, that is, of the pubic hair, would be admissable (*Beit ha-Behirah*, 176). In the only attempt to deal with the complexity of the rabbinic discussions on the physical signs of puberty that I am aware of, Bamberger contents himself with noting that "these physiological evidences were virtually disregarded by the halakhah [and] the gemara does not fully harmonize these two approaches" ("Qetanah, Na'arah, Bogereth," 292). The later halakhic development, personified for Bamberger by Maimonides, manages to bracket out the reliance on women's testimonies entirely, whereas in the gemara both approaches are debated, but not reconciled into one consistent system. However, Bamberger does not deal with the talmudic texts in great detail.

41. Rashi does not discuss who it would be that would perform the examinations during this period. He merely elaborates on why *women* may not perform the examination then. Hence, Rashi (bNid 48b ad loc.) comments that "women are *not* competent [halakhic witnesses] to be relied on, in order to make girls of doubtful status [with respect to their status as minors or adults] permissible on their testimony, and to rule that the girl has turned into a legal adult, so that she can perform the ceremony of *halitzah*. And since Rabbi Yehuda holds the opinion that during the period of puberty, just like after that period, the two pubic hairs are an indicating sign of her legal status [with respect to her age], we do not believe them [the examining women]." According to Rashi then, in cases where we have to rely on the testimony of physical evidence, women—just as in most other halakhic circumstances—are halakhically not admissible as reliable witnesses.

42. It is noteworthy, though, that when the Bavli (bNid48b) cites the baraita, it again differs decisively from our version in the Tosefta: א״ר אליעזר בר׳ צדוק כך היו מפרשין ביבנה ואמרו כיון שבא התחתון שוב אין משגיחין על עליון—"Rabbi Eliezer [this should be El'azar] son of Zaddoq said: thus they interpreted in Yavneh: once the lower sign appears, they do not consider the upper one." Here the court in Yavneh is only *interpreting*, that if the lower sign, that is, the pubic hairs, comes first, the search for the upper sign is rendered superfluous. The court could still take recourse to women's examination and merely fulfill the function of interpreting the result.

43. I would like to emphasize that I am not making a chronological argument. Whether or not the opening anonymous principle is historically an earlier one is not essential to my argument. Whether we read the text synchronically or diachronically, the text in its present form still follows a rhetorical movement toward restriction. For a diachronic analysis of the different layers in Mishnah and Tosefta see the introduction of A. Goldberg, "The Mishna—A Study Book of Halakha."

44. With Shmu'el's statement the Talmud offers an additional answer to the Mishnah's question. In rabbinic literature he is known for his medical knowledge. See for instance bB.M.85b; also J. Preuss, *Biblical and Talmudic Medicine*, 21.

45. The verse is often split up differently, so that "forever" refers to the previous part of the verse: "you may keep them [the non-Israelite] slaves as a possession for your children after you, for them to inherit as property forever. Such you may treat as slaves" (Levine, *Leviticus*, 180).

46. The midrash of Lev. 25:46, which Shmu'el adduces as a "proof" for the propriety of his behavior, has an abbreviated parallel form in Sifra, Behar 5:7: לעולם בהם תעבודו אין לך בהם אלא עבודה בלבד—" 'these you may put to work forever' [implies] you can only employ them for work."

47. It goes without saying that the rabbinic concept of shame needs to be historicized. To my knowledge, no study of the range of meanings of shame in rabbinic culture has been done yet. For instance, the association of nakedness, and specifically female nakedness, with shame has a quite different meaning in rabbinic culture than in early Christianity, where nakedness inevitably evoked the story of the fall and thus sinfulness (Miles, *Carnal Knowledge*).

48. Compare for instance bTaanit 21b, the story of Abba the cupper, whose merit is that he devised a way in which he could let blood and yet not look at the woman patient: ואית ליה לבושא דאית ביה קרנא דהוות בועא כי כוזילתא כי הוות אתיא ליה איתתא הוה מלביש לה כי היכי דלא ניסתכל בה—"and he had a garment in which there was fastened a cup (for receiving the blood) which (garment) was cut in at the shoulder. And when a woman came he would dress her in this garment in a way that he would not look at her."

49. This can, of course, also be read as part of the larger rabbinic project of taking control or establishing themselves as the legitimate inheritors and interpreters of the biblical traditions.

50. The rare Aramaic term is מרבינתיה. Derivatives of this term appear mostly in the Targumim, where it comprises several meanings, such as educator or teacher (Targ. Prov. II, 17) or nurse and foster-mother (Targ. Yer. Gen 25:8). Rashi explains it as אומנת, a female pedagogue or educator. Nevertheless, Abaye calls her consistently "my mother."

51. Similarly, however, Jacob Neusner in his history of the Jewish community in Babylonia quotes the remedies of Abaye's mother primarily to corroborate his historiographical point that "between the time of Abaye (died 338) and that of Rav Papa (died 376), fears of witchcraft [most commonly repeated in connection with medical remedies] had so increased that academic discussions were affected" (*History of the Jews in Babylonia*, 3:348). Neusner assumes that the "academic discussions" of the rabbis, as a cultural segment above the others, had a certain rationality to them, which was undermined and corroded by the omnipresent superstitious fear pervasive in the external cultural world. Thus, both Preuss and Neusner present Abaye's

mother as the internal "other" of rabbinic discourse rather than as an integrative part of talmudic literature. She is just the personification of the *vox populi* or of some uncontrollable fear of the supernatural and as such forces herself upon the otherwise academic or scientific discourse of the rabbis.

52. This is a common phenomenon of androcentric hermeneutics and historiography. The work of Elisabeth Schüssler Fiorenza, Bernadette Brooten, Ross Shephard Kraemer and many other feminist scholars has attempted to reveal the strategies of such scholarship and to undo its presumptions. Similarly, Galit Hasan-Rokem's work discusses the problematic application of Western paradigms such as the distinction between folk tradition and high culture to rabbinic literature. She writes: "Even the most open and most self-reflexive works of recent scholars . . . conceive of Talmudic-Midrashic texts as academic responses to a dogma-oriented, more or less known corpus of texts. . . . This results in a mapping of influences which focuses on specific texts notwithstanding the fact that very often we may not be able to determine the specific texts or the direction of influence. The truth is, however, that the ancient literary poly-system, in which folk literature and oral tradition fill a central function, is in principle as well as pragmatically irretrievable. It seems to me that what is at work in most scholarship on Rabbinic literature is a projection of Western scholastic and academic models of discourse which focus on the written modes of expression in favor of the oral ones" ("Narratives in Dialogue," 127–28). In her own work on midrashic literature she rejects this juxtaposition and shows how rabbinic narratives are often complex webs of mythological, legendary, and other folkloristic discourses from various cultural spheres (ibid., 118; see also *The Web of Life*).

53. See Gafni (*The Jews of Babylonia*, 164–65) on the difference between the Babylonian and the Palestinian Talmuds regarding issues such as witchcraft, astrology, and medicine. The Babylonian Talmud presents much more fantastic literary material than the Palestinian Talmud. Nineteenth-century *Science of Judaism* scholars praised the Palestinian over and against the Babylonian Talmud for its presumed immunity from the superstition of the masses. However, Saul Lieberman has already debated the difficulty of making such an ideological comparison between the two Talmuds: "It is fundamentally an error to generalize and say that in Palestinian Talmudo-Midrashic literature fewer 'superstitions' are found than in the Babylonian" (110). He points out: "The Palestinian Talmud is much shorter than the Babylonian. There is much of Halakhic material in the latter, recorded in the name of Palestinian sages, of which there is no trace in the Palestinian Talmud. Moreover, many passages in that Talmud have so far remained obscure, and we may hope, that, in the course of time, when these will be elucidated, more facts and ideas bearing on Palestinian 'superstitions' will also be revealed" (*Greek in Jewish Palestine*, 110–11).

54. The Aramaic term איספלנית is a derivative of the Greek σπληνίον, or Latin *splenium* (Krauss, *Griechische und Lateinische Lehnwörter*, 90). An important question to consider is whether this loan word indicates an intertext, that is, that the

rabbis knew the medical literature emerging in the surrounding culture, or whether this was just a common term in the general culture. In his *Greek in Jewish Palestine* Lieberman has shown the pervasiveness of Greek terms in rabbinic literature and has carefully discussed the implications for how much "Greek wisdom" the rabbis in Palestine knew. Medicine, which Lieberman does not discuss in his studies, would be one of the branches of Hellenistic sciences with which some rabbis might have been familiar. A more comprehensive comparison of rabbinic and Greek medicinal literature, than the current context allows for, would be required before a more general answer to this question can be established.

55. The Aramaic term קירא is an import from Latin *cera* (wax) (Krauss, *Griechische und Lateinische Lehnwörter*, 538). Soranus, the Greek medical writer of the Roman imperial period, made a prescription quite similar to that of Abaye's mother: "For itching of the body application of heat is helpful, as well as plenty of ointment made of refined olive oil to which a little wax is added, so that the oil becomes thicker and remains longer on the body" (Temkin, *Soranus' Gynecology*, 122). And "also it is sometimes advisable to anoint the body with Etruscan wax melted together with olive oil before swaddling. For this softens and warms the body and futhermore it somehow nourishes and whitens it" (108).

56. Rashi explains that, since one of the threads might grow into the flesh while the wound is healing, the חלוק, when it is pulled off, might tear off the tip of the penis and cause genital mutilation.

57. The *Arukh ha-shalem*, a talmudic dictionary from the eleventh century, explains the obscure verb form מנשתיה as "to urinate," להשתין. This reading is supported by the Munich manuscript of the Babylonian Talmud, which has ולינשתין מייא. Rashi, however, explains it: "his breath is not visible, because his heartbeat is not normal" and that "one should fan him with a fan." See also Preuss (*Biblical and Talmudic Medicine*, 403), who translates: "a child that does not breathe should be moved to-and-fro."

58. Another obscure verb, which the *Arukh ha-shalem* explains as the breath not coming out of its nose, and Rashi similarly: "its breath does not enter and exit easily." See Preuss (403), who translates: "if the infant does not cry, it should be rubbed with its own placenta."

59. See for instance Soranus's chapter "On the Care of the Newborn" (Temkin, *Soranus' Gynecology*, 79–128).

60. Ann Hanson observes similarly for one of the Hippocratic writers: "In separating himself from female practitioners he considers outside his Hippocratic tradition, this medical writer not only gives voice to Hippocratic professionalism, which saw itself as different from previous medical traditions, but also draws attention to women's unskillful and unlettered habits" ("Continuity and Change," 81).

61. With many other sayings on issues like magical practices and recipes for fever she is one voice along with the rabbis. See, for instance, bA.Z. 28b on remedies for

ailment of the ear, bEruv 29b on remedies for ailment of the heart, bGit 69b/70a a collection of general health care, and bShab 66b on incantations against fever.

62. He lived at the end of the second century and came to Palestine from Babylon.

63. It should be noted that here it is surprisingly the woman who circumcises her baby son.

64. Only the second part of this baraita has its source in the Tosefta and is cited throughout rabbinic literature. See Shir Ha-Shirim Rabbah 7:2, bHul 47b, pYeb 6:6, 7d. In some manuscripts of the Tosefta and in the version of the Palestinian Talmud "the Babylonian" is missing in the naming of the baby; see Lieberman (*Tosefta ki-Fshuta*, 251).

65. With the exception of bHul 47b, which also presents both parts of the baraita, the red baby and the green baby. However, I would argue that the editor of the gemara of Hullin already knows the version of the baraita as it appears in Tractate Shabbat, rather than quoting a tannaitic baraita in front of him but lost to us. The context in which the baraita is quoted in Hullin is the question of the color of lungs of sacrificial animals: if the lungs of the animal are green, rather than red, would it still be a fit sacrifice? It seems to me that the context in Tractate Shabbat really seems to be the more original context of the baraita.

66. See H. Eilberg-Schwartz, who argues that, beginning with Moses Mendelssohn, Jewish reformers and early scholars of the Wissenschaft adopted strategies from Christian thinkers to make Judaism more respectable in terms of the contemporary discourse: "Mendelssohn argued that Judaism was both a religion of reason and a divinely revealed legislation that had never been abrogated. But this defense of Judaism proved problematic almost immediately. It provided the basis for Kant's argument that Judaism did not qualify as a religion since its deity commanded outward observance, a conception of God that contradicted a religion of reason. Mendelssohn's disciples responded to Kant's criticism by endeavoring to show that the God of Judaism was purely an ethical God and that the outward observances were secondary accretions to the core. In this way, the strategies used to protect Christianity were appropriated by Jewish thinkers and remained an important way of explaining the primitive elements of Judaism among proponents of Jewish Reform and advocates of Wissenschaft des Judentums throughout the nineteenth and into the twentieth century" (*The Savage in Judaism*, 60).

## CHAPTER 6

1. More recently, see also Schottroff and Wacker, eds., *Von der Wurzel getragen* (1996), a German collection of essays that deal with this dynamic in Christian feminist literature.

2. For a recent discussion of the politics of marriage in Paul's correspondence see

Boyarin's *A Radical Jew*, especially chapter eight, "There Is No Male and Female" (180–201).

3. Castelli points out that "the theme of the pains of marriage is common in the hellenistic rhetorical tradition and it became a useful trope in the construction of the notion of virginity in the fourth century literature" ("Virginity and Its Meaning for Women's Sexuality," 68). See her article for references to Chrysostom, Jerome, Gregory of Nyssa, and Eusebius of Emesa. Of the "fathers" Jerome, who is quite eloquent on illustrating the horror of marriage and child-rearing and for whom the only good of marriage was to produce virgins for the church, is the most extreme when it comes to the denigration of marriage (Clark, " 'Adam's Only Companion,' " 144). This, and his advice to other men to avoid women's lascivious company, stands in stark contrast to his warm friendships with women (Miller, "The Blazing Body," 23). Jerome develops this view of marriage most systematically in his rejoinder to Jovinian, who against the Pauline tradition had praised marriage as an equal divine gift, in spite of being an ascetic himself (Clark, " 'Adam's Only Companion,' " 144). See, however, also Pat Cox Miller's analysis of Jerome's theory of sexuality in his famous letter to Eustochium ("The Blazing Body," 21–45). Jerome's opening sentence in his rejoinder to Jovinian is to the point: "The debate between Jovinian and myself is this: He reards marriage as equal to virginity, whereas I regard it as inferior" (Faivre, *The Emerence of the Laity*, 201). However, Jerome's extremism does in no way represent a majority Christian view, as is illustrated by the hesitating reception of his remarks against Jovinian among the Roman Christian community (Brown, *The Body and Society*, 377; Faivre, *The Emergence of the Laity*, 201). With respect to the Jovinian controversy Kate Cooper emphasizes that "in the 380s the conservatives still held sway. They saw the social dangers of too enthusiastic a reception for the ascetics' ideal" (*The Virgin and the Bride*, 82). In fact, "since the Jovinian controversy of the 390s, more than one Christian writer had come to be troubled by the self-congratulation of certain factions within the ascetic movement" (114).

4. In Elizabeth Castelli's path-breaking articles, "Virginity and Its Meaning for Women's Sexuality in Early Christianity" and " 'I Will Make Mary Male': Pieties of the Body and Gender Transformation of Christian Women in Late Antiquity." See also Boyarin (*A Radical Jew*, 180–201).

5. The earliest "monastic" community in that sense is the famed community of Therapeutae and Therapeutrides, a Jewish ascetic community that Philo "describes" in his *Vita Contemplativa*, in which women played a significant part (Kraemer, "Monastic Jewish Women"; Schüssler Fiorenza, *In Memory of Her*, 224; Brown, *The Body and Society*, 39) though it has not and perhaps cannot be clarified whether Philo dreams up an ideal community or indeed describes an actual community. With the beginning of the monastic movement women's convents were often established alongside the monasteries of men, often by female relatives of the founders of the neighboring male monasteries (Faivre, *The Emergence of the Laity*, 198–99). At the

end of this development stand the communities of virgins which Theodoret describes at the beginning of the fifth century (Castelli, "Virginity and Its Meaning," 79; Elm, *"Virgins of God"*).

6. She uses the hagiographical story of Helia, presumably written by Theodora from Spain, one of Jerome's correspondents. According to Salisbury, freedom of thought here manifests itself in using Jerome's texts while at the same time omitting Jerome's extremely restricting guidelines for women who chose a virginal life (*Churchfathers, Independent Virgins*, 74–82). In other words, Salisbury traces those moments when women who chose a Christian life as virgins did indeed take their virginal autonomy seriously, and did not shift from their parental or marital submission to a submission to the "fathers" of the church.

7. This freedom manifests itself primarily in all those hagiographies of women who reject their parents' choice of a bridegroom in favor of a life as a virgin, most famously Constantine the Great's daughter (Salisbury, *Churchfathers, Independent Virgins*, 60–73). These hagiographies concern mostly aristocratic women from a background of higher social standing. In such cases the stories then serve to emphasize the intensified difficulties the virgins had to surmount, since here the important politics of family alliances were threatened. However, Ross Kraemer has pointed to the advantage of virginal life also for "marginal women" who could not fulfill the social expectation of childbearing, as for example for barren women (cited in Castelli, "Virginity and Its Meaning," 84).

8. See also Gillian Cloke, who writes that "if women were essentially sinful because essentially sexual, the first and most obvious need was to negate that aspect of their nature—or to stand it on its head. If 'woman represents the flesh and the passions' [Origen, *In Exod*, PG 12.305], then 'he is truly male who ignores sin, which is to say female fragility' [Origen, *In Levit*, PG 12.188]" (*"This Female Man of God,"* 33).

9. For a similar argument see Boyarin (*A Radical Jew*, 196–97) who cites Castelli approvingly. He juxtaposes women under the reign of rabbinic Judaism with Christian women: "To be sure, Christian women had possibilities for living lives of much greater autonomy and creativity than their rabbinic Jewish sisters, but always on the stringent condition and heavy price of bodily renunciation" (1994, 197). See also Cloke in her *"This Female Man of God."*

10. Boyarin formulates Paul's hierarchical rhetorics of sexual choices as a "two-tiered system of thought regarding sexuality: celibacy as the higher state but marriage as a fully honorable condition for the believing Christian" (*A Radical Jew*, 192), though for Paul marriage attains its honor primarily as "a defense against lust and fornication" (192; compare Brown, *The Body and Society*, 55).

11. See, however, the studies of the attractiveness of an ascetic life of study for men by Biale (*The Eros and the Jews*), Boyarin (*Carnal Israel*), and Fraade ("Ascetical Aspects").

12. On the increasingly intensifying merger of the image of the monk with the

image of the clergy see Faivre (*The Emergence of the Laity in the Early Church*, esp. 197–205).

13. In her recent study of the rise of the virginal ideal, Kate Cooper has importantly focused on the consequences of its introduction for married (Christian) women. She has moved married women onto the stage of analysis by "abandoning the generic category of 'women's experience,'" thus enabling us to reflect on "the conditions for experience in various groups of women" (*The Virgin and the Bride*, 85). This, of course, is exactly the point of this current chapter. Cooper suggests, correctly in my opinion, that the model for studying the tensions arising from the introduction of the virginal ideal in late antique Christian literature is in need of revision: "The distinction [ . . . ] is not really between authentic and compromised models of Christianity—it is between two very different conceptions of the body social" (93), what she calls the separatist view and the civic view. Whereas, according to Cooper, the former develops religious ideals as a means of distinguishing the chosen few from the masses, the latter envisions the whole of society to be united by those ideals. Importantly for my current argument, she emphasizes that "the historical success of the separatist view should not blind us to the integrity of the civic view of religion among late Roman Christians" (93). Concluding the book with an analysis of the *Liber ad Gregoriam*, an anonymous sixth century devotional manual addressed to a Latin-speaking *matrona* in the imperial household, Cooper writes: "We should, I hope, be warned against an easy acceptance of the early Christian literature of continence and rejection of family as a literature of women's autonomy. To such an equation, the question must be put: which women? A second, more far-reaching question follows: what could autonomy itself have meant to a population so deeply committed to the values of group and dynasty?" (143). Jewish women would, then, be in situation quite similar to the Roman *matronae*.

14. Gillian Cloke presents a list of statements by Palladius, Gregory of Nazianzus, Augustine, Paulinus of Nola, and Jerome on women who had in their eyes become men (*"This Female Man of God,"* 214–16). Based on the pervasiveness of this trope she concludes that women's virtue was "directly and proportionally linked with a perceived ability to cast off the qualities and trappings of their tainted gender" (213). And, even more strongly, "every one of the many who achieved fame through piety was held to 'surpass her sex'—never, be it noted, to elevate the expectations that might be held of their sex" (220). Therefore, it is important to emphasize the distinction between the discursive annihilation of the female body of difference and the abolishing of gender difference altogether, for as Castelli has argued: "'Becoming male' marks for these thinkers the transcendence of gendered differences, but it does so only by reinscribing the traditional gender hierarchies of male over female, masculine over feminine" ("'I Will Make Mary Male,'" 33).

15. The only study that deals with this question directly that I am aware of

is Shaye Cohen's, in his recent article on "Menstruants and the Sacred." See also Geburgis Feld ("'Wie es eben Frauen ergeht,'" 29–43).

16. On the dispute over the dating of Easter and the liturgical calendar see Robert Wilken (*John Chrysostom and the Jews*, 76) who points out that in spite of the regulation of the Council of Nicea in 325 a diversity of practice existed until at least the early fifth century. Wilken's crucial observation is that in the fourth century "even though the emperor was a Christian, the culture was still informed by traditional pagan values, and Christians had no reason to suppose that a Christian emperor was to be a permanent feature of the Roman Empire" (xvii). Thus he claims, at least for the example of the city of Antioch at the end of the fourth century, that it "was still a pagan city, for those features of its life that transmitted and nurtured the values of its citizens and molded the character of its young people—education, social custom, literature, art and architecture, legends and myths—were still untouched by Christianity." This amounts to the "striking feature of the fourth century that the Church had created no schools for the education of the young" (24), partially since Christian literature was still in its infancy in the fourth century.

17. Cooper, in fact, devotes her last chapter to the devotional literature of the fifth and sixth centuries, which dealt in various forms with "the pastoral problem of addressing the *matrona* who felt herself excluded by the rising prestige of asceticism" (*The Virgin and the Bride*, 115).

18. For a discussion of the dating of the document see the introduction of Vööbus to his translation, on which I am relying, as well as R. H. Connolly's translation (1929) and G. Strecker's analysis ("On the Problem of Jewish Christianity," 244). Of the Greek original only remnants are preserved, primarily in the Apostolic Constitutions, a fourth-century compilation of church rules (Vööbus, *The Didascalia*, 23; Connolly, *Didascalia*, xi). Two early translations of the work exist. The Syriac translation, on which Vööbus relies for his English rendition, stems from the fourth century and is deemed to be older than the Latin translation (Connolly, xvii, Vööbus, 28). As far as the manuscript tradition of the Syriac translation is concerned, Vööbus distinguishes between an earlier version and a later recension. The earliest manuscripts date from the eighth to ninth centuries (Connolly, xi; Vööbus, 13). The time of the (incomplete) Latin translation, whose manuscript tradition is older than that of the Syriac translation (end of the fifth century), can, according to Vööbus, not be established with certainty, though "scholarly opinion has suggested that the origin of the translation must be a century older than the manuscript itself" (Vööbus, 30; Connolly, xix). Of the two translations the Latin one is the more literal (Connolly, xix; Vööbus, 29), most likely for linguistic reasons, since Latin is a language similar in character to the original Greek, as opposed to Syriac as a Semitic idiom. For certain important passages I will therefore subsequently refer to the Latin text as edited by Tidner. The transcription of the Syriac into Hebrew letters is based on Vööbus's edition of the Syriac version.

19. The literary genre of the Didascalia has been variously described as Church Order, along with the Didache and the Apostolic Tradition of Hippolytus. However, already Connolly pointed out that "in its aims and in the character of its contents it stands apart from most of the other documents of this class, for it deals hardly at all with formal legislation" (*Didascalia*, xxvii). He calls it instead "an elementary treatise on Pastoral Theology." Heggelbacher, on the other hand, insists that the Didascalia is regarded as a book in law in both Palestine and Syria (*Geschichte des frühchristlichen Kirchen rechts*, 5).

20. This is the title of the main body of the text (Vööbus *The Didascalia*, 9). The table of contents preceding the text is entitled "didascalia, i.e. the teaching of the holy apostles" (Vööbus, 1). The Syriac as well as the Latin version merely transliterates the Greek term. Connolly (xxviii) surmises that the choice of Didascalia was determined by the fact that the more obvious word for doctrine, *Didache*, was already in requisition for the title of an older work, which, however, presumes that the author of the Didascalia knew the Didache. The commonly used title of the work is the Latinized form, i.e. *Didascalia Apostolorum*.

21. In his analysis of the similarities between rabbinic, and specifically tannaitic texts and the Didascalia as to certain rules of conduct, Marmorstein already speculated that "it is not impossible that the writer of the Didascalia was born a Jew, and as such indebted to the Rabbis in more than one instance" ("Judaism and Christianity," 233). Due to the chronological closeness of the Didascalia and tannaitic literature, the writer "may or may not have sat at the feet of the masters of Usha or Sepphoris, Tiberias or Meron" (233), though Marmorstein admits that similarity in rules of conduct does not necessarily indicate a literary-traditional dependence. Georg Strecker, on the other hand, contends that even though the Didascalia betrays a detailed acquaintance with Jewish customs and teachings, this does not necessarily have to be explained by the assumption that the author had been of Jewish origin: "such a hypothesis cannot be based upon observations that in reality do nothing more than to identify various items of information" ("On the Problem of Jewish Christianity," 251). Rather, Strecker claims, "it is more probably the case that there was an active relationship between Christians and Jews in the author's world" (251). However, Strecker ignores the above passage. It is, then, incomprehensible to me how Strecker can come to the conclusion that "in spite of the apparent close connection between the Jewish Christian 'heretics' and the community of the author, it is not to be assumed that they actually belong to the community of the Didascalia" (255).

22. Primarily by those who have produced critical editions and translations. Further, however, the document has played a significant role in the context of the historiography of what has come to be called *Jewish Christianity*, thus prominently in the classic studies by Marcel Simon (*Verus Israel*) and Georg Strecker ("On the Problem of Jewish Christianity"), but also by A. Marmorstein ("Judaism and Christianity"). Jean Danielou's monumental work, *The Theology of Jewish Christianity*,

hardly deals with the Didascalia. The phenomenon of so-called Jewish Christianity has been widely discussed by scholars of early Christianity throughout this century, with increasing intensity and decreasing agreement on the meaning of the term or its representative value. It has become so problematic that a recent article has been entitled "The Phenomenon of Early Jewish-Christianity: Reality or Scholarly Invention?" (Joan Taylor). I will return to this debate further down, when we have to ask how it could be meaningful to consider the women of the Didascalia within the framework of a supposed "Jewish Christianity."

23. See Karen Torjesen's recent *When Women Were Priests* and Charlotte Methuen's essay "Widows, Bishops and the Struggle for Authority in the Didascalia Apostolorum."

24. Methuen, however, hints that "the possibility that women held positions of authority in the stream of Jewish Christianity opposed by the Didascalia cannot be excluded" ("Widows, Bishops," 211).

25. Methuen carefully distinguishes between the more restrictive role granted to the deaconesses and the role of the widows. She argues that the author regarded the authority of the widows as something that needed to be contained, to be replaced in part by the order of the deaconesses who were subject to the male bishop's authority.

26. I am thinking here primarily of the book of Acts, which is post-Paul. For a further discussion of the literature and the so-called *agrapha* of Christian discourse which the Didascalia uses, see Strecker ("On the Problem of Jewish Christianity," 246–49).

27. The literature on the apostolic council abounds. For a brief analysis of the dating and historicity of our two sources, as well as a bibliography, see Betz (*Galatians*, 81–83). More recently James Dunn (*Jesus, Paul, and the Law*, 129–82) has pointed out that whereas the scholarly literature has mostly dealt with the relationship between Acts and Galatians, hardly any work has been done on the issues of the conflict themselves (129), a situation he attempts to rectify by approaching the analysis with cultural-anthropological questions. Aside from the direct responses to Dunn's article, other scholars have subsequently taken up the question along his lines (Jack Sanders, "Jewish Christianity"; Boyarin, *A Radical Jew*, 113–16).

28. Of course, here the author uses the term "catholic," which he transcribes from Greek into Syriac, in the Greek sense of "universal."

29. τῷ ἔθει τῷ Μωυσέως. Some manuscripts, however, have καί τῷ ἔθει Μωυσέως περιπατῆτε, that is, this side of the conflict would demand of non-Jews who join the Apostolic communities, circumcision and conduct according to the customs of Moses. The Didascalia's retelling of Acts 15 most likely relies on this manuscript tradition (Vööbus, *The Didascalia*, 215).

30. There is a long and extensive debate on the cause-and-effect relationship between the conflict in Antioch and the apostolic council in Jerusalem, especially

since Paul's presentation of the sequence of events in his letter to the Galatians differs profoundly from Acts 15. However, the endeavor to understand "what really happened" in the mid-first century is of no immediate consequence for our analysis of the conflict which the Didascalia faces in the early third century. The Didascalia itself is not interested in the historicity of the events, but uses Acts 15 as a literary staging for dealing with its own conflict while ignoring Paul's account in Galatians 2 completely. The Didascalia in general hardly ever makes use of the Pauline corpus and, according to Strecker ("On the Problem of Jewish Christianity," 249, note 21), it is not even demonstrable that it had at its disposal all of Paul's New Testament letters.

31. The phrase "keeping away from meats" seems to allude to the laws of *kashrut*, however inexactly, since *kashrut* is not about vegetarianism. However, the Didascalia also formulates the concern about food regulations as "distinction of food" [פורשא דמאכלתא; escarum descretiones] (Vööbus, *The Didascalia*, 223), or refers to those who said "that one was bound to withhold from swine only, but might eat those things which the Law pronounces clean" [דמן חזירא בלחוד היב אנש דנכלא נפשה ואילין דמהא נמוסא נאכול וננזור איך דבנמוסא דלא אנש נאכול בשרא] (213), which would come closer to the practices of *kashrut*. Hence, Strecker rightly observes against some scholars that the Didascalia does not address "a vegetarian Jewish Christianity that rejected marriage, the eating of meat, and the Old Testament," a group to which the Christian heresiologist Epiphanius attests, but which he seems to merely invent ("On the Problem of Jewish Christianity," 253). It is somewhat hard to imagine what could be Jewish about a Jewish Christianity that rejects the "Old Testament."

32. Justin Taylor deals with the Didascalia as a reader of Acts 15. In defense of modern source and literary criticism Taylor argues that the Didascalia already saw literary problems in Acts 15, which modern scholars of Acts attempt to solve by taking Acts 15 apart into its various sources. The various difficulties of the text then are explained by the argument that the redactor of Acts 15 did not adequately weld his sources together. Hence the role of Paul and Barnabas in the account of Acts 15 is rather strange, since they—as the Antiochene delegates—do not play any significant part in the council itself, even though Acts presents the Antiochene conflict as the reason for the council. Thus, Taylor points out that the compiler of the Didascalia recognized that Paul and Barnabas are superfluous to the narrative and "quietly omitted" them from his retelling ("Ancient Texts and Modern Critics," 378). Taylor's point of dealing with the Didascalia as an ancient reader of Acts 15 is indeed important, but not primarily for the purpose of underscoring contemporary source criticism. Rather, it is important for the analysis of why and how the Didascalia uses Acts 15 as a narrative staging for its own argument in the conflictual situation of its own contemporary community, and why it entirely ignores Paul.

33. On the argumentative strategies against the Sabbath as a day of significance for the community the Didascalia addresses, see especially Marcel Simon in his classic *Verus Israel* (310–18). Simon's account of the conflict in the community of the

Didascalia is, however, highly problematic, especially with respect to its rhetorics. For a recent critical assessment see M. S. Taylor's *Anti-Judaism and Early Christian Identity* (1995).

34. The Latin translation reads "qui vero observantes . . . custodiunt consuetudinaria naturaliter, seminis sui cursus et adproximationes mulierum" (Tidner, *Didascaliae*, 91). This formulation apparently addresses the men in the community, if not because of the male pronouns, at least because of the circumscription of intercourse as the "approach of women."

35. The Tosefta is, of course, a Palestinian text. However, the Galilee of the rabbis in the third century and northern Syria are neighboring regions. Heggelbacher points out that the Didascalia was regarded as a book of law in both Palestine and Syria (*Geschichte des frühchristlichen Kirchen rechts*, 4).

36. This passage has recently been analyzed by D. Boyarin in the context of discussing the prohibition of women's Torah study in rabbinic culture (*Carnal Israel*, 180–81). He uses this passage to demonstrate that Palestinian textual traditions were more permissive toward women's study than Babylonian traditions. Thus "this text takes it as a matter of course that women are permitted to study all of these branches of Torah, and the only issue dealt with is whether they are permitted to do so in certain physiological situations" (180).

37. The Latin phrase is *consuetudinaria naturaliter*, the natural habits (Tidner, 91).

38. The Latin phrase here is "si enim speras te."

39. אנתי דין או אנתתא אן איך דאמרא אנתי דביומתא דמרדיתכי ספיקתי (Vööbus, 258). The Latin phrase is "tu autem, o mulier, sicuti dicis, etiamsi in diebus sessionis tuae vacua sis . . ." (Tidner, 95).

40. סכלתא נטורתא סריקתא נטרא אנתי (Vööbus, 257). The Latin reads "vana observas et vana custodis" (Tidner, 93)—in vain you observe and in vain you take heed.

41. In his introduction Vööbus points out that "over against this simple statement, the other [Syriac] recension displays changes which make the meaning of the passage specific and concrete speaking of the indwelling of the Holy Spirit in baptism and in the eucharist" (Vööbus, 57). By theological simplicity Vööbus seems to refer to making the community as a whole the receptacle of the Holy Spirit, whereas the confinement of the Holy Spirit to only the rituals of baptism and eucharist is the theological refinement. Elsewhere, the text signifies the rite of baptism as receiving the fellowship of the Holy Spirit (114).

42. To the Didascalia the leadership of the community is the metaphor of the Trinity: the bishop represents God, the deacon represents Christ, and the deaconess represents the Holy Spirit (Vööbus, 100).

43. Elsewhere the Didascalia specifies that "to those who have believed from the [Jewish] people or from the gentiles, forgiveness of their evil words has been granted through baptism" (Vööbus, 221). The emphasis lies on the inclusion of the gentiles in the people of God, since it emphasizes that "sins are forgiven by baptism also to those

who from the gentiles draw near and enter the holy church of God" (183). In spite of its elaborations on the signification of the rite of baptism, however, the Didascalia does not seem to consider circumcision as the possible rival rite of entry into the community. Circumcision had played a much greater role for Paul in his dispute with those who understood the Christian community as a Jewish community that believed in Jesus. In the Didascalia's situation of conflict, therefore, there do not seem to be those from "among the people" who insisted on circumcision.

44. Some manuscripts, which Vööbus categorizes with the second recension, add that blasphemy consists in denying the indwelling of the Holy Spirit in the rituals of baptism and eucharist (Vööbus, 221, note 23). See note 18 above. The theme of blasphemy against the Holy Spirit most likely derives from Matthew, where Jesus says to the Pharisees accusing him of performing exorcisms by the power of the "Beelzebul the ruler of the demons [εν τω Βεελζεβουλ αρχοντι των δαιμονιων]" (Matthew 12:23) rather than by the power of God: "Therefore I tell you, people will be forgiven for every sin and blasphemy, but blasphemy against the Spirit will not be forgiven. Whoever speaks a word against the Son of Man will be forgiven, but whoever speaks against the Holy Spirit will not be forgiven, either in this age or in the age to come" (Matthew 12:31–32).

45. Recent works on the role of women, and especially on the question of ordination of women in early Christianity, have made extensive use of this passage. But it is differently evaluated by various scholars. The more positive assessment of this passage reads it as indicating that the deaconesses in the early Church were more than "aides" to the male clergy and that they instead functioned as equals (Ide, *Woman as Priest*, 47) or at least quasi equals (Laporte, *The Role of Women*, 115). The more negative assessment, on the other hand, argues that the main gist of the Didascalia is to adopt the monarchic model as the ideal system for the church. The bishop takes the place of the king and centralizes authority functions in his office (Faivre, *The Emergence of the Laity*, 85; Torjesen, *When Women Were Priests*, 146–51). Hence, the role of the deaconess as an instructor of women at baptism is merely that of godmother or sponsor (Faivre, 101) and by far not as extensive as that of the male deacon (Gryson, *The Ministry of Women*, 42). Faivre argues that in fact the office of the deaconess was instituted as a means of control of women in a community in which widows had a highly visible and authoritative function. This would seem to be corroborated by the Didascalia's insistence that the power to bestow baptism on the convert remains exclusively with the bishop, for "if it were lawful to be baptized by a woman, our Lord and teacher Himself would have been baptized by Mary His Mother" (Vööbus; see Torjesen, 148).

46. The Syriac term here is the "second law" or "second nomos," derived from the Greek term for law. In Latin this term is *secundatio*, in Greek δευτερωσις.

47. On the Didascalia's concept of the *deuterosis* see also Simon (*Verus Israel*, 88–91), Marmorstein (*Judaism and Christianity*, 231) and Connolly (lvii–lxix). In the

Didascalia the term refers to a section of biblical law. The meaning of the Greek term shifts later on in patristic literature, when from the fourth century on it refers to rabbinic oral tradition, and specifically the Mishnah. For references to patristic literature see Simon, 88–91. Hence, the Greek term functioned as the translation of the Hebrew term Mishnah (89), though the rabbis themselves do not imply a secondariness of the Mishnah to the Torah. See, however, the explanation of the Hebrew term Mishnah by Natan ben Jechiel in his eleventh-century *Arukh ha-shalem*: "Or (differently vocalized) as *mishneh*, since it is second vis-à-vis the Torah, and in Greek is therefore called *deuterosis*" (Kohut, 5:278; see Stemberger, *Einleitung*, 114). Simon claims that the Greek term was created for Greek-speaking Jews by Greek-speaking rabbis when the Mishnah began to acquire the force of law, which happens right around the time of the Didascalia's composition. "It is from the Jews that the author of the Didascalia borrows the word, but when he applies it to the second revelation on Sinai, it is by wresting the original meaning of the word" (*Versus Israel*, 89). In the hands of the Didascalia's author the term acquires a pejorative meaning. Simon conjectures that the Didascalia was aware of the rabbinic assertion that the Mishnah is an integral part of the divine revelation on Mount Sinai: "He thus identifies the point of departure with the second code delivered at the renewal of the covenant. It is this second code which the Mishnah explains and expands" (90). Hence, even though explicitly the author only employs the term for biblical legislation, it logically and most likely intentionally implied the repudiation of the Mishnah.

48. As a heading for the chapter in which the argumentation with the women appears, several manuscripts provide the following: "Chapter 26 teaches what is the law and what is the second legislation; and a warning to all Christians that they should flee the bonds of the second legislation and should not seek to carry them ..." (Vööbus, 223, note 1). Later on the author insists that "now while you have the Gospel—you yield to the Law, the renewal of the Law and the seal; seek nothing else, (anything) more than the Law and the prophets. Indeed, the second legislation is dissolved, but the Law is made firm" (237). For the latter phrase the Latin version reads: "Secundatio enim destructa est, lex autem confirmata est" (Tidner, 90). Again, the writer emphasizes: "The law therefore is indissoluble, but the second legislation is temporary, and is dissoluble" (Vööbus, 224).

49. The rhetorical construction of the juxtaposition of the "true" and the "false" Law reminds one, of course, of Paul's strategy in his argument with those who continue with biblically ordained ritual observance as a marker of the Christian community. Paul develops his notion of the true Law, or the "Law of faith" (Gal 3:27) which for him is the basis of the universal community of God in Christ, in distinction from the false Law of the observances of physical rites, which established the ethnic community of the Jews. Boyarin writes, "the true Law is the spiritual, allegorical, inward interpretation of the external which is only its sign.... Through the true meaning of the Law, which was revealed in the crucifixion and resurrection of Christ

as a hermeneutic key and as a mysterious transformation, I have died to the old (mis)understanding of the Law as the outward observance which makes one (so I thought) a real Jew" (Boyarin, *A Radical Jew*, 123). But, as Boyarin emphasizes in his analysis of Paul's letter to the Galatians, for Paul the freedom from the Law as the outward observance does not mean anarchy. Rather, according to Paul "the whole law is fulfilled in one word, 'You shall love your neighbor as yourself'" (Gal. 5:14). This summary of the whole Torah and its Laws in one ethical/spiritual principle is the "law of Christ," the Christian understanding of the Law. The argument of the Didascalia, then, would seem to be structurally similar to Paul's, only that here the ten commandments replace the love of one's neighbor in Paul's letter to the Galatians. Among the few who have dealt with the relationship between Paul and the Didascalia, Connolly had claimed that "the author's treatment of the problem of the Old Law is doubtless influenced by St. Paul, and especially by the Epistle to the Galatians" (lx). However, the Didascalia never directly quotes from Paul's letter to the Galatians, nor from any other of the Pauline Epistles, of which one can at most find "traces," "influence," or "reminiscences" (Connolly, lxii), mostly evidenced by quoting some of the same biblical verses that Paul uses for his argument. Even Connolly himself remarks that the Didascalia "differs widely from St. Paul in his estimate of the purpose and value of the ceremonial law" (lxi). It seems to me that a renewed analysis of the difference between Paul and the Didascalia would be instructive as to the latter's place in the struggle of early Christian self-definition, especially in light of recent cultural analyses of Paul.

50. He cites Deuteronomy 27:26: "Cursed is everyone who does not uphold the words of this Torah, by doing it." This verse has been made famous for Christian polemic literature by Paul in his letter to the Galatians (Gal. 3:10–12). However, whereas the Didascalia argues that the second legislation cannot be fulfilled, because the Temple has been destroyed, Paul of course lived at a time when the Temple still existed. Again, the Didascalia does not cite Paul here in spite of using the same verse. For a discussion of Paul's use of this difficult verse, see Boyarin, *A Radical Jew*, 137–43.

51. Simon quotes a Christian text, the *Dialogue of Timothy and Aquila*, which does indeed go so far as to exclude at least the entire book of Deuteronomy from the canon: "He denies to it all status of inspired scripture. 'The fifth book is Deuteronomy, which was not dictated by the mouth of God but deuteronomized by Moses. This is why it was not deposited in the ark, that is to say, the ark of the covenant'" (*Verus Israel*, 90).

52. Vööbus remarks that here the Syriac text is corrupt and needs to be corrected from the citation of the Didascalia in the Apostolic Constitutions, which reads "you have the glorious law of the Lord God" [τὸν ἔνδοξον κυρίου τοῦ θεοῦ νόμον] (15, note 14). The Latin, which reads "and of laws and commandments you have the glorious law of the Lord," corresponds with the Greek citation. This emendation

would seem to make sense, since the book of Exodus is not the only book of law in the Torah, and at that not the most legal one compared with Leviticus, Numbers, and Deuteronomy. In oral communication, Boyarin suggests that the use of the term ספרא evokes perhaps Leviticus; the halakhic midrashic commentary of the rabbis is actually called thus. This term may subsequently have been misunderstood by a glossator who added מפקנא.

53. This is Vööbus's translation. The term סקובלא, however, derives from the Greek σκύβαλα, meaning "refuse," "garbage" or "trash." Compare Paul's use of this rhetorical device in Philippians 3:8.

54. According to Vööbus, the Didascalia here bases itself on the gospel of Matthew (244, note 227). The Latin term for that part of Jesus' garment, *fimbria*, would indicate that much, since that is the term that appears in the Vulgate of Matthew. At the same time it also appears in Luke's version of the story. Be that as it may, for the Didascalia's argument it does not matter on which gospel its author bases himself.

55. Jesus and the woman seem to be alone: both the crowds and the disciples disappear from the narrative stage. Matthew leaves out Mark's commentaries on the narrative development (Theissen, *Urchristliche Wundergeschichten*, 137).

56. Mark 5:26: καὶ πολλὰ παθοῦσα ὑπὸ πολλῶν ἰατρῶν καὶ δαπανήσασα τὰ παρ αὐτῆς πάντα καὶ μηδὲν ὠφεληθεῖσα ἀλλὰ μᾶλλον εἰς τὸ χεῖρον ἐλθοῦσα— "She had endured much under many physicians, and had spent all that she had; and she was no better, but rather grew worse" (NRSV). Luke 8:43: [ἰατροῖς προσαναλώσασα ὅλον τὸν βίον] οὐκ ἴσχυσεν ἀπ' οὐδενὸς θεραπευθῆναι "[and though she had spent all she had on physicians], no one could cure her" (NRSV).

57. Mark 5:28: ἐὰν ἅψωμαι κἂν τῶν ἱματίων αὐτοῦ σωθήσομαι—"If I but touch his cloak, I will be made well". Matthew 9:21 ἐάν μόνον ἅψωμαι τοῦ ἱματίου αὐτοῦ σωθήσομαι—"If I only touch his cloak I will be made well." Luke and Matthew further specify the part of Jesus' garment which the woman touches, that is ἥψατο τοῦ κρασπέδου τοῦ ἱματίου αὐτοῦ (Matthew 9:20; Luke 8:44). The κράσπεδον can mean the hem of his garment, but is used in the Septuagint for the fringes which the Israelites are commanded to wear at the corner of their garments (Num. 15:38f; Deut. 22:12). The distinction is important only for those who use this narrative to make an argument with respect to how strictly Jesus followed Mosaic law. However, it has only minor relevance for the following reading.

58. Matthew puts the healing at the end of the story, after Jesus' pronouncement to the woman.

59. Luke 8:46: ἥψατό μού τις ἐγὼ γὰρ ἔγνων δύναμιν ἐξεληλυθυῖαν ἀπ' εμοῦ— "Someone touched me; for I noticed that power had gone out from me" (NRSV).

60. Mark 5:31 καὶ ἔλεγον αὐτῷ οἱ μαθηταὶ αὐτοῦ βλέπεις τὸν ὄχλον συνθλίβοντά σε καὶ λέγεις τίς μου ἥψατο—"And his disciples said to him: You see the crowd pressing in on you; how can you say, 'Who touched me?'" (NRSV). Luke 8:45:

εἶπεν ὁ Πέτρος (mss: και οι συν αυτω) ἐπιστάτα οἱ ὄχλοι συνέχουσιν σε καὶ ἀποθλίβουσιν—"Peter (some manuscripts add: and those who were with him) said: Master, the crowds surround you and press in on you" (NRSV).

61. Mark 5:33: ἡ δὲ γυνὴ φοβηθεῖσα καὶ τρέμουσα, εἰδυῖα ὃ γέγονεν αὐτῇ— "But the woman, knowing what had happened to her, came in fear and trembling, fell down before him, and told him the whole truth." Luke 8:47 ἰδοῦσα δὲ ἡ γυνὴ ὅτι οὐκ ἔλαθεν, τρέμουσα ἦλθεν καὶ προσπεσοῦσα αὐτῷ δί ἥν αἰτίαν ἥψατο αὐτοῦ ἀπήγγειλεν ἐνώπιον παντὸς τοῦ λαοῦ καὶ ὡς ἰάθη παραχρῆμα—"When the woman saw that she could not remain hidden, she came trembling; and falling down before him, she declared in the presence of all the people why she had touched him, and how she had been immediately healed" (NRSV).

62. Marla Selvidge, *Woman, Cult and Miracle Recital;* and Peter Trummer, *Die blutende Frau.*

63. The articles are too numerous to be listed here. For a survey, however, see Selvidge. In addition to Selvidge's survey see also von Kellenbach's list of references (*Anti-Judaism*, 112), mostly to West German Christian feminist New Testament scholars.

64. See O. Weinreich, *Antike Heilungswunder* (1909).

65. Similarly Gnilka (*Das Matthäusevangelium*, 215): "Gemaess dem hier vorliegenden Wunderverstaendnis, das hellenistisch konzipiert ist, kam das Wunder durch eine von Jesus ausgehende Kraft zustande [According the the hellenistic concept of miracles, present here, the miracle came about by an energy exuding from Jesus]." Witherington takes the narrative elements which are typical for stories of miraculous healings in antiquity as an incentive to reflect on whether the story is merely a fictional account composed from such literary means, or whether it has a historical kernel. He insists on the latter; he accepts "the nucleus of the story as revealing something of Jesus' views of women" (*Women in the Ministry of Jesus*, 72), whereas the genre elements are merely Mark's embellishments of the historical account in front of him.

66. καὶ παρεκάλουν αὐτὸν ἵνα κἂν τοῦ κρασπέδου τοῦ ἱματίου αὐτοῦ ἅψονται. The term for the fringe of his garment here—τὸν κράσπεδον τοῦ ἱματίου—appears in the the story of the woman with a blood-flow only in Matthew's and Luke's version, whereas Mark only knows about her touching of his garment.

67. Rudolf and Martin Hengel again refer to Otto Weinreich's analysis of ancient legends of healing, which observes that healing by touch is also a common element in hellenistic healing stories ("Die Heilungen Jesu," 347). New Testament scholars often make the point that the story intends to differentiate between some "magic touch" and the woman's touching of Jesus as an act of faith. When Jesus tells the woman at the end of the story that "your faith had made you well" he is understood as reinterpreting her act. Thus, the readers of the story are supposed to understand that it was not the touch in and by itself which healed the woman, but her faith (Guehlich,

*Mark 1–8:26*, 299; Kertelge, *Das Markusevangelium*, 115; Gnilka, *Das Matthäusevangelium*, 1:213). Other New Testament commentaries also recognize the magical element of a healing by touch, but here faith and magic are not competitors. The trust in the healing magic of the touch enhances her faith (Schmithals 1979, 294).

68. For an account of the story see the Loeb Classical Library edition, 1932, 2:175–76. See also Selvidge, *Woman, Cult and Miracle Recital*, 20.

69. The English translation of the *Life of Anthony*, from which I quote here, is published in *Nicene and Post-Nicene Fathers*, ed. Ph. Schaff and H. Wace, 211–12. For questions concerning the date and the author of this work, see ibid. (188–93; see also Selvidge, *Woman, Cult and Miracle Recital*, 20). The story of how Constantine's daughter Constantina became a consecrated virgin begins with recounting how she was advised by St. Agnes to believe in "Jesus the Christ, the son of God, who grants health," whereupon she was healed from her leprosy instantaneously (Salisbury, *Churchfathers, Independent Virgins*, 61).

70. The term Mark employs to describe the woman's affliction (Mark 5:29). It can be used in both in physical and spiritual senses, and would best be rendered as "affliction" in English.

71. Selvidge comments on Jerome's allegorization that "as a type of gentile, the heroine lost her identity. Jerome ignored the meaning and significance of this passage for Mark's earliest auditing and reading publics" (*Woman, Cult and Miracle Recital*, 18). However, in this judgment she ignores the fact that the story does precisely allow for such a reading, because the woman with the blood-flow remains ethnically undefined.

72. Compare Mark 5:25: γυνὴ οὖσα ἐν ῥύσει αἵματος δώδεκα ἔτη (Luke 8:43).

73. Compare Matthew: 9:20 γυνὴ αἱμορροοῦσα.

74. Selvidge's method notwithstanding. She argues that the predominance of the term for blood flow in Lev. indicates that "the Greek translation of Leviticus seems to exhibit a preference for the vocabulary used in Mark to describe or diagnose the condition of the woman in Mark 5:24–34" (*Woman, Cult and Miracle Recital*, 48). Her point that of "the seventeen times ῥύσις is used in the LXX, fifteen are found only in Lev." (48) seems to work with the assumption that intertexual or linguistic connections are quantifiable. More convincing is her point that the term for "the source of her blood" (Mark 5:29) is found in LXX only in Lev., that is, Lev. 12:7 and in Lev. 20:18.

75. Milgrom prefers the former reading. The difference between the Hebrew versions lies between the use either בה or בם.

76. Ever since Billerbeck's collection of rabbinic sources as a "background" for the gospels, the reference to this passage has made its entry into the New Testament commentary literature. The problem of this treatment of mishnaic law, both in terms of historical methodology and cultural-political terms, is an old one and will not be rehearsed here.

77. Trummer even argues that she does not merely render Jesus impure, but that she makes him guilty: "At any rate, this woman demands a lot from Jesus with her bleeding, even too much, since she endangers him with her impurity, renders him guilty along with her, guilty himself" (*Die blutende Frau*, 85). This infliction of guilt he explains based on Lev. 5:3 (121). However, he completely misunderstands the verse since the verse sets up a case in which someone "who touches human impurity [such as the zavah]—any such impurity whereby one becomes impure—and, though he has known it the fact escapes him but (thereafter) he feels guilt" as a consequence of which such a person would have to bring an offering of purification to the Temple (Lev. 5:6). In his careful analysis of this text Milgrom explains this case as referring to someone who "has contracted impurity knowingly, even deliberately, but has forgotten to purify himself within the prescribed time limits. If he subsequently remembers and feels guilt, he must confess his wrong and expiate it by a purification offering" (*Leviticus 1–16*, 313). Thus Trummer is wrong when he argues that "he who does not realize his impurity by touch has to bring a sacrifice once he becomes aware of it" (121). In our story, Jesus would only be obligated to bring a sacrifice if he neglected to purify himself, of which we learn nothing in the story. But he certainly does not incur any form of guilt merely by being touched.

78. Many New Testament scholars, however, reject the interpretation of the woman's fear as a sign of her guilt complex. Theissen considers that she might have been afraid that her act could be misinterpreted as either the intent to rid herself of her sickness by transferring it to Jesus, or as some love magic (*Urchristliche Wundergeschichten*, 137; cited by Pesch, *Das Markusevangelium*, 304 and Gnilka *Das Matthaeusevangelium I*, 216), which seems an unlikely interpretation to me. Guehlich rejects all these suggestions and proposes that "this description expresses her reaction of awe at what had happened to her" (*Mark 1*, 298; also Schmithals *Das Evangelium nach Markus*, 294). Most convincing I find Trummer's reference to the only other use of this pairing of fear and trembling at the end of Mark's gospel where it describes the women's reaction when they are told that Jesus has risen from the dead (Mark 16:8). Thus, fear is in the gospel of Mark always the reaction when the significance of Jesus is recognized. Hence, Trummer argues "die erfolgte Heilung bringt der Frau zum Bewusstsein, dass sie sich in der Person Jesu nicht getaeuscht hatte, sondern dass sie sogar noch Grösseres erwarten konnte, als sie vermuten durfte" [her healing indicates to the woman that she was not mistaken in the person Jesus, but that she could expect even greater things than she had expected] (1991, 98).

79. Selvidge writes "The woman had touched him. According to Jewish tradition, she had potentially defiled him. 'He shows no indignation at the ritual defilement, but ignores it; for the woman is seen not as an unclean object but as a human being suffering. . . . He does not attack the demands of the cult worship directly, he merely ignores them as irrelevant when they distract from the essential relationship between

man and God'" (*Woman, Cult and Miracle Recital*, 92). The quote stems from Irene Breannan, "Women in the Gospels," *New Blackfriars* 52 (1971, 296). This is the center of Selvidge's argument that this story was written to free early Christian women from the social bonds of niddah. Similarly Ruether, who contends that "Jesus' reaction to the woman with a hemorrhage shows his deliberate discarding of this taboo" (*New Woman/New Earth*, 64).

80. Professor Daryl Schmidt kindly called my attention to Paula Fredriksen's recent discussion of Marcus Borg's work on the historical Jesus. Her criticism in her article "Did Jesus Oppose the Purity Laws?" (*Bible Review* 1995, 19–47) underlines my current claim here, though she does not specifically deal with the story of the woman with a blood-flow. She refutes Borg's contention that Jesus imagines "a community shaped not by ethos and politics of purity, but by the ethos and politics of compassion" (quoted in "What You See Is What You Get," 20). She notes that "the opposition between compassion (Jesus) and purity (first-century Judaism, especially as associated with Jerusalem) is a leitmotif of Borg's scholarship" (45 fn1). Borg's effort, while to be commended for its effort to present a Jesus in his Jewish cultural environment, thus repeats the majority New Testament scholarship with respect to our story, i.e. the confusion of impurity with sin or even transgression. Refuting Borg's confusion of impurity with social distinctions, Fredriksen then emphasizes that, first, impurity is not sin, second, it does not correspond to social class, and third, that it is gender-blind (23), the latter meaning that both men and women can contract a status of impurity vis-à-vis the Temple.

81. Gnilka's commentary that the woman's fear and trembling is caused by the thought that her act might have been misunderstood as wanting to approach or come on to Jesus as a beautiful woman (*Das Matthaeusevangelium*, 216), has no basis in the story whatsoever. Where does the presumed beauty of the woman come from all of a sudden, if not from the commentator's fantasy?

82. There are several factors that account for that. First of all, of course, the fact that for most of the Order of Purities, including the mishnaic tractate that deals with the impurity of irregular discharges, we do not have a Talmud. Second, the main concern of the tractate for which we do have a Talmud, that is, Tractate Niddah, is about the biblical prohibition of sexual contact between a woman in her menstruation and her husband. Here the transfer of impurity by touch (of something and not of somebody) comes into play only concerning the priestly share of food, which the menstruant woman, as well as other people in a status of impurity, would invalidate. The third factor is, of course, that in post-Temple times the transfer of the status of impurity becomes irrelevant.

83. Ironically, the very fact that she was milling around in the masses could also be read as an indication that (Jewish) women who were *zavot* could move around freely in the streets (von Kellenbach, *Anti-Judaism in Feminist Religious Writings*, 62).

I have already attempted to argue in the first chapter that women with a regular menstruation were not subjected to ostracism or banishment from public life, except from the temple, as long as it still stood.

84. Shaye Cohen, however, argues that "Dionysius is transferring to Christianity the pollution categories of Leviticus 15," based on Dionysius' application of Temple terminology to the church, since the woman who is not "pure in both soul and body shall be prevented from approaching the holy and the holy of holies" ("Menstruants and the Sacred," 288). Nonetheless, Dionysius does not reason that the menstruous woman should not do that because Lev. 15 rules in that manner. They should not do so as "pious and faithful" women. He might perhaps allude to concerns that stem from the traditions based on Lev. 15, but he certainly treats them rather discriminately: "as to those who are overtaken by an involuntary flux in the night-time, let such follow the testimony of their own conscience, and consider themselves as to whether they are doubtfully minded in this matter or not" (Ross Kraemer, *Maenads, Martyrs, Matrons, Monastics*, 43). As far as the man and his "impurity" is concerned, he should act according to his own conscience, whereas the woman and her "impurity" are not given such a choice. Hence, his motivation to exclude the women from the Eucharist and from church must lie elsewhere than in his attachment to the regulations of Lev. 15.

85. For the regulations concerning sexual behavior in general, and the prohibition of sexual relations during the wife's menstrual period in medieval Christian literature, see the comprehensive work of James Brundage (*Law, Sex, and Christian Society in Medieval Europe*). In all cases in which menstruation is raised, only once does he discuss the origin of the prohibition, that is, in the context of the penitential literature: "This prohibition was based on the purity rules of the Mosaic law, perhaps augmented by a belief in the terrifying physical effects of contact with menstrual fluid described in the *Natural History* of the elder Pliny" (156). But he only speculates on the origins. An exception seems to be the opinion of one Huguccio at the end of the 12th century who considers the possibility of menstrual sex. Huguccio writes during a period when canon law began to come into its own, independent from theology. He notes that if the wife sought sexual intercourse during her menstruation, her husband could refuse, unless there was imminent danger that she might commit fornication (283).

86. Gregory the Great, pope from 590 till 604, writes in his answers to the inquiries of a certain Augustine, one of the early missionaries to the British Isles and the first bishop of Canterbury: "A woman's periods are not sinful, because they happen naturally. But nevertheless, because our nature is itself so depraved that it appears to be polluted even without the consent of the will, the depravity arises from sin, and human nature itself recognizes its depravity to be a judgment upon it," cited in Bede's *Ecclesiastical History* (1994, 49). Gregory's answers to Augustine provide

another important example of how Christians later dealt with their heritage of the levitical system of purity and impurity, and specifically those concerning menstruation. In Gregory's answer it is not menstruation as such which is a source of pollution, but it is more generally a sign of the depravity of human nature. We can also observe a development in early medieval Jewish culture parallel to the foregrounding of menstrual repugnance in Christian literature. An extra-halakhic text such as the *Baraita de-Niddah* of the early post-Talmudic period is an expression of blatant misogyny when, among other things, it suggests that a sage who partakes of food prepared by a menstruant will forget his learning. For a brief discussion see Sh. Cohen ("Menstruants and the Sacred," 281) who observes that "the belief that a menstruant poses a danger to those around her appears in Jewish sources for the first time in the sixth or seventh century C.E." Cohen then speculates that "its emergence and acceptance then may be the result either of outside influence (whether Christian or Islamic) or of new perceptions of the woman within Jewish society" (ibid.).

87. Barkley points out that Rufinus "admits to having changed the text of the Homilies on Leviticus more than the other homilies on the Pentateuch" (*Origen's Homilies on Leviticus: 1–16*, 21), so that Origen's original expression has been lost to us. But at the same time he contends that "the genuineness of the thought remains. To not use the Latin texts would invite the criticism of Henri de Lubac who argues that rejecting them on the basis of textual criticism is 'too much an invitation to laziness and simple lack of inquiry' " (23). The distinction between what might have been Origen's genuine expression and what is Rufinus's embellishment, abbreviation, or explanation does not concern me here, since my interest here is not what Origen in this case really said, but what happens hermeneutically to the book of Leviticus.

88. Origen here builds on the famous passage in Paul's second letter to the Corinthians (2 Cor. 3:7–18). For an extensive discussion of that passage and its significance for Paul's thinking, see Boyarin, *A Radical Jew*, 97–105.

89. This hermeneutic distinction is classic Origen, and the basis of all of his sophisticated allegorical readings. His method of biblical interpretation is most systematically developed in Book Four of *De Principiis* (Barkley, *Origen's Homilies on Leviticus*, 14), where he writes as a scholar. There he develops a tripartite hermeneutical scheme of the historical/literal/bodily sense, the moral or pneumatic sense and the mystical or psychic one, in parallel to the Platonic anthropological composition of body, soul, and spirit (Crouzel, *Origen*, 69–73; Barkley 15; Boyarin *Intertextuality*, 109). For a literary critical analysis of Origen's application of his methodology to the Song of Songs in comparison with the midrashic reading of the rabbis, see Boyarin 1990, 108–10. In the homilies he applies this methodology to preaching.

90. For the Latin text I am using W. A. Baehrens (1920), who edited a critical edition of the homilies in Rufinus' translation.

91. Strecker ("On the Problem of Jewish Christianity," 255) calls them Jewish-Christians, but not because of their background in Jewish tradition, but because of their continuing close ties to Judaism which "go far beyond mere 'Judaizing.'"

92. One of the most convincing articles is Joan Taylor's on "The Phenomenon of Early Jewish-Christianity: Reality or Scholarly Invention?" (1990, 313–334). Taylor reviews the history of the term in scholarly literature, from the beginning of its use in the Tübingen school by F. C. Baur, to whom Jewish Christianity, led by Peter, presented the thesis, which merged with its antithesis, a Gentile Christianity, led by Paul into the synthesis of Catholic Christianity. From Baur onwards the term is primarily used as describing a theology, till Robert Kraft pointed out that such a category was crafted "without consideration of whether any historical groups consciously adhered to such a theology" ("In Search of 'Jewish Christianity,'" 86, quoted in Taylor, 314). Thus Taylor proceeds to argue persuasively that "the beliefs and practices of Jews within the Church would have varied as much as did Christian Gentiles' beliefs and practices, and there is no reason to doubt that both ethnic groups participated in the full spectrum of possible attitudes. There is no sure way of dividing the Christian Jews from the Gentiles in theological terms" (314).

93. This term ἰουδαΐζω turns the adjective or adverb for Jewish into a verb by adding -ιζω, otherwise a common phenomenon in Greek. In Christian literature it has its origin in Paul's letter to the Galatians (Gal 2:14), a hapax legomenon in the New Testament. For an extended debate of the term and its possible implications see Dunn 1990, 149–50. Betz (*Galatians*, 112) states that "it is not quite synonymous with ἰουδαϊκῶς ζῇς" a phrase which Paul uses in the same verse, and which also means "to live like a Jew." Instead, Betz claims that "it seems to describe the somewhat artificial behavior of the new converts," though he does not provide any support for this. Paul employs the term ἰουδαιζεῖν when he accuses Peter of forcing non-Jewish converts "to live Jewishly" (ἰουδαΐζειν), while he himself, a Jewish man, "lives according to a gentile manner and not according to a Jewish manner" (ἐθνικῶς καὶ οὐχὶ ἰουδαϊκῶς ζῇς, Gal. 2:14). The two terms as descriptive terms do seem to be synonymous. Both Paul's as well as Josephus's use of the term (Bell. 2, 17:10 and 2, 18:2) is more descriptive, referring to non-Jews who live like Jews, according to Jewish customs. For other references see Dunn (*Jesus, Paul, and the Law*, 149–50) and Betz (112). In early patristic literature, however, and especially in Chrysostom's sermons against the Jews (Wilken 1983), it acquires an increasingly polemical ring. Subsequently, in Christian historiography the term has turned into a heresiological term, referring to those who not merely (continue to) live according to Jewish customs, but who—by defining their Christian-ness through Jewish practices—threaten the integrity, and hence the orthodoxy of Christianity. Hence, the "Judaizers" come to designate that distinct group of people who try to lure others into their "misconceptions." Not only do they live like Jews, in accordance with Jewish customs, but they try to convince others to do so. Their image in scholarly literature has often the tinge of

infiltrators. The English term is therefore not a neutral or merely descriptive term, but takes on the later polemical connotation. However, the problematic term once married to this sense, should—against Marcel Simon's classic and now somewhat dated analysis of the text (*Versus Israel*, 1948)—not be applied to the people against whom the Didascalia argues, especially since the text itself never uses this term. This will be further elucidated in the following discussion.

94. The Latin translation, however, states the complete opposite: Itaque, cum naturalia profluunt uxoribus vestris, nolite convenire illis sed sustinete eas et scientes propria membra esse diligete sicut propria membra esse (Tidner, *Didascaliae*, 99). Vööbus comments that the strong prohibition of the Latin "indicates that something is wrong with the text in Syriac. Since a deliberate change cannot come into account here we must reckon with an accidental loss of the missing part of the text" (Vööbus, 244, fn 229). It is somewhat curious that whereas usually he prefers the Syriac over the Latin version, here he conjectures for no compelling reason that the Latin version is the more reliable. However, Cohen holds that "the Latin translator was so offended by it that he emended it out of existence" ("Menstruants and the Sacred," 290). Against Vööbus he argues, to my mind convincingly, that the Syriac version fits the argument of the paragraph, whereas the Latin does not (298, note 60).

# BIBLIOGRAPHY

Adler, Rachel. "Feminist Folktale of Justice: Robert Cover as a Resource for the Renewal of Halakha." *Conservative Judaism* 45 (1993): 40–56.

———. "In Your Blood, Live: Re-Visions of a Theology of Purity." *Tikkun* 8:1 (1993): 38–41.

———. "The Virgin in the Brothel and Other Anomalies: Character and Context in the Legend of Beruriah." *Tikkun* 3:6 (1988): 28–32, 102–5.

———. "Tum'ah and Taharah: Ends and Beginnings." In *The Jewish Woman*, ed. E. Koltun, 63–71. New York: Schocken Books, 1976.

Adorno, Theodor W. *Negative Dialectics*. Trans. E. B. Ashton. New York: Seabury Press, 1973.

Albeck, H. *Mehqarim ba-baraita ve-Tosefta ve-yahsan la-Talmud*. Jerusalem: Mosad ha-Rav Kook, 1944.

———. *Shishah Sidrei Mishnah 1–6*. Jerusalem: Mosad Bialik, 1988.

Albeck, H., and J. Theodor. *Midrash Bereshit Rabba: Critical Edition with Notes and Commentary*. Jerusalem: Wahrmann Books, 1965.

Alon, Gedalyahu. "The Boundary of the Halkahot of Purity." *Jews, Judaism and the Classical World*, pp. 148–76 [Hebrew].

———. "The Impurity of Foreigners." In *Jews, Judaism and the Classical World: Studies in the History of Israel in the Times of the Second Temple and the Talmud*. Tel Aviv: Ha-Kibbuz Me'uhad, 1958, pp. 121–47 [Hebrew].

Arava, Rachel. "Precious Shall Be Their Blood": Women's Perception and Experience of Menstruation in Traditional Judaism. M.A. Thesis, University of California–Berkeley, 1990.

Archer, Leonie. "Bound by Blood: Circumcision and Menstrual Taboo in Post-

Exilic Judaism." In *After Eve*, ed. Janet M. Soskice, 38–62. London: Collins Marshall Pickering, 1990.

———. *Her Price Is Beyond Rubies: The Jewish Woman in Graeco-Roman Palestine.* JSOT Suppl. Series 60. Sheffield: Sheffield Academic Press, 1989.

———. " 'In Thy Blood Live': Gender and Ritual in the Judaeo-Christian Tradition." In *Through the Devil's Gateway: Women, Religion and Taboo*, ed. Alison Joseph. London: SPCK, 1990, pp. 22–50.

Aspegren, Kerstin. *The Male Woman: A Feminine Ideal in the Early Church*, ed. Renee Kieffer. Stockholm: Almqvist & Wiksell International, 1990.

Baehrens, Walter. *Homilien zum Hexateuch in Rufins Uebersetzung, Origenes Werke 6.* Leipzig: J. C. Hinrichs'sche Buchhandlung, 1920.

Baker, Cynthia. "Bodies, Boundaries, and Domestic Politics in a Late Ancient Marketplace." *Journal of Medieval and Modern Studies* 26:3 (1996): 391–419.

Bakhtin, Mikhail. *Rabelais and His World*. Bloomington: Indiana University Press, 1984.

Bal, Mieke. *Lethal Love: Feminist Interpretations of Biblical Love Stories*. Bloomington: Indiana University Press, 1987.

———. *Murder and Difference: Gender, Genre and Scholarship on Sisera's Death*. Bloomington: Indiana University Press, 1988.

———. *Death and Dissymmetry: The Politics of Coherence in the Book of Judges*. Chicago: University of Chicago Press, 1988.

Bamberger, Bernard. "Qetanah, Na'arah, Bogereth." *Harvard Theological Review* (1973): 281–94.

Barkley, Gary Wayne, *Origen's Homilies on Leviticus: 1–16*. The Fathers of the Church 83. Washington, D.C.: Catholic University of America Press, 1990.

Baskin, Judith. "Rabbinic Reflections on the Barren Wife." *Harvard Theological Review* 82:1 (1989): 101–14.

———. "The Separation of Women in Rabbinic Judaism." In *Women, Religion and Social Change*, ed. Yvonne Y. Haddad and Ellison B. Findly. Albany: State University of New York Press, 1985.

Baskin, Judith R., ed. *Jewish Women in Historical Perspective*. Detroit: Wayne State University Press, 1991.

Batmartha, Ina Johanne. "Machen Geburt und Monatsblutung die Frau "unrein"? Zur Revisionsbeduerftigkeit eines missverstandenen Diktums." In Schottroff and Wacker, eds. *Von der Wurzel getragen: Christlich-feministische Exegese in Auseinandersetzung mit Antijudaismus*, 43–61. Leiden: Brill, 1996.

Baur, Walter. *Orthodoxy and Heresy in Earliest Christianity*. Philadelphia: Fortress Press, 1971.

Bede. *The Ecclesiastical History of the English People*. Oxford: Oxford University Press, 1994.

Betz, Hans Dieter. *Galatians: A Commentary on Paul's Letter to the Churches in Galatia.* Philadelphia: Fortress Press, 1979.

Biale, David. *The Eros and the Jews: From Biblical Israel to Contemporary America.* New York: Basic Books, 1992.

———. *Power and Powerlessness in Jewish History.* New York: Schocken, 1986.

Biale, Rachel. *Women and Jewish Law: An Exploration of Women's Issues in Halakhic Sources.* New York: Schocken, 1984.

Bialik, H. N. "Halakhah and Aggadah." In *Collected Works*, 207–13. Tel Aviv: Hotsa'at Va'ad ha-Yovel, 1933 [Hebrew].

Boid, Iain Ruairidh McMhanaim. *Principles of Samaritan Halakhah.* Studies in Judaism in Late Antiquity 38. Leiden and New York: Brill, 1989.

Bokser, B. M. "An Annotated Bibliographical Guide to the Study of the Palestinian Talmud." *Aufstieg und Niedergang der Römischen Welt* II/19.2: 139–256.

———. *Samuel's Commentary on the Mishnah: Its Nature, Forms, and Contents.* Leiden: Brill, 1975.

Bordo, Susan. *Unbearable Weight: Feminism, Western Culture and the Body.* Berkeley and Los Angeles: University of California Press, 1993.

Boyarin, Daniel. *Carnal Israel: Reading Sex in Talmudic Culture.* Berkeley and Los Angeles: University of California Press, 1993.

———. "The Eye in the Torah: Ocular Desire in Midrashic Hermeneutic." *Critical Inquiry* 16 (1990): 532–50.

———. *Intertextuality and Reading the Midrash.* Bloomington: Indiana University Press, 1990.

———. "Language Inscribed by History on the Bodies of Living Beings: Midrash and Martyrdom." *Representations* 25 (winter 1989): 139–51.

———. "On the Status of the Tannaitic Midrashim." *Journal of the American Oriental Society* 112:3 (1992): 455–65.

———. "Placing Reading: Ancient Israel and Medieval Europe." In *Ethnography of Reading*, ed. Jonathan Boyarin, 10–38. Berkeley and Los Angeles: University of California Press, 1993.

———. *A Radical Jew: Paul and the Politics of Identity.* Berkeley and Los Angeles: University of California Press, 1994.

———. *Unheroic Conduct: The Rise of Heterosexuality and the Invention of the Jewish Man.* Berkeley and Los Angeles: University of California Press, 1997.

Braidotti, Rosi. "Embodiment, Sexual Difference, and the Nomadic Subject." *Hypatia* 8:1 (1993): 1–13.

———. "Of Bugs and Women: Irigaray and Deleuze on the Becoming-Woman." In *Engaging With Irigaray: Feminist Philosophy and Modern European Thought*, ed. Carolyn Burke, Naomi Schor, Margaret Whitford, 111–40. New York: Columbia University Press, 1994.

———. "Organs Without Bodies." *differences* 1:1 (1988): 147–61.

———. "Sexual Politics as a Nomadic Political Project." In *Nomadic Subjects: Embodiment and Sexual Difference in Contemporary Feminist Theory*, 146–73. New York: Columbia University Press, 1994.

Brooten, Bernadette. *Love Between Women: Early Christian Responses to Female Homoeroticism*. Chicago: University of Chicago Press, 1996.

———. *Women Leaders in the Ancient Synagogue*. Brown Judaic Studies 36. Chico, Calif.: Scholars Press, 1982.

Brown, Peter. *The Body and Society: Men, Women and Sexual Renunciation in Early Christianity*. Lectures on the History of Religions, vol. 13. New York: Columbia University Press, 1988.

———. "The Saint as Exemplar." *Representations* 2 (1983): 1–25.

Brown, Raymond. "Not Jewish Christianity and Gentile Christianity but Types of Jewish/Gentile Christianity." *Catholic Biblical Quarterly* 45:1 (1983): 74–79.

Brown, Wendy, "Feminist Hesitations, Postmodern Exposures." *differences* 3:1 (1991): 63–85.

Brundage, James. *Law, Sex, and Christian Society in Medieval Europe*. Chicago: University of Chicago Press, 1991.

Buckley, Thomas, and Alma Gottlieb, eds. *Blood Magic: The Anthropology of Menstruation*. Berkeley and Los Angeles: University of California Press, 1988.

Butler, Judith. *Bodies That Matter: On the Discursive Limits of Sex*. New York and London: Routledge, 1993.

———. *Gender Trouble: Feminism and the Subversion of Identity*. London: Routledge, 1990.

Cameron, Averil, and Amelie Kuhrt, eds. *Images of Women in Antiquity*. London and Canberra: Croom Helm, 1983.

Carson, Anne. "Putting Her in Her Place: Woman, Dirt, and Desire." In *Before Sexuality: The Construction of Erotic Experience in the Ancient Greek World*, ed. D. Halperin, J. Winkler, and F. Zeitlin, 137–71. Princeton: Princeton University Press, 1990.

Castelli, Elizabeth. "'I Will Make Mary Male': Pieties of the Body and Gender Transformation of Christian Women in Late Antiquity." In *Body Guards: The Cultural Politics of Gender Ambiguity*, ed. Julia Epstein and Kristina Straub, 29–50. New York: Routledge, 1991.

———. "Virginity and Its Meaning for Women's Sexuality in Early Christianity." *Journal of Feminist Studies in Religion* 2 (1986): 61–88.

Cixous, Hélène, and Catherine Clément. *The Newly Born Woman*. Minneapolis: University of Minnesota Press, 1991 [orig. French 1975].

Clark, Elizabeth. "'Adam's Only Companion': Augustine and the Early Christian Debate on Marriage." *Recherches Augustiniennes* 21 (1986): 139–62.

———. *Ascetic Piety and Women's Faith: Essays on Late Ancient Christianity.* Lewiston, N.Y.: Edwin Mellen Press, 1986.
Clark, Gillian. *Women in Late Antiquity: Pagan and Christian Life-Styles.* Oxford: Clarendon Press, 1994.
Cloke, Gillian. *"This Female Man of God": Women and Spiritual Power in the Patristic Age, A.D. 350–450.* London and New York: Routledge, 1995.
Cohen, Aryeh. *Rereading Talmud: Gender, Law, and the Poetics of Sugyot.* Atlanta, Ga.: Scholars Press, 1998.
Cohen, Shaye. "Solomon and the Daughter of Pharaoh: Intermarriage, Conversion and the Impurity of Woman." *Journal of Ancient Near East Society* 16–17 (1984–1985): 23–37.
———. "Menstruants and the Sacred in Judaism and Christianity." In *Women's History and Ancient History*, ed. Sarah B. Pomeroy, 273–99. Chapel Hill: University of North Carolina Press, 1991.
Conley, Verena Andermatt. *Hélène Cixous: Writing the Feminine.* Lincoln: University of Nebraska Press, 1984.
Connolly, R. Hugh. *Didascalia Apostolorum: Syriac Version Translated and Accompanied by the Verona Latin Fragments.* Oxford: Clarendon Press, 1929.
Cooper, Kate. *The Virgin and the Bride: Idealized Womanhood in Late Antiquity.* Cambridge, Mass.: Harvard University Press, 1996.
Crouzel, Henri. *Origen: The Life and Thought of the First Great Theologian.* Trans. A. S. Worrall. San Francisco: Harper and Row, 1989.
Danielou, Jean. *Théologie du Judéo-Christianisme.* Paris: Desclee, 1958. Trans. J. A. Baker as *The Theology of Jewish Christianity.* London: Darton, Longman, and Todd, 1964.
De Lange. *Origen and the Jews.* Cambridge: Cambridge University Press, 1976.
De Lauretis, Teresa, ed. *Feminist Studies, Critical Studies.* Bloomington: Indiana University Press, 1985.
———. *Technologies of Gender.* Bloomington: Indiana University Press, 1987.
Dean-Jones, Lesley. "The Cultural Construct of the Female Body in Classical Greek Science." In *Women's History and Ancient History*, ed. Sarah Pomeroy, 111–38. Chapel Hill: University of North Carolina Press, 1991.
———. *Women's Bodies in Classical Greek Science.* Oxford: Clarendon Press, 1994.
Delaney, Janice, Mary Jane Lupton, Emily Toth. *The Curse: A Cultural History of Menstruation.* New York: Dutton, 1976.
Dinari, Yedidyah. "The Customs of Menstrual Impurity: Their Origin and Development." *Tarbiz* 49 (1979–80): 302–24 [Hebrew].
———. "The Profanation of the Holy by the Menstruant Woman and 'Takanot Ezra.'" *Te'uda* 3 (1983): 17–38 [Hebrew].
Douglas, Mary. "The Anthropologist and the Believer." Henry Rapoport Lecture, 1993 [unpublished].

———. *Purity and Danger: An Analysis of the Concepts of Pollution and Taboo.* London and New York: ARK Paperbacks, 1966 [repr. 1989].
duBois, Page. *Sowing the Body: Psychoanalysis and Ancient Representations of Women.* Chicago: University of Chicago Press, 1988.
Dunn, James. *Jesus, Paul, and the Law: Studies in Mark and Galatians.* Louisville: Westminster/John Knox Press, 1990.
Eider, Rabbi Shimon D. *Halachos of Niddah.* Lakewood, N.J.: Feldheim, 1981.
Eilberg-Schwartz, Howard. *God's Phallus and Other Problems for Men and Monotheism.* Boston: Beacon Press, 1994.
———. *The Savage in Judaism: An Anthropology of Israelite and Ancient Judaism.* Bloomington: Indiana University Press, 1990.
Eilberg-Schwartz, Howard, ed. *People of the Body: Jews and Judaism from an Embodied Perspective.* Albany: State University of New York Press, 1992.
Elliger, Karl. *Leviticus. Handbuch zum Alten Testament*, Erste Reihe 4. Tübingen: J. C. B. Mohr, 1966.
Elm, Susanna. *"Virgins of God": The Making of Asceticism in Late Antiquity.* New York: Oxford University Press, 1996.
Epstein, J. N. *Der gaonische Kommentar zur Ordnung Tohoroth.* Berlin: Mayer und Müller, 1915 [repr. Jerusalem 1982].
———. *Introduction to Tannaitic Literature: Mishna, Tosephta and Halakhic Midrashim.* Ed. E. Z. Melamed. Jerusalem: Magnes, 1957 [Hebrew].
———, *Introduction to the Text of the Mishnah.* Jerusalem: Magnes, 1948 [Hebrew].
Eshkoli, A. Z. "Halakha and Customs Among the Falasha Jews in the Light of Rabbinic and Karaite Halakha." *Tarbiz* 7 (1936): 121–25 [Hebrew].
Faivre, Alexandre. *The Emergence of the Laity in the Early Church.* New York: Paulist Press, 1990 [orig. French ed. 1984].
Feld, Geburgis. "' . . . Wie es eben Frauen ergeht.' (Gen. 31, 35): Kulturgeschichtliche Überlegungen zum gegenwaertigen Umgang mit der Menstruation der Frau in Gesellschaft und Theologie." In *Von der Wurzel getragen: Christlich-feministische Exegese in Auseinandersetzung mit Antijudaismus*, ed. L. Schottroff and M.-T. Wacker, 29–43. Leiden: Brill, 1996.
Feldman, David M. *Marital Relations, Birth Control and Abortion in Jewish Law.* New York: Schocken, 1968.
Fonrobert, Charlotte. "Women's Bodies, Women's Blood: On the Politics of Gender in Rabbinic Judaism." Ph.D. Dissertation, Berkeley: Graduate Theological Union, 1995.
Foucault, Michel. *The Order of Things.* New York: Vintage Books, 1970.
Fraade, Stephen. "Ascetical Aspects of Ancient Judaism." In *Jewish Spirituality from the Bible through the Middle Ages*, ed. Arthur Green, 253–88. New York: Crossroads, 1986.
Frankel, Z. *Mavo ha-Yerushalmi.* Breslau: Schletter, 1870 [repr. Jerusalem 1967].

Frederiksen, Paula. "Did Jesus Oppose the Purity Laws?" *Bible Review* 11:3 (June 1995): 19–47.

———. "What You See Is What You Get: Context and Content in Current Research on the Historical Jesus." *Theology Today* 52:1 (1995): 75–98.

Fuss, Diana. *Essentially Speaking: Feminism, Nature and Difference*. New York: Routledge, 1989.

Gafni, Isaiah. *The Jews of Babylonia in the Talmudic Era: A Social and Cultural History*. Jerusalem: The Zalman Shazar Center for Jewish History, 1990 [Hebrew].

Gallop, Jane. *Thinking Through the Body*. New York: Columbia University Press, 1988.

Gatens, Moira. *Feminism and Philosophy: Perspectives on Difference and Equality*. Cambridge: Polity Press, 1991.

Gnilka, Joachim. *Das Matthaeusevangelium I. Teil (1:1 - 13:58)*. Herders Theologischer Kommentar zum Neuen Testament. Freiburg and Basel: Herder, 1986.

Goldberg, Abraham. "The Babylonian Talmud." In *The Literature of the Sages 1*, ed. Schmuel Safrai, 323–45. Philadelphia: Fortress Press, 1987.

———. "The Mishna—A Study Book of Halakha." In *The Literature of the Sages 1*, ed. Shmuel Safrai, 211–63. Philadelphia: Fortress Press, 1987.

Goldenberg, Naomi. *Resurrecting the Body: Feminism, Religion and Psychotherapy*. New York: Crossroads, 1989.

Goodblatt, David M., *Rabbinic Instruction in Sasanian Babylonia*. Leiden: Brill, 1975.

Goodman, Martin. "Nerva, The Fiscus Judaicus and Jewish Identity." *Journal for Roman Studies* 79 (1989): 40–44.

Green, Monica. "The Transmission of Ancient Theories of Female Physiology and Diseases through the Early Middle Ages." Ph.D. Dissertation, Princeton University, 1985.

———. "Women's Medical Practice and Health Care in Medieval Europe." *Signs* 14 (1988/89): 434–73.

Greenberg, Blu. *Women and Judaism: A View from Tradition*. Philadelphia: JPS, 1982.

Greenberg, Moshe. "The Etymology of נדה '(Menstrual) Impurity.'" In *Solving Riddles and Untying Knots: Biblical, Epigraphic and Semitic Studies in Honor of Jonas Greenfield*, ed. Z. Zevit, S. Gitin, and M. Sokoloff, 69–79. Winona Lake, Ind.: Eisenbrauns, 1995.

Grosz, Elizabeth. *Sexual Subversions: Three Feminist French Writers*. Sydney: Allen & Unwin, 1989.

———. *Volatile Bodies: Toward a Corporeal Feminism*. Bloomington: Indiana University Press, 1994.

Gruzman, Meir. "On the Halakhic Development Which Led the Blood of Defloration to Be Treated as Ritually Unclean." *Sidra* 5 (1989): 47–63 [Hebrew].

Gryson, Roger. *The Ministry of Women in the Early Church*. Collegeville, Minn.: The Liturgical Press, 1976.

Guehlich, Robert A. *Mark 1—8:26*. Word Biblical Commentary 34A. Dallas: Word Books, 1989.

Hahn, Ferdinand. "Die Verwurzelung des Christentums im Judentum." *Kerygma und Dogma* 34 (1988): 193–209.

Halperin, David M. "Why Is Diotima a Woman? Platonic Eros and the Figuration of Gender." In *Before Sexuality: The Construction of Erotic Experience in the Ancient Greek World*, ed. D. Halperin, J. Winkler, and F. Zeitlin, 257–309. Princeton: Princeton University Press, 1990.

Hann, Robert. "Judaism and Jewish Christianity in Antioch: Charisma and Conflict in the First Century." *Journal of Religious History* 14:4 (1987): 341–60.

Hanson, Ann Ellis. "Continuity and Change: Three Case Studies in Hippocratic Gynecological Therapy and Theory." In *Women's History & Ancient History*, ed. S. Pomeroy, 73–111. Chapel Hill: University of North Carolina Press, 1991.

———. "The Medical Writers' Women." In *Before Sexuality: The Construction of Erotic Experience in the Ancient Greek World*, ed. D. Halperin, J. Winkler, and F. Zeitlin, 309–39. Princeton: Princeton University Press, 1990.

Haraway, Donna. *Simians, Cyborgs, and Women: The Reinvention of Nature*. New York: Routledge, 1991.

Harrington, Hannah K. *The Impurity Systems of Qumran and the Rabbis: Biblical Foundations*. SBL Dissertation Series 143. Atlanta: Scholars Press, 1993.

Hartin, Patrick. "Jewish Christianity: Focus on Antioch in the First Century." *Scriptura* 36 (1991): 38–50.

Hasan-Rokem, Galit. "Narratives in Dialogue: A Folk Literary Perspective on Interreligious Contacts in the Holy Land in Rabbinic Literature of Late Antiquity." In *Sharing the Sacred: Religious Contacts and Conflicts in the Holy Land*, ed. A. Kofsky and G. G. Stroumsa, 109–31. Jerusalem: Yad Izhak Ben Zvi, 1998.

———. *The Web of Life—Folklore in Rabbinic Literature*. Tel Aviv: Am Oved, 1996 [Hebrew].

Hauptman, Judith. *The Development of the Talmudic Sugya: The Relationship Between Tannaitic and Amoraic Sources*. Lanham, Md.: University Press of America, 1988.

———. "Feminist Perspectives on Rabbinic Texts." In *Feminist Perspectives on Jewish Studies*, ed. Lynn Davidman and Shelly Tenenbaum, 40–62. New Haven: Yale University Press, 1994.

———. "Images of Women in the Talmud." In *Religion and Sexism*, ed. Rosemary Ruether, 184–212. New York: Simon and Schuster, 1974.

———. *Rereading the Rabbis: A Woman's Voice*. Boulder, Colo.: Westview Press, 1998.

Hayes, Christine E. *Between the Babylonian and Palestinian Talmuds: Accounting* for Halakhic Difference in Selected Sugyot from Tractate Avodah Zarah. New York and Oxford: Oxford University Press, 1997.

Heggelbacher, Othmar. *Geschichte des frühchristlichen Kirchenrechts bis zum Konzil von Nizäa 325.* Freiburg/Schweiz: Universitätsverlag, 1974.

Hengel, Martin, and Rudolf Hengel. "Die Heilungen Jesu und medizinische Denken." In *Der Wunderbegriff im Neuen Testament*, ed. Alfred Suhl, 338–74. Darmstadt: Wissenschaftliche Buchgesellschaft, 1980 [orig. ed. 1959].

Heschel, Susannah, ed. *On Being a Jewish Feminist.* New York: Schocken, 1983.

Hoffmann, D. *Das Buch Levitikus.* Berlin: Poppelauer, 1905.

Holtz, Traugott. "Der antiochenische Zwischenfall (Galater 2:11–14)." *New Testament Studies* 32 (1986): 344–61.

Hort, F. J. A. *Judaistic Christianity.* London: Macmillan, 1894.

Ide, Arthur Frederick. *Woman as Priest, Bishop and Laity in the Early Catholic Church to 440 A.D.* Texas: Ide House, 1984.

Ilan, Tal. *Jewish Women in Greco-Roman Palestine.* Peabody, Mass.: Hendrickson Publishers, 1996.

———. *Mine and Yours Are Hers: Retrieving Women's History from Rabbinic Literature.* Leiden: Brill, 1997.

Irigaray, Luce. *An Ethics of Sexual Difference.* Ithaca: Cornell University Press, 1993 [orig. French: 1984].

———. *Speculum of the Other Woman.* Ithaca: Cornell University Press, 1985 [orig. French ed. 1974].

———. *This Sex Which Is Not One.* Ithaca: Cornell University Press, 1985 [orig. French ed. 1977].

Jacobs, Louis. *The Talmudic Argument.* Cambridge: Cambridge University Press, 1984.

Jaffee, Martin S. "The Babylonian Appropriation of the Talmud Yerushalmi: Redactional Studies in the Horayot Tractates." In *New Perspectives on Ancient Judaism*, ed. J. Avery-Peck, 4:3–27. Lanham, Md.: University Press of America, 1989.

———. "The Mishnah in Talmudic Exegesis: Observations on Tractate Maaserot of the Talmud Yerushalmi." In *Approaches to Ancient Judaism IV*, ed. W. S. Green, 137–57. Chico, Calif.: Scholars Press, 1983.

Jardine, Alice. *Gynesis: Configurations of Woman and Modernity.* Ithaca: Cornell University Press, 1985.

Jastrow, Marcus. *A Dictionary of the Targumim, the Talmud Babli and Yerushalmi, and the Midrashic Literature.* New York: Judaica Press, 1992 [repr.].

Jerome. *Select Letters.* Trans. F. A. Wright. Cambridge, Mass.: Harvard University Press, 1991.

Joy, Morna. "Levinas: Alterity, the Feminine, and Women—A Meditation." (unpublished paper)

Kamesar, Adam. *Jerome, Greek Scholarship, and the Hebrew Bible: A Study of the Quaestiones Hebraicae in Genesim*. Oxford: Clarendon Press, 1992.

Kaplan, Marion. "Tradition and Transition—The Acculturation, Assimilation and Integration of Jews in Imperial Germany—A Gender Analysis." *Leo Baeck Year Book* 27 (1982): 3–37.

Kellenbach, Katharina von. *Anti-Judaism in Feminist Religious Writings*. Atlanta, Ga.: Scholars Press, 1994.

Kelly, J. N. D. *Jerome: His Life, Writings, and Controversies*. New York: Harper and Row, 1975.

Kertelge, Karl. *Das Markusevangelium*. In *Die Neue Echter Bibel*. Würzburg: Echter Verlag, 1994.

Kinzig, Wolfram. " 'Non-Separation': Closeness and Co-Operation Between Jews and Christians in the Fourth Century." *Vigiliae Christianae* 45 (1991): 27–53.

Klijn, A. F. "The Study of Jewish Christianity." *New Testament Studies* 20:4 (1974): 419–32.

Knohl, Israel. *The Sanctuary of Silence: The Priestly Torah and the Holiness School*. Philadelphia: Fortress Press, 1995.

Kohut, A., ed. *Arukh ha-Shalem 1–9*. Vienna 1878–1937 [repr. New York: Pardes, 1955].

Koltun, Elisabeth. *The Jewish Woman: New Perspectives*. New York: Schocken, 1976.

Kraeling, Carl. "The Jewish Community at Antioch." *Journal of Biblical Literature* 51 (1932): 130–60.

Kraemer, David. *The Mind of the Talmud: An Intellectual History of the Bavli*. Oxford: Oxford University Press, 1990.

Kraemer, Ross. *Her Share of the Blessing*. Oxford and New York: Oxford University Press, 1992.

———. "Monastic Jewish Women in Greco-Roman Egypt: Philo Judaeus on the Therapeutrides." *Signs* 14 (1989): 342–70.

Kraemer, Ross, ed. *Maenads, Martyrs, Matrons, Monastics: A Sourcebook on Women's Religion in the Greco-Roman World*. Philadelphia: Fortress Press, 1988.

Kraft, Robert. "In Search of 'Jewish Christianity' and its 'Theology': Problems of Definition and Methodology." In *Judéo-Christianisme: Recherches historiques et théologiques offertes en homage au J. Danielou*, 81–92. Paris: Recherches de Science Religieuse, 1972.

———. "The Multiform Jewish Heritage of Early Christianity." In *Christianity, Judaism and Other Graeco-Roman Cults* 3, ed. Jacob Neusner, 174–99. Leiden: Brill, 1975.

Krauss, Samuel. *Griechische und Lateinische Lehnwörter im Talmud, Midrasch und Targum*. Berlin: 1898–99 [repr. Hildesheim: Olm Verlag, 1987].

———. *Talmudishe Archäologie: Grundisse der Gesamtwissenschaft des Judentums V*. Leipzig: G. Fock G.m.b.h., 1911.

Kriegel, Stanley K. "Jewish Christianity: Definitions and Terminology." *New Testament Studies* 24 (1978): 410–15.

Kristeva, Julia. *Powers of Horror: An Essay on Abjection*. Trans. Leon S. Roudiez. New York: Columbia University Press, 1982.

Laporte, Jean. *The Role of Women in Early Christianity*. Studies in Women and Religion 7. New York and Toronto: Edwin Mellem Press, 1982.

Laqueur, Thomas. *Making Sex: Body and Gender from the Greeks to Freud*. Cambridge, Mass.: Harvard University Press, 1990.

Levinas, Emmanuel. "Judaism and the Feminine." In *Difficult Freedom: Essays on Judaism*, 30–38. Baltimore: Johns Hopkins University Press, 1990.

———. *Nine Talmudic Readings*. Trans. Annette Aronowicz. Bloomington: Indiana University Press, 1985.

Levine, Amy-Jill. "Second Temple Judaism, Jesus, and Women: Yeast of Eden." *Biblical Interpretation* 2:1 (1994): 8–33.

———. *"Women Like This": New Perspectives on Jewish Women in the Greco-Roman World*. Atlanta, Ga.: Scholars Press, 1991.

Levine, Baruch. *Leviticus*. JPS Commentary. Philadelphia and New York: Jewish Publication Society, 1989.

Lieberman, Saul. *Greek in Jewish Palestine*. New York: Jewish Theological Seminary of America, 1965.

———. *Hellenism in Jewish Palestine: Studies in the Literary Transmission, Beliefs and Manners of Palestine in the First Century*. New York: Jewish Theological Seminary of America, 1962.

———. "The Knowledge of Halakhah by the Author (or Authors) of the Heikhaloth" (Appendix). In *Apocalyptic and Merkavah Mysticism*, ed. Ithamar Gruenwald, 241–45. Leiden: Brill, 1980.

———. *Tosefet Rishonim 1–4*. Jerusalem: Bamberger and Wahrmann, 1937–39 [Hebrew].

———. *The Tosefta*. New York: The Jewish Theological Seminary, 1973 [Hebrew].

———. *Tosefta ki-Fshuta: A Comprehensive Commentary on the Tosefta 1–8*. New York: Jewish Theological Seminary, 1955–83 [Hebrew].

Lieberman, Saul. *Greek in Jewish Palestine/Hellenism in Jewish Palestine*. New York: Jewish Theological Seminary of America, 1994.

Lloyd, G. R. E. *Science, Folklore, and Ideology*. Cambridge: Cambridge University Press, 1983.

Luz, Ulrich. *Das Evangelium nach Matthäus 8–17*. Evangelisch-Katholischer Kommentar zum Neuen Testament. Gütersloh: Neukirchen, 1989.

Malina, Bruce J. "Jewish Christianity or Christian Judaism: Toward a Hypothetical Definition." *Journal for the Study of Judaism* 7:1 (1976): 46–57.

Manuli, Paola. "Fisiologia e patologia del femminile negli scritti ippocratici dell' antica ginecologia greca." In *Hippocratica: Actes du colloque hippocratique de Paris*. Paris: CNRS, 1980.

Margulies, Mordecai. *Midrash Wayyikra Rabbah: A Critical Edition*. New York and Jerusalem: The Jewish Theological Seminary, 1993.

Marmorstein, A. "Judaism and Christianity in the Middle of the Third Century." *Hebrew Union College Annual* 10 (1937): 223–65.

Martin, Emily. "Body Narratives, Body Boundaries." In *Cultural Studies*, ed. Lawrence Grossberg, Cary Nelson, Paula Treichler, 409–23. New York: Routledge, 1992.

Mayer, Günter. *Die jüdische Frau in der hellenistisch-römischen Antike*. Stuttgart and Berlin: Verlag W. Kohlhammer, 1987.

Meacham, Tirzah Zechurah. "Mishnah Tractate Niddah with Introduction: A Critical Edition with Notes on Variants, Commentary, Redaction and Chapters in Legal History and Realia." Ph.D. Dissertation, Hebrew University, Jerusalem, 1989.

Meiri, Menahem ben Solomon. *Beit ha-Behirah*. Ed. Abraham Sofer. Jerusalem: Makhon ha-Talmud, 1970 [Hebrew].

Mendes-Flohr, Paul, ed. *The Jew in the Modern World: A Documentary History*. New York and Oxford: Oxford University Press, 1980.

Methuen, Charlotte. "Widows, Bishops and the Struggle for Authority in the Didascalia Apostolorum." *Journal of Ecclesiastical History* 46:2 (1995): 197–213.

Metzger, David, ed. *Hidushei ha-Rashba al Massekhet Niddah*. Jerusalem: Mosad ha-Rav Kook, 1989.

Miles, Margret. *Carnal Knowledge: Female Nakedness and Religious Meaning in the Christian West*. New York: Vintage Books, 1991.

Milgrom, Jacob. *Leviticus 1–16: A New Translation with Introduction and Commentary*. The Anchor Bible. New York/London: Doubleday/The Anchor Bible, 1991.

———. "The Priestly Impurity System." In *Proceedings of the Ninth World Congress of Jewish Studies*, 121–27. Jerusalem: World Union of Jewish Studies, 1986.

Miller, Patricia Cox. "The Blazing Body: Ascetic Desire in Jerome's Letter to Eustochium." *Journal of Early Christian Studies* 1:1 (March 1993): 21–45.

Mimouni, Simon C. "Pour une Définition Nouvelle du Judéo-Christianisme Ancien." *New Testament Studies* 38 (1992): 161–86.

Minh-ha, Trinh T., *Women, Native, Other*. Bloomington: Indiana University Press, 1989.

Munck, J. "Jewish Christianity in Post-Apostolic Times." *New Testament Studies* 6 (1960): 103–16.

Muraoka, T. *A Grammar of Biblical Hebrew*. Rome: Editrice Pontificio Istituto Biblico, 1991.

Murray, Robert. "Jews, Hebrews and Christians: Some Needed Distinctions." *Novum Testamentum* 24:3 (1982): 194–208.

Myers, Jody Elizabeth. "The Myth of Matriarchy in Recent Writings on Jewish Women's Spirituality." *Jewish Social Studies* N.S. 4:1 (fall 1997): 1–27.

Neusner, J. "From Scripture to Mishnah: The Origins of the Mishnaic Tractate Niddah," *Journal of Jewish Studies* 29 (1978): 135–48.

———. *A History of the Jews in Babylonia*, vols. 1–5. Leiden: Brill, 1965–70.

———. *A History of the Mishnaic Law of Purities*, vols. 15–16, 21–22. Leiden: Brill, 1976–77.

———. *The Idea of Purity in Ancient Judaism*. Leiden: Brill, 1973.

Noth, Martin. *Leviticus: A Commentary*. Philadelphia: Westminster Press, 1965 [English].

Oppenheimer, Aharon. *Babylonia Judaica in the Talmudic Period*. In collaboration with Benjamin Isaac and Michael Lecker. Wiesbaden: L. Reichert, 1983.

Ouaknin, Marc-Alain. *The Burnt Book: Reading the Talmud*. Princeton: Princeton University Press, 1995.

Pardes, Ilana. *Countertraditions in the Bible*. Cambridge, Mass.: Harvard University Press, 1992.

Pesch, Rudolf. *Das Markusevangelium I. Teil: Einleitung und Kommentar zu Kapitel 1, 1–8, 26*. Herders Theologischer Kommentar zum Neuen Testament. Freiburg and Basel: Herder, 1976.

Peskowitz, Miriam. "Engendering Jewish Religious History" (unpublished).

———. "Family/ies in Antiquity: Evidence from Tannaitic Literature and Roman Galilean Architecture." In *The Jewish Family in Antiquity*, Brown Judaic Series 289, ed. Shaye Cohen, 9–39. Atlanta, Ga.: Scholars Press, 1993.

———. *Spinning Fantasies: Rabbis, Gender, and History*. Berkeley and Los Angeles: University of California Press, 1997.

———. "Spinning Tales: On Reading Gender and Otherness in Tannaitic Texts." In *The Other in Jewish Thought and History*, ed. L. J. Silberstein and Robert Cohn, 91–121. New York and London: New York University Press, 1994.

Plaskow, Judith. "Jewish Theology in Feminist Perspective." In *Feminist Perspectives on Jewish Studies*, ed. Lyn Davidman and Shelly Tenenbaum, 62–85. New Haven: Yale University Press, 1994.

———. *Standing Again at Sinai: Judaism from a Feminist Perspective*. San Francisco: Harper and Row, 1990.

Prell, Riv-Ellen. "The Vision of Woman in Classical Reform Judaism." *Journal of the American Academy of Religion* 50:4 (1982): 575–89.

Preuss, Julius. *Biblical and Talmudic Medicine*. Trans. F. Rosner. Northvale, N.J.: J. Aronson, 1993 [orig. German ed. 1911].

Profet, Margie. "Menstruation as a Defense Against Pathogens Transported by Germs." *Quarterly Review of Biology* 68:3 (1993): 335–81.

Rebenich, Stefan. *Hieronymus und sein Kreis: prosopographische und sozialgeschichtliche Untersuchungen*. Stuttgart: F. Steiner, 1992.

Reinhart, A. Kevin. "Impurity/No Danger." *History of Religions* 30:1 (1990): 1–24.

Rich, Adrienne. "Compulsory Heterosexuality and Lesbian Existence." In *Powers of*

*Desire*, ed. Ann Snitow, Christine Stansell, and Sharon Thompson, 177–205. New York: Monthly Review Press, 1983.

———. *On Lies, Secrets, and Silence.* New York: Norton, 1979.

Roth, Joel. "The Concepts of De-Oraita and De-Rabanan." In *The Halakhic Process*, 13–49. New York: The Jewish Theological Seminary, 1986.

Rousselle, Aline. "Observation feminine et idéologie masculine: Le corps de la femme d'après les médecins grecs." *Annales ESC* 35 (1980): 1089–1115.

———. *Porneia: On Desire and the Body in Antiquity.* Oxford: Basil Blackwell, 1988 [orig. French ed. 1983].

Ruether, Rosemary. "Misogynism and Virginal Feminism in the Fathers of the Church." In *Religion and Sexism*, ed. R. R. Ruether, 150–83. New York: Simon and Schuster, 1974.

———. "Mothers of the Church: Ascetic Women in the Later Patristic Age." In *Women of Spirit: Female Leadership in the Jewish and Christian Traditions*, ed. R. R. Ruether and Eleanor McLaughlin, 71–99. New York: Simon and Schuster, 1979.

———. *New Women/New Earth.* New York: The Seabury Press, 1975.

———. "Women's Body and Blood: The Sacred and the Impure." In *Through the Devil's Gateway: Women, Religion and Taboo*, ed. Alison Joseph, 7–22. London: SPCK, 1990.

Salisbury, Joyce. *Churchfathers, Independent Virgins.* London and New York: Verso, 1991.

Sand, Alexander. *Das Evangelium nach Matthaeus.* Regensburg: Verlag Friedrich Pustet, 1985.

Sanders, E. P. *Jewish Law from Jesus to the Mishnah.* Philadelphia: Trinity Press International, 1990.

———. *Judaism: Practice and Belief 63 B.C.E.–66 C.E.* Philadelphia: Trinity Press International, 1992.

———. *Paul and Palestinian Judaism: A Comparison of Patterns of Religion.* Philadelphia: Fortress Press, 1977.

Sanders, Jack. "Jewish Christianity in Antioch Before the Time of Hadrian: Where Does Identity Lie?" *SBL Seminar Paper Series* 31 (1992): 346–61.

Scarry, Elaine. *The Body in Pain.* Oxford and New York: Oxford University Press, 1985.

Schaff, Ph., and H. Wace, eds. "Life of Anthony." In *Nicene and Post-Nicene Fathers of the Christian Church*, 2nd Series, vol. 4. Grand Rapids, Mich.: Wm. B. Eerdmans, 1891.

Schechter, Salomon, ed. *Aboth de Rabbi Nathan.* London and Frankfurt: Nutt and Kauffman Knöpfelmacher, 1887 [repr. Jerusalem 1979].

Schmithals, Walter. *Das Evangelium nach Markus, Kapitel 1–9,1.* Oekumenischer Taschenbuch-Kommentar zum Neuen Testament 2/1. Gütersloh: Gerd Mohn, 1979.

Schor, Naomi. "This Essentialism Which Is Not One: Coming to Grips with Irigaray." In *Engaging With Irigaray: Feminist Philosophy and Modern European Thought*, 57–78. New York: Columbia University Press, 1994.

Schor, Naomi, Carolyn Burke, and Margaret Whitford, eds. *Engaging With Irigaray: Feminist Philosophy and Modern European Thought*. New York: Columbia University Press, 1994.

Schottroff, Luise. *Befreiungserfahrung: Studien zur Sozialgeschichte des Neuen Testaments*. Theologische Bücherei 82. Munich: Chr. Kaiser Verlag, 1990.

Schottroff, Luise, and Marie-Theres Wacker, eds. *Von der Wurzel getragen: Christlich-feministische Exegese in Auseinandersetzung mit Antijudaismus*. Leiden: E. J. Brill, 1996.

Schüssler Fiorenza, Elisabeth. *In Memory of Her: A Feminist Theological Reconstruction of Christian Origins*. New York: Crossroads, 1985.

Scott, James C. *Domination and the Arts of Resistance: Hidden Transcripts*. New Haven: Yale University Press, 1990.

Scott, Joan W., "Deconstructing Equality-Versus-Difference: Or, the Uses of Poststructuralist Theory for Feminism." *Feminist Studies* 14:1 (1988): 33–50.

———. "Gender: A Useful Category of Historical Analysis." *American Historical Review* 91 (1986): 1053–75.

Scott, Lynn T. "Not Merely Chattel: Women as Guardians of Holiness in the Mishnah's Society." In *Recovering the Role of Women: Power and Authority in Rabbinic Jewish Society*, 23–37. Atlanta, Ga.: Scholars Press, 1992.

Selvidge, Marla. *Woman, Cult and Miracle Recital: A Redactional Critical Investigation on Mark 5:24–34*. London and Toronto: Associated University Presses, 1990.

Simon, Marcel. "Réflexions sur le Judéo-Christianisme." In *Christianity, Judaism and Other Graeco-Roman Cults*, vol. 2, ed. Jacob Neusner, 53–76. Leiden: Brill, 1975.

———. *Verus Israel: A Study of the Relations Between Christians and Jews in the Roman Empire (135–425)*. The Littman Library of Jewish Civilization. Oxford: Oxford University Press, 1986 [orig. French ed. 1948].

Sireling, Linda. "The Jewish Woman: Different and Equal." In *Through the Devil's Gateway: Women, Religion and Taboo*, ed. Alison Joseph, 87–96. London: SPCK, 1990.

Slonim, Rivkah. *Total Immersion: A Mikvah Anthology*. Northvale, N.J., and London: Jason Aaronson, 1996.

Smith, Sidonie. *Subjectivity, Identity, and the Body: Women's Autobiographical Practices in the Twentieth Century*. Bloomington: Indiana University Press, 1993.

Spivak, Gayatri Chakravorty. *In Other Worlds*. New York and London: Routledge, 1988.

———. *The Post-Colonial Critic: Interviews, Strategies, Dialogues*. New York and London: Routledge, 1990.

Stemberger, Günter. *Einleitung in Talmud und Midrasch*. Munich: C. H. Beck, 1992.

Stern, David. "Midrash and Indeterminacy." *Critical Inquiry* 15 (1988): 132–61.

Stiegman, Emero. "Rabbinic Anthropology." In *Aufstieg und Niedergang der Römischen Welt* 19:2, ed. H. Temporini and W. Haase, 488–579. Berlin: Walter de Gruyter, 1977.

Strecker, Georg. "Judenchristentum." *TRE* 17 (1988): 310–25.

———. "On the Problem of Jewish Christianity." Appendix, *Orthodoxy and Heresy in Earliest Christianity*, ed. Walter Bauer, 241–85. Philadelphia: Fortress Press, 1971.

Sussman, Yacov, "A Study of the History of Halakhah and the Dead Sea Scrolls." *Tarbiz* 59 (1989): 11–76 [Hebrew].

Swartz, Michael D. " 'Like the Ministering Angels': Ritual and Purity in Early Jewish Mysticism and Magic." *AJS Review* 19:2 (1994): 135–67.

Swidler, Leonard. *Women in Judaism: The Status of Women in Formative Judaism*. Metuchen, N.J.: The Scarecrow Press, 1976.

Taylor, Joan. "The Phenomenon of Early Jewish-Christianity: Reality or Scholarly Invention?" *Vigiliae Christianae* 44 (1990): 313–34.

Taylor, Justin. "Ancient Texts and Modern Critics: Acts 15, 1–34." *Revue Biblique* 99:2 (1992): 373–78.

Taylor, Miriam S. *Anti-Judaism and Early Christian Identity: A Critique of the Scholarly Consensus*. Leiden: E. J. Brill, 1995.

Temkin, O. (trans.). *Soranus' Gynecology*. Baltimore: Johns Hopkins University Press, 1991.

Theissen, Gerd. *Urchristliche Wundergeschichten: Ein Beitrag zur formgeschichtlichen Erforschung der synoptischen Evangelien*. Studien zum Neuen Testament 8. Gütersloh: Gerd Mohn, 1974.

Thurston, Bonnie Bowman. *The Widows: A Women's Ministry in the Early Church*. Philadelphia: Fortress Press, 1989.

Tidner, Erik. *Didascaliae Apostolorum Canonum Ecclesiasticorum Traditionis Apostolicae Versiones Latinae*. Berlin: Akademie-Verlag, 1963.

Tigay, Jeffrey H. "Examination of the Accused Bride in 4Q159: Forensic Medicine at Qumran." *Journal of the Ancient Near Eastern Society* 22 (1993): 129–34.

Torjesen, Karen Jo. *When Women Were Priests: Women's Leadership in the Early Church and the Scandal of Their Subordination in the Rise of Christianity*. San Francisco: Harper, 1993.

Trummer, Peter. *Die blutende Frau: Wunderheilung im Neuen Testament*. Freiburg and Basel: Herder, 1991.

Umansky, Ellen. "Creating a Jewish Feminist Theology." In *Weaving the Vision: New Patterns in Feminist Spirituality*, ed. Judith Plaskow and Carol P. Christ, 187–99. San Francisco: Harper and Row, 1989.

Umansky, Ellen, and Dianne Ashton, eds. *Four Centuries of Jewish Women's Spirituality*. Boston: Beacon Press, 1992.

Urbach, Ephraim. *The Sages: Their Concepts and Beliefs.* Cambridge, Mass.: Harvard University Press, 1987.
Valler, Shulamit. *Women and Womanhood in the Stories of the Babylonian Talmud.* Tel Aviv: Hakibbutz Hemeuhad Publishing House, 1993 [Hebrew].
Vööbus, Arthur. *The Didascalia Apostolorum in Syriac I + II*, CSCO 401–2, 407–8. Louvain: Secrétariat du Corpus SCO, 1979 [with English trans.].
Wasserfall, Rachel. "Menstruation and Identity: The Meaning of Niddah for Moroccan Women Immigrants to Israel." In *People of the Body: Jews and Judaism from an Embodied Perspective*, ed. H. Eilberg-Schwartz, 309–28. Albany: State University of New York Press, 1992.
Wegner, Judith Romney. *Chattel or Person? The Status of Women in the Mishnah.* New York and Oxford: Oxford University Press, 1988.
———. "The Image and Status of Women in Classical Rabbinic Judaism." In *Jewish Women in Historical Perspective*, ed. Judith R. Baskin, 68–94. Detroit: Wayne State University Press, 1991.
Weil, Kari. *Androgyny and the Denial of Difference.* Charlottesville: University Press of Virginia, 1992.
Weinreich, Otto. *Antike Heilungswunder: Untersuchungen zum Wunderglauben der Griechen und Römer.* Religionsgeschichtliche Versuche und Vorarbeiten. Giessen: Alfred Töpelmann, 1909.
Weiss, I. H. *Sifra.* Vienna, 1862 [repr. New York: Om Publishing, 1947].
Weissler, Chava. "Mitzvot Built into the Body: Tkhines for Niddah, Pregnancy, and Childbirth." In *People of the Body: Jews and Judaism from an Embodied Perspective*, ed. H. Eilberg-Schwartz, 101–17. Albany: State University of New York Press, 1992.
———. "Women's Studies and Women's Prayers: Reconstructing the Religious History of Ashkenazic Women." *Jewish Social Studies* New Series 1 (1995): 28–47.
Wilken, Robert. *John Chrysostom and the Jews: Rhetoric and Reality in the Late Fourth Century.* Berkeley and Los Angeles: University of California Press, 1983.
———. *Judaism and the Early Christian Mind: A Study of Cyril of Alexandria's Exegesis and Theology.* New Haven: Yale University Press, 1971.
Williams, Michael A. *Rethinking "Gnosticism": An Argument for Dismantling a Dubious Category.* Princeton: Princeton University Press, 1996.
Winkler, John. *The Constraints of Desire: The Anthropology of Sex and Gender in Ancient Greece.* London: Routledge, 1989.
Wire, Antoinette Clark. *The Corinthian Women Prophets: A Reconstruction Through Paul's Rhetoric.* Philadelphia: Fortress Press, 1990.
Witherington, Ben. *Women and the Genesis of Christianity.* New York and Sydney: Cambridge University Press, 1990.
———. *Women in the Earliest Church.* Cambridge: Cambridge University Press, 1988.
———. *Women in the Ministry of Jesus: A Study of Jesus' Attitudes to Women and*

*Their Roles as Reflected in His Earthly Life.* Cambridge: Cambridge University Press, 1984.

Woolf, Virginia. *A Room of One's Own.* New York: Harcourt, Brace and World, 1957 [first published 1929].

Zeitlin, Froma I. "Signifying Difference: The Case of Hesiod's Pandora." In *Playing the Other: Gender and Society in Classical Greek Literature,* 53–87. Chicago and London: Chicago University Press, 1996.

Zuckermandel, M. S. *Tosephta Based on the Erfurt and Vienna Codices.* Jerusalem: Bamberger and Wahrman, 1937.

# INDEX OF PRIMARY SOURCES

**BIBLICAL**

Leviticus
| | |
|---|---|
| 5:3 | 294 |
| 11:29–47 | 237 |
| 12:7 | 294 |
| 13 | 200, 265 |
| 15 | 20, 46, 56, 179, 193, 200 |
| 15:2–15 | 44, 184 |
| 15:2 | 44, 48–49, 53 |
| 15:7 | 46 |
| 15:13 | 105, 232 |
| 15:15 | 45 |
| 15:16–18 | 44 |
| 15:17 | 45 |
| 15:18 | 46 |
| 15:19–24 | 44 |
| 15:19 | 44, 49, 70–71, 74, 81–82, 98, 104, 180 |
| 15:20–22 | 248 |
| 15:24 | 46 |
| 15:25–30 | 45 |
| 15:25 | 104–5 |
| 15:27 | 193 |
| 15:28 | 104 |
| 15:30 | 45 |
| 15:31 | 19 |
| 16:6 | 63 |
| 18 | 20, 46 |
| 18:19 | 20, 46, 86 |
| 20:18 | 20, 46, 50 |
| 21:1 | 200 |
| 25:46 | 149 |

Deuteronomy
| | |
|---|---|
| 22:12 | 291 |
| 25:5–9 | 272–73, 290 |
| 27:26 | 290 |

1 Kings
| | |
|---|---|
| 6:8 | 235 |

Isaiah
| | |
|---|---|
| 49:12 | 224 |

Jeremiah
| | |
|---|---|
| 2:22 | 255 |

Ezekiel
| | |
|---|---|
| 7:19–20 | 223 |
| 36:17 | 223 |

Psalms
| | |
|---|---|
| 45:14 | 68 |

Proverbs
| | |
|---|---|
| 7:9 | 241 |
| 18:8 | 234 |
| 26:22 | 234 |
| 30:20 | 238 |

Job
| | |
|---|---|
| 15:34 | 224 |

Ezra
| | |
|---|---|
| 9:11 | 223 |

**NEW TESTAMENT**

Matthew
- 5:18 — 182
- 9:20 — 186, 188, 291, 293
- 11:28 — 167, 183
- 12:23 — 288
- 12:31–32 — 288
- 12:43–45 — 177

Mark
- 5:25–34 — 186, 188
- 5:25 — 293
- 5:26 — 291
- 5:28 — 291
- 5:29 — 293
- 5:31 — 291
- 5:33 — 292

Luke
- 8:42–48 — 186, 188
- 8:43 — 293
- 8:44 — 291
- 8:45 — 292
- 8:46 — 292
- 9:43 — 291

Acts
- 2:17 — 199
- 15:1 — 171
- 15:2 — 171
- 15:5 — 172
- 15:25 — 170

2 Corinthians
- 3:14 — 199
- 3:17–18 — 297

Galatians
- 2:1–10 — 170
- 2:14 — 298
- 3:10–12 — 290
- 3:27 — 289
- 4:4–5 — 202
- 5:14 — 290

**RABBINIC**

*Mishnah*

mKeritot
- 1:1 — 24
- 7:6 — 24

mMikvaot
- 2:2 — 88, 252

mNegaim
- 1:1 — 108
- 1:2 — 108
- 2:4 — 265
- 2:5 — 125, 264–65

mNiddah
- 1:1 — 85, 99, 251
- 1:3 — 139
- 2:2 — 75
- 2:5 — 28, 50, 237
- 2:6 — 106
- 2:7 — 106
- 4:1 — 269
- 4:2 — 270
- 5:1 — 53, 244, 254
- 5:3 — 270
- 5:6 — 269
- 5:7 — 272
- 5:8 — 143
- 5:9 — 143, 148, 272
- 6:1 — 143, 272
- 6:11–12 — 143, 272
- 7:2 — 90
- 7:4 — 224
- 8:1 — 28, 244
- 8:2 — 117
- 8:3 — 113
- 8:4 — 75
- 9:1 — 75, 244
- 9:3 — 80
- 9:6 — 259

mOhalot
- 1:8 — 58

mSanhedrin
- 7:2 — 239

mShabbat
- 2:6 — 24, 32
- 19:2 — 153

mShevuot
- 2:4 — 228

mSotah
- 3:4 — 273

mTerumah
- 3:1 — 90, 252

| mYevamot | | |
|---|---|---|
| 12:6 | 273 | |
| 13:1ff | 273 | |
| mYoma | | |
| 1:1 | 63 | |
| mZavim | | |
| 2:2 | 259 | |
| 5:1 | 193–94 | |

*Tosefta*

| tBerakhot | | |
|---|---|---|
| 2:13 | 19, 173, 204 | |
| tEduyot | | |
| 1:5 | 263 | |
| tMikvaot | | |
| 1:16 | 252 | |
| tNiddah | | |
| 1:5f | 139 | |
| 1:8–9 | 269 | |
| 3:9 | 50 | |
| 3:11 | 106 | |
| 4:3 | 259 | |
| 4:13 | 236 | |
| 5:1 | 269 | |
| 5:2 | 270 | |
| 5:4 | 138 | |
| 5:5 | 270 | |
| 5:14 | 273 | |
| 5:15–17 | 271 | |
| 6:2–7 | 143 | |
| 6:2 | 272–73 | |
| 6:4 | 143 | |
| 6:5–6 | 272 | |
| 6:8–9 | 144, 274 | |
| 6:17 | 117 | |
| 7:4 | 80, 117 | |
| 7:6 | 245 | |
| 7:7 | 245 | |
| 8:2 | 137 | |
| 8:4 | 234 | |
| 8:10 | 259 | |
| tShabbat | | |
| 15:8 | 156 | |
| tTerumah | | |
| 4:7 | 90, 252 | |

*Palestinian Talmud*

| pGittin | |
|---|---|
| 9:10 | 50, 262 |
| 8:10, 49c | 270 |
| pKetubbot | |
| 2:5, 26c | 26 |
| pNiddah | |
| 1:1, 48d | 250, 253 |
| 2:4, 50a | 50–52 |
| 2:6, 50a | 110, 258 |
| 2:7, 50b | 258 |
| pPeah | |
| 1:1, 15c | 274 |
| pShabbat | |
| 19:1, 16d | 263 |
| pYevamot | |
| 6:1, 7b | 237 |
| 1:6, 3a | 274 |

*Babylonian Talmud*

| bAvodah Zarah | |
|---|---|
| 7a | 263 |
| 28b | 278 |
| bBava Batra | |
| 96a | 252–53 |
| bBava Metzia | |
| 59b | 145 |
| bBekhorot | |
| 45a | 57, 239 |
| bBerakhot | |
| 22b | 225 |
| 61a | 238 |
| 63b | 263 |
| bEruvin | |
| 29b | 279 |
| bGittin | |
| 31b | 251 |
| 69b–70a | 279 |
| bHullin | |
| 16b | 238 |
| 27a | 229 |
| 44b | 263 |
| 47b | 279 |
| 70a | 237 |
| bKeritot | |
| 2a | 24 |

bKetubbot
- 4b — 24, 227
- 10a–b — 59–60
- 13a — 238
- 61a — 227
- 61b — 24
- 65b — 238

bKiddushin
- 31b — 151
- 79a — 252

bMakkot
- 23b — 239

bMeilah
- 17a — 39

bMenahot
- 34a — 235

bNedarim
- 20a–b — 145

bNiddah
- 2a–3b — 84
- 2b — 88, 93, 252, 254
- 3a — 90, 97, 237, 254–55
- 4b — 99, 250
- 9a–10b — 269
- 9b — 138
- 10b — 138–39, 141
- 16b — 55
- 17b — 51
- 19b — 110
- 20a — 110–11, 258
- 20b — 116, 118–19, 126, 261
- 21b — 244
- 31b — 25, 33, 269
- 40a — 244, 254
- 41b — 54, 56, 237, 244
- 45b — 271
- 47a — 149
- 48b — 144–45, 274
- 56a — 253
- 57a — 246
- 57b — 70–74, 76–78, 244, 255
- 58a — 248
- 59a — 112
- 59b — 245
- 65b–66a — 137, 261–62

bPesahim
- 111a — 34–35

bRosh Hashanah
- 26a — 18

bSanhedrin
- 93b — 262
- 108b — 269
- 113a — 229

bShabbat
- 31b — 24
- 32a–34a — 32–35
- 65a–b — 271
- 66b — 279
- 88a — 229
- 134a — 155, 156
- 152a — 230

bSotah
- 5a — 229
- 42b — 224

bYevamot
- 76a — 270

bYoma
- 75a — 238

*Extra-Canonical Tractates*

Avot di-Rabbi Nathan B
- 9, 13a — 31, 229

*Midrash*

Bereshit Rabbah
- 18:1 — 30–31, 227, 271
- 18:3 — 57

Leviticus Rabbah
- 14:4 — 240
- 30 — 262

Sifra Tazria
- Behar — 264
- Metzora — 276

Tanhuma Ki Tissa — 13

Noah
- 1:14b — 30

# GENERAL INDEX

Abaye, 99, 227n32, 255n70
Abaye's mother, 151–58, 213, 278n55
Adler, R., 221n1, 222n9, 263n49, 264nn51,53
Adorno, T., 217n4
Albeck, H., 236n37, 267n16
Alfasi, 157
Ambrose, 164
Amoraim, 14, 54, 248n34
Androcentrism, 8, 65, 69, 100, 212, 230n53
Aristotle, 41, 44, 58, 231n5, 240n59
Avot di-Rabbi Nathan, 31–32, 229n42

Baker, C., 223n16, 232n6, 236n36, 238n49
Bal, M., 70, 104, 119, 121, 219nn12,16, 249n40
Bamberger, B., 274n40
Baptism, 175–77, 204, 287n41, 287–88nn43,44,45
Baraita, 14, 57, 58, 75, 79, 89–90, 135, 141, 156–57, 252n52, 253n53, 279nn64,65, 296n86
Baskin, J., 32, 221n1, 230n49
Beauvoir, S. de, 42, 218n7
Bede, 296n86
Beit Midrash, 5, 7, 211–12, 239n55
Benjamin, W., 4, 253n56
Betz, H. D., 298n93
Biale, D., 232n11, 281n11

Biale, R., 148, 222n4,9, 225n23, 258n20, 271n29
Blood: Colors, 28, 103–6, 108–9, 229n38, 257nn8,11; of Desire, 116–17, 261n39; Flow, 71, 75, 94–95, 254nn59,60, 268n18; Stain, 28, 75, 80, 103–7, 112–15, 117–18, 243n7, 245nn17,20, 247, 257nn5,8, 258nn15,21; Virginal, 116
Body: Examination of, 137–51; and Impurity, 43–46; Instrumentalization, 57, 69; Male, 42, 44–46, 56; Medicalized, 42; Metaphors of Interior 65; and Objectification, 100; Sensation, 71–72, 76–78, 97; Women's, 3, 42, 44–67, 69, 137–151
Boid, I. R., 257n11
Bokser, B., 227n27, 244n10
Boyarin, D., 32, 34–38, 148, 204, 218n9, 219n11, 225n22, 229n46, 230nn47,53, 231n1, 233nn15,17, 239n55, 257n6, 261n37, 267n14, 279n2, 280n4, 281nn9,10,11, 287n36
Braidotti, R., 218n6
Brooten, B., 270n28
Brown, P., 162, 164, 280n3
Buckley, T., 129, 224n17
Butler, J., 231n3, 256n72

Carson, A., 62, 231n5, 241n69
Castelli, E., 162–65, 280nn3,4,5

Cixous, H., 66, 212
Clark, E., 162, 280n3
Cloke, G., 163–164, 281n8, 282n14
Cohen, A., 243n1
Cohen, S., 19, 204, 208, 222n11, 225n22, 256n3, 282n15, 296n86
Connolly, R. H., 207, 283n18, 288n47, 289n49
Cooper, K., 166, 280n3, 282n13, 283n17

Danielou, J., 284n22
Dean-Jones, L., 63, 95, 132, 230n50, 231n5, 235n35, 241n69, 266n10
Desire, 116, 119, 142, 261n39, 270n28
Deuterosis, 182–85, 209, 288nn46, 289n48
Didache, 284nn19,20
Didascalia Apostolorum, 11–12, 213–14; and Apostolic Authorship 170–72, 285–86nn29,30,32; and Holy Spirit, 174–79, 287n41; and Jewish-Christians 206–9, 286n31; and Women, 166–69, 203–6
Dinari, Y., 19, 222n11, 224n20
Dionysius, 196, 209, 296n85
Discourse: Authors of, 7; Counterdiscourse, 67, 69–70; Halakhic, 36, 73, 100; Medical, 235; of Niddah, 69; Rupture, 68–72, 83, 97–100; Talmudic, 85
Douglas, M., 107
duBois, P., 41, 54
Dunn, J., 285n27, 298n93

Eider, Rabbi S., 229nn38,39, 257n8
Eilberg-Schwartz, H., 238n46, 279n66
Elliger, K., 233n16
Epstein, I., 222n11, 267n16
Eucharist, 204, 287n41, 288n44, 296n84
Exteriority, 50, 54–56

Faivre, A., 162, 167, 280n3, 281n12, 288n45
Feldman, D., 271n29
Folklore, 36, 152, 158, 277n52
Foucault, M., 107

Gafni, I., 260n35, 277n53
Galen, 8, 42, 130, 135, 235n35, 265n3
Goodblatt, D., 218n8
Gottlieb, A., 129, 224n17

Green, M., 134, 267n11
Greenberg, B., 221n2, 247n28
Greenberg, M., 16–19, 222, 223n12
Gregory the Great, 296n86
Grosz, E., 45, 96, 231n2, 254n62
Gryson, R., 288n45
Gynecology: Greco-Roman, 8–9, 42, 61–63, 130, 155; Hippocratic, 8–9, 61–63, 95, 130–32, 241n69, 265n3; Medieval, 134; Rabbinic, 134–35

Halperin, D., 158
Hanson, A., 55, 61–62, 131, 142, 266n8, 278n60
Harrington, H., 222n11, 226n24, 232n10
Hasan-Rokem, G., 36, 230n51, 267n12, 277n52
Hauptman, J., 26, 135, 227n30, 228nn34,36, 229n39, 247n28, 250n45, 256n4, 257n5, 259n27, 267n15,16
Hayes, C., 212, 250n45
Heggelbacher, O., 284n19, 287n35
Hengel, M., 190, 292n67
Hillel, 85–87, 95, 97–99, 249nn41,42, 250n45, 270n24

Ide, A. F., 164, 288n45
Ifra Hormiz, 116–17, 260–61
Ilan, T., 263n46, 273n36
Imma Shalom, 145
Impurity: of an Animal, 90, 237n42, 253n57, 255n63; of Birth, 200; Language of, 228n37; and Leprosy, 200; Men's, 23, 48–49, 232nn10,11, 256n4; Menstrual, 20–29, 37, 243n7, 244n10, 245n20, 255n70; Retroactive, 85–91, 101, 139, 251nn46,47; of Semen, 44–46, 233n14; Status of, 77–78, 85–91, 106, 180, 236n37, 243n7, 247n33, 248n34, 268n18; Tohorot, 23; Women's, 48–50, 232n11
Indagatio Corporis, 142–47
Interiority, 48–56, 68, 235nn29,31,33
Irigaray, L., 66, 218n6, 242n77, 254n62

Jacobs, L., 251n47
Jaffee, M., 250n45
Jardine, A., 65–66

**324** GENERAL INDEX

Jerome, 115, 164, 260nn32,33,34, 280n3, 282n14, 293n71
Jesus and the Woman with a Blood-Flow, 186–98, 291nn55,56,57, 292
Jewish Christianity, 206–9, 284n22; in the Didascalia, 204; Women's, 206
Jovinian, 164
Judaizing Christians, 207

Karaites, 257n11
Kellenbach, K. von, 161, 189–90, 220n22, 292n63, 295n83
Kraemer, D., 82, 243n3
Kraemer, R., 32, 233n15, 280n5, 296n84
Kraft, R., 298n92
Krauss, S., 238n50, 239n56, 277n54, 278n55
Kristeva, J., 66

Laporte, J., 167, 288n45
Lapsus, 121
Laqueur, T., 231n5, 240n59, 241n69
Levinas, E., 65, 67, 242n76
Levine, B., 48, 222nn6,10, 225n23, 233nn13,17
Lieberman, S., 268n18, 274n37, 277nn53,54, 279n64
Lloyd, G. R. E., 42, 265nn3,4, 266nn5,6,9

Maimonides, 52, 145, 268n18, 274n40
Marmorstein, A., 284n22, 288n47
Meacham, T. Zechurah 52, 234n24, 237nn38,45, 261n39
Meiri, 52, 86, 140, 235n31, 247n33, 268n18, 274nn38,40
Menstruation: and Eucharist, 204, 288n44; Menarche, 138, 143; Menstrual Huts, 129, 224n17; Sexual Prohibition, 20–22, 24–27, 46–48, 233n15, 259n23. See also Mitzvat Niddah
Merleau-Ponty, M., 254n62
Metaphor, 40–41, 50–52, 54, 60, 101, 234nn22,24, 235n32, 241n68
Methuen, C., 167–68, 285nn24,25
Milgrom, J., 48, 222nn5,6,8, 225n23, 232nn9,10, 233nn12,17, 234n20, 256nn1,3
Miqveh, 15, 87–89, 91, 93–96, 221n3, 251n48
Modesty, 150
Myers, J., 221n3

Neusner, J., 226n24, 249n41, 258n12, 260nn35,36, 262n44, 276n51
Niddah: Etymology, 16–19, 222–23; Mitzvat Niddah, 29–36

Origen, 196, 198–203, 297nn87,88,89
Ouaknin, M.-A., 220n19, 221nn28,30
Ovaries, 52, 241n69

Pardes, I., 38, 220n18
Paul, 38, 161–63, 169, 171–72
Peskowitz, M., 217n2, 219nn13,15, 244n11, 253n56, 265n2
Pliny, 35, 230n50, 296n85
Pregnancy, 57, 58
Preuss, J., 57, 134, 143, 234nn23,24, 235nn32,35, 237nn38,43, 238n51, 256n3, 258n17, 268n17, 276n44, 278n58
Profet, M., 237n40
Puberty, Signs of, 143, 148–150, 268n18, 269n19, 272nn30,31, 273n35, 274n39,40, 275nn41,42
Purity, 2, 23; Family Purity, 29, 229n39; and Pharisees, 226n24; Purification, 180–81

Qumran, 222n11, 274n38

Rabbah, 99–100
Rabbi Aqiva, 18, 113–14, 224n19, 259nn27,28, 263n47
Rabbi Meir, 25, 75, 236n37, 264n58
Rabeinu Asher, 157
Rashi, 19, 59, 89, 145, 222n11, 227n31, 228n33, 229n44, 253n53, 255nn65,70, 260n36, 264n55, 270nn23,26, 275n41, 276n50
Rav Ashi, 80–82, 111, 247n32, 248n35, 249n36, 265n59
Roth, J., 247n31, 259n24
Rousselle, A., 63, 132–33, 235n35, 265n3
Ruether, R., 162, 194
Rufus, 42, 130–32, 297n87

Salisbury, J., 162, 281nn6,7, 293n69
Samaritans, 220n21, 257n11, 269n22
Sanders, E.P., 226n24, 232n10
Sanders, J., 206
Scarry, E., 72

Schor, N., 218, 242n77
Schottroff, L., 194
Schüssler Fiorenza, E., 161, 163, 280n5
Scott, J. C., 263n50
Selvidge, M., 189, 195, 292nn62,63, 293nn68,69,74
Septuagint, 232n7
Shame, 149, 276n47
Shammai, 85–95, 97–99, 249nn41,42, 250nn44,45, 253n57, 255n69
Sherira Gaon, 249n38
Shmu'el, 25–26, 57, 70–84, 97, 149–50, 212, 227n32, 228n35, 243n6
Simon, M., 284n22, 286n33, 288n47, 290n51, 298n93
Smell, 115–17, 262n40
Soranus, 42, 62, 130–32, 155, 242n71, 278n59
Stern, D., 249n37
Stiegman, E., 231n4
Strecker, G., 170–71, 283n18, 284n22, 285n28, 286n31, 298n91
Symptom, 70, 119

Tannaim, 14
Taylor, Joan, 284n22, 298n92
Taylor, Justin, 286n32
Taylor, M. S., 286n33
Taste, 115–16
Temkin, O., 62, 235n35, 278nn55,59
Temple, 2, 20, 50, 128, 225n23, 227n29
Terumah, 50, 88–89, 234n26, 252n50
Theissen, G., 291n55
Tidner, E., 184–85, 287nn34,40
Torjesen, K., 167, 285n23, 288n45

Tosafot, 76, 78, 227n27, 234nn24,27, 240n63, 247n29, 255n67, 263n48
Tosfei Rosh, 75
Touch, 21, 193, 195
Trickster, 120
Trummer, P., 194, 294nn77,78

Urbach, E., 32, 220n23, 238n51, 249n42
Uterus, 52

Vagina, 52, 237, 238n46, 241n69
Valler, S., 240n61
Virginity, 161–65, 280nn3,4, 282n13; of Mary, 201–2
Vision, 54–55, 109–11, 114–15, 212, 254n62
Vööbus, A., 167, 170, 172, 177–78, 180, 182, 184–85, 208, 283n18, 287n41. *See also* Didascalia Apostolorum

Wegner, J., 32, 222n4, 233n15, 257n10, 271n29
Wilken, R., 283n16
Winkler, J., 111
Wire, A. C., 169, 205, 220n20
Witherington, B., 194, 292n65
Women: Commandments of, 24, 30–31, 233n15; Identity of, 38; Invisibility of, 129; Space of, 68, 129; Voice of, 5, 151–52, 159

Yalta, 118–28, 213, 262n44, 263, 264nn51,53

Zara'at, 121, 258n14
Zavah, 105, 193–94, 256n4
Zeitlin, F., 61, 242n72

**CONTRAVERSIONS:**

**JEWS AND OTHER DIFFERENCES**

---

Gabriella Safran, *Rewriting the Jew: Assimilation Narratives in the Russian Empire*
Galit Hasan-Rokem, *The Web of Life: Folklore in Rabbinic Literature*
Charlotte Elisheva Fonrobert, *Menstrual Purity: Rabbinic and Christian Reconstructions of Biblical Gender*
James A. Matisoff, *Blessings, Curses, Hopes, and Fears: Psycho-Ostensive Expressions in Yiddish*, second edition
Benjamin Harshav, *The Meaning of Yiddish*
Benjamin Harshav, *Language in Time of Revolution*
Amir Sumaka'i Fink and Jacob Press, *Independence Park: The Lives of Gay Men in Israel*
Alon Goshen-Gottstein, *The Sinner and the Amnesiac: The Rabbinic Invention of Elisha ben Abuya and Eleazar ben Arach*
Bryan Cheyette and Laura Marcus, eds., *Modernity, Culture, and 'the Jew'*
Benjamin D. Sommer, *A Prophet Reads Scripture: Allusion in Isaiah 40–66*
Marilyn Reizbaum, *James Joyce's Judaic Other*

The authorized representative in the EU for product safety and compliance is:
Mare Nostrum Group
B.V Doelen 72
4831 GR Breda
The Netherlands

www.ingramcontent.com/pod-product-compliance
Lightning Source LLC
Chambersburg PA
CBHW021801220426
43662CB00006B/149